Patient Safety in Dialysis Access

Contributions to Nephrology

Vol. 184

Series Editor

Claudio Ronco Vicenza

Patient Safety in Dialysis Access

Volume Editors

Matthias K. Widmer Bern
Jan Malik Prague

58 figures, 48 in color and 35 tables, 2015

Illustrations
Janine Heers Zürich

KARGER Basel · Freiburg · Paris · London · New York · Chennai · New Delhi · Bangkok · Beijing · Shanghai · Tokyo · Kuala Lumpur · Singapore · Sydney

Contributions to Nephrology
(Founded 1975 by Geoffrey M. Berlyne)

Matthias K. Widmer, MD
Universitätsklinik für Herz- und
Gefässchirurgie
Inselspital
CH–3010 Bern (Switzerland)

Jan Malik, MD, PhD
3rd Department of Internal Medicine
First Faculty of Medicine
Charles University and General
University Hospital
U nemocnice 1
CZ–128 08 Prague (Czech Republic)

Library of Congress Cataloging-in-Publication Data

Patient safety in dialysis access / volume editors, Matthias K. Widmer, Jan Malik.
p. ; cm. -- (Contributions to nephrology, ISSN 0302-5144 ; vol. 184)
Includes bibliographical references and indexes.
ISBN 978-3-318-02705-1 (hard cover : alk. paper) -- ISBN 978-3-318-02706-8 (electronic version)
I. Widmer, Matthias K., editor. II. Malik, Jan, 1968- , editor. III. Series: Contributions to nephrology ; v. 184. 0302-5144
[DNLM: 1. Renal Dialysis. 2. Vascular Surgical Procedures--methods. 3. Kidney--surgery. 4. Patient Safety. W1 CO778UN v.184 2015 / WJ 378]
RC901.7.P48
617.4'61059--dc23
2014047410

Bibliographic Indices. This publication is listed in bibliographic services, including Current Contents® and Index Medicus.

Disclaimer. The statements, opinions and data contained in this publication are solely those of the individual authors and contributors and not of the publisher and the editor(s). The appearance of advertisements in the book is not a warranty, endorsement, or approval of the products or services advertised or of their effectiveness, quality or safety. The publisher and the editor(s) disclaim responsibility for any injury to persons or property resulting from any ideas, methods, instructions or products referred to in the content or advertisements.

Drug Dosage. The authors and the publisher have exerted every effort to ensure that drug selection and dosage set forth in this text are in accord with current recommendations and practice at the time of publication. However, in view of ongoing research, changes in government regulations, and the constant flow of information relating to drug therapy and drug reactions, the reader is urged to check the package insert for each drug for any change in indications and dosage and for added warnings and precautions. This is particularly important when the recommended agent is a new and/or infrequently employed drug.

www.karger.com
Printed in Germany on acid-free and non-aging paper (ISO9706) by Kraft Druck, Ettlingen
ISBN 978–3–318–02705–1
e-ISBN 978–3–318–02706–8
ISSN 0302–5144
e-ISSN 1662–2782

KARGER 125 YEARS

Contents

Foreword

Twenty-five years ago, the field of patient safety, apart from a number of early pioneers, did not exist, and the lack of attention to medical accidents could reasonably be described as negligent. Major progress has now been made in assessing the nature and scale of harm. The findings of the major record review studies are widely accepted, and numerous other studies have catalogued the nature and extent of surgical adverse events, infections, adverse drug events and other safety issues. Analyses of incidents are now routinely performed, albeit often in a framework of accountability rather than in the spirit of reflection and learning.

Substantial progress has been made in many clinical areas in understanding the causes of error and harm. Surgery, for instance, was long ago identified as the source of a high proportion of preventable adverse events. A decade ago, most of these would have been considered unavoidable or ascribed, generally incorrectly, as due to poor individual practice. Studies of process failures, communication, teamwork, interruptions and distractions have now identified multiple vulnerabilities in systems of surgical care. Many groups are now moving beyond the undoubted gains of checklists to a more sophisticated understanding of surgical teamwork in both the operating theatre and the wider health care system. A considerable number of interventions have shown that errors can be reduced and processes made more reliable in many other areas of health care. Interventions such as computer order entry, standardisation and simplification of processes and systematic handover have all been shown to improve reliability, and in some cases reduce harm, in specific contexts.

We are also learning that safety needs to be approached differently according to context. Each clinical activity poses its own particular risks to patients and the solutions must be customised and adapted for each setting. Some settings benefit from tight procedures and standardisation, whereas others require more flexible approaches to the management of risk and crisis.

Dialysis is of enormous benefit to patients and their families but, like other effective treatments, also poses risks. This book brings our understanding of patient safety to bear on the processes and systems of dialysis access, examining both the nature of the risk to patients and the means of managing them effectively. The book will surely be greatly welcomed by dialysis patients, families and all those who care for them.

Charles Vincent, London
Professor of Psychology
University of Oxford
Emeritus Professor Clinical Safety Research
Imperial College London

Preface

Patients with end-stage renal disease and its comorbidities have a high risk of suffering adverse events during their continuous treatment as in- or outpatients. Furthermore, dialysis access creation and maintenance are prone to complications. Therefore, specific strategies and various techniques to promote a patient safety initiative are of genuine interest.

Even 15 years after the publication of *To Err Is Human: Building a Safer Health System* by the Institute of Medicine, doctors and nurses are not always aware of the consequences of unsafe behavior. Today, we face the fact that knowing about the right thing is not a guarantee of doing the right thing. With this book, we aim to raise health care professionals' awareness of the aspects of patient safety, which combines medical education with evidence-based medicine. We are convinced that preventive strategies are key to avoid harm and to improve the outcome of the treatment of the growing number of patients with chronic kidney failure.

We are grateful that so many authors from different countries have contributed to this book. They give us a diversified insight into important concepts and technical tricks, which are essential to create and maintain a functional dialysis access. With checklists in our mind, we can be more precise in the timing and in the process of dialysis access creation. Besides simulation training, we also need a better focus on interdisciplinary and interprofessional communication. We are convinced that these efforts lead to more satisfaction amongst health care professionals and result in an improved medical outcome for our patients.

We thank the Vascular Access Society (www.vascularaccesssociety.com), the Vascular International School (www.vascular-international.org) and several industrial sponsors for their support when we started this patient safety project.

Please share your contributions with us at patientsafetyvas@insel.ch.

Matthias K. Widmer, Bern
Jan Malik, Prague

Acknowledgements

The volume editors gratefully acknowledge the support by the following sponsors:

Vascular Access Society
Maastricht, The Netherlands

Vascular International Foundation and School
Fürigen, Switzerland

Bio Nova International
North Melbourne, Australia

GE Healthcare
Prague, Czech Republic

Jotec Sales AG
Muri, Switzerland

MAQUET GETINGE GROUP
Hilversum, The Netherlands

MCM MEDSYS AG
Solothurn, Switzerland

Vascutek Deutschland GmbH, a Terumo Company
Spreitenbach, Switzerland

Widmer MK, Malik J (eds): Patient Safety in Dialysis Access.
Contrib Nephrol. Basel, Karger, 2015, vol 184, pp 1–12
DOI: 10.1159/000365497

Patient Safety: What Is It All about?

David Schwappach

Swiss Patient Safety Foundation, Zürich, and Institute of Social and Preventive Medicine, University of Bern, Bern, Switzerland

Abstract

Patient safety is a major concern in health care systems worldwide. Patients with serious conditions, multimorbidity, and with intense and fragmented health care utilization, like end-stage renal disease (ESRD) patients, are at increased risk for suffering adverse events. In this chapter, the fundamental terms and concepts of patient safety are introduced. Essential epidemiological data relating to the frequency of adverse events and medical errors are provided. The chapter reports important safety threats for ESRD patients and describes examples of key innovations which contribute to patient safety. Recommendations and risk reduction strategies to improve care of ESRD patients are presented.

Recommendations to Improve Patient Safety

- Patients with end-stage renal disease (ESRD) are at increased risk for adverse events and medical errors.
- Important safety threats for ESRD patients are wrong site access surgery, infections of access site, needle infiltration, venous needle dislodgements, clotting, medication error (in particular dose omissions), and falls following hemodialysis.
- Staff noncompliance and failures to follow protocols and procedures are the main sources of errors and adverse events.
- Interdisciplinary 'safety teams' should be installed to assess and monitor risks and implement evidence-based risk reduction strategies.

Introduction

Patient safety is a major concern in health care systems worldwide and has gained increasing attention since the Institute of Medicine published its report *To Err Is Human* in 1999 [1]. Based on extrapolations of study data, this report estimated that approximately 44,000–98,000 Americans die annually due to adverse events in health care. Patients with serious conditions, multimorbidity, and with intense and fragmented health care utilization, like end-stage renal disease (ESRD) patients, are at increased risk for suffering adverse events. It is thus vital that clinicians caring for ESRD patients make patient safety a top priority and cooperate on safety with their colleagues within and across other clinical specialties inside and outside the hospital. In this chapter, we will introduce the fundamental terms and concepts of patient safety and present readers an overview of essential data. We describe examples of important innovations which contribute to patient safety and briefly discuss future needs and developments.

Terms and Definitions

In brief, *patient safety* refers to the absence of errors and preventable adverse events associated with health care. Interventions, activities and policies which reduce the frequency or consequences of preventable adverse events thus improve patient safety. This definition of patient safety introduces two important terms: adverse events, and medical errors. *Adverse events* have two major characteristics: a patient has been harmed and this harm was caused by the medical management rather than the underlying condition or progression of disease. The term adverse event describes that an unintended and undesirable outcome occurred; it does not necessarily involve error. An allergic reaction to a drug is a common adverse event. Clearly, we have an unintended injury, but as long as the allergy was unknown to care providers, no error occurred when the drug was prescribed or administered. *Medical error* is defined as the failure of a planned action to be completed as intended (error of execution) or the use of a wrong plan to achieve an aim (error of planning). Medical errors have the potential to cause undesirable outcomes but do not require a link to actual subsequent harm. In fact, the vast majority of errors do not result in iatrogenic injury. Prescribing a patient with known allergy penicillin because the information is overseen during prescribing is an error. But the error may be detected by the administering nurse before the error reaches the patient and thus harm can be avoided. Adverse events, i.e. harm, caused by error are – by definition – preventable and are

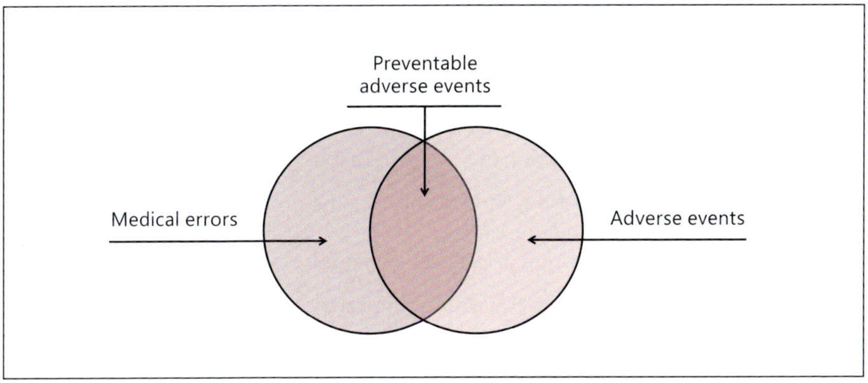

Fig. 1. Concept of medical errors, adverse events and preventable adverse events.

thus called 'preventable adverse events'. A *preventable adverse event* is defined as harm resulting from error in medical management. Figure 1 conceptualizes the terms and how they are interconnected. Patient safety is mainly concerned with preventable adverse events.

Different classifications of error (sub)types emerged in the last years which are *not* mutually exclusive. All types of errors have in common that they are unintentional behaviors. Contrary, violation of rules describes intentional, willful behavior. Useful distinctions amongst errors are between slips/lapses and mistakes, errors at the sharp and at the blunt end, and errors of omission and commission. Slips and lapses are both skill-based errors, whereas mistakes are decision-making failures, for example, making a poor judgment. *Slips and lapses* are failures of schematic behavior and occur in familiar tasks which are conducted with little attention. Common causes of slips and lapses are fatigue or stress. In contrary, *mistakes* are failures in attentional behaviors requiring thought, analysis, planning or problem solving. Mistakes are often caused by lack of knowledge, experience or training. Typically, mistake happens when we do something wrong believing it to be right. Historically, mistakes have received much more attention than slips and lapses, though it is believed that the latter are much more frequent. Slips/lapses and mistakes require quite different treatments. For example, more or better education and supervision is a common and often appropriate 'antidote' to mistakes, but ineffective in the prevention of slips. Errors can occur at the sharp and at the blunt end. The former are often called 'active failures', whereas the latter are termed 'latent conditions'. Errors at the sharp end describe actions committed by the person closest to the patient, whereas organizational failures and poor process design occur at the blunt end. Errors at the sharp end are easier to detect but are often only the last failure in

Table 1. Important terms and examples

Term	Example
Error	Passing incorrect information during hand-off Prescription of a drug to a patient with known allergy
Error subtypes Slip/lapse	Forgetting hand disinfection before touching a patient's wound dressings Confusion of look-alike syringes
Mistake	Choosing the wrong surgical technique Using the wrong formula to calculate a medication dose adjustment
Error of commission	Access not taped/bandaged appropriately after dialysis Heparin ordered when contraindicated
Error of omission	Failure to provide preoperative antibiotic prophylaxis Not ordering renal diet
Error at the blunt end (latent conditions)	Management decision to have the surgical count performed by only one technician (no double check) Equipment designed with poor display design making it hard to identify numbers
Error at the sharp end (active failures)	Unintentionally retained foreign objects in the body (e.g. surgical sponge) Error in programming an infusion pump
Adverse event	Allergic drug reaction Postoperative infection
Preventable adverse event	Wrong site surgery Allergic drug reaction to a drug in a patient with known allergy

the error chain and preceded by one or more latent failures at the blunt end. Finally, errors can be classified as acts of *commission* and acts of *omission*. Errors of commission describe 'doing something wrong', whereas errors of omission involve a failure to do required actions. Acts of commission are usually easier to recognize and thereby received much more attention, but errors of omission are more common. Table 1 presents some examples.

Health Care as a Risk: The Magnitude of the Safety Problem

Different methodological approaches exist to assess the frequency of adverse events or medical errors. The 'state of the art' methodology for assessing errors is observation and document analysis. With observation, health care professionals are ‘shadowed’ during their tasks, and any deviations from standards are recorded. This resource-intensive approach has been followed to estimate the frequency of medication errors in particular. Chedoe et al. [2] used ethnographic observation to detect medication preparation and administration errors on a neonatal intensive care unit. With an incidence of 49%, these errors were quite common. 0.3% medications contained severe and 26% moderate errors. A similar error rate (48%) was found by Taxis and Barber [3] when they observed errors in preparing and administering intravenous drugs in a German hospital. Document analysis has typically been used to detect physicians’ prescription errors in written orders.

Contrary to errors, adverse events are usually not detectable by observation. The gold standard methodology for assessing the frequency of adverse events is retrospective record review with at least two stages. Patients’ charts are usually screened for potential incidents by trained nurses (stage 1) and then reviewed by qualified expert physicians (stage 2). Physician reviewers also rate events in terms of preventability and severity. Numerous studies in different countries have been conducted using this approach in the last years. These studies revealed adverse event rates of 5–15% of all acute care hospital admissions [4–8]. Approximately 50% of events were deemed preventable [5]. Based on these studies, it has been estimated that ca. 0.1%, i.e. one out of 1,000, patients admitted to hospital will die due to preventable adverse events [4]. Hauck and Zhao [9] modelled the risk of adverse events based on administrative hospital episode data of more than 200,000 patients admitted to Australian hospitals. Based on these data, a hospital stay carries a 5.5% risk of an adverse drug reaction, 17.6% risk of infection, and 3.1% risk of ulcer for an average episode. In a recent retrospective record review analysis in 10 hospitals in North Carolina, reviewers found 25.1 harms per 100 patient admissions. Notably and despite all patient safety efforts, there was no significant change over time in the rate of harms during the past 5 years [10].

Some countries have also established mandatory reporting systems for ‘never events’. These are serious events which are deemed as largely preventable and every health care system should strive for zero frequency. Examples of never events are wrong site surgery, wrong application route of chemotherapy agents, and mistakenly left instruments after surgery. In the UK, 762 of these never events occurred during 2009–2012 (http://www.england.nhs.uk/ourwork/patientsafety/never-events/). Such data help to monitor ‘the tip of the iceberg’ and to establish safety measures for the prevention of severe patient harm and death.

Patients and citizens have also been surveyed about their experiences with the safety of medical care. In the ‘Commonwealth Fund’s 2010 International Survey of the General Public’s Views of their Health Care System’s Performance’, citizens of 11 countries were asked to report about medical errors [11]. Across

Table 2. Summary of important safety threats to ESRD patients

Wrong site access surgery (rare but serious)
Needle infiltration
Venous needle disconnections/dislodgements (rare but potentially dangerous)
Clotting in the hemodialysis circuit or lines
Medication errors, in particular omissions
Infection of access
Falls (following hemodialysis)

countries, medical error during the last 2 years was reported by 11% of patients but with marked differences between countries. Perceived poor care coordination was the single most important risk factor for reporting errors. Similar studies have been conducted to assess the frequency of infection during or after hospital stay or errors in chemotherapy treatment [12–14]. Despite the tragedy associated with all these incidents, medical errors also come at high financial cost. In a recent study, the annual cost of measurable medical errors with patient harm was estimated at USD 17.1 billion in 2008. Postoperative surgical infections were the most costly error and accounted for USD 3,364 million [15].

Specific Safety Threats for Patients on Hemodialysis

Though a large and increasing number of patients with ESRD undergo hemodialysis and the technology is well established, only limited data are available about the specific safety hazards associated with the treatment. As ESRD patients often suffer serious comorbidities and have intense and fragmented health care utilization with multiple providers involved and thus a high level of exposure, it is likely that these patients are at elevated risk for medical errors. Table 2 summarizes important safety threats to ESRD patients.

Like all surgical patients, patients undergoing vascular access surgery are at risk for wrong site surgery. Wrong site surgery, i.e. *wrong* site, *wrong* patient, or *wrong*-procedure surgery, is rare but is devastating and a true 'never event'. Of the total of 375 reports of wrong site surgery the Pennsylvania Patient Safety Authority received during the years 2004–2010, 7 reports involved the wrong vascular access device [16]. Five of the cases indicated confusion between subcutaneous venous access ports and Hickman or Broviac intravenous catheters. One report indicated confusion between a dialysis catheter and an intended port and another confusion between a dialysis catheter and an intended arteriovenous fistula. The Authority concludes that insertion of the correct vascular access device from among all the potential options appears to be the most common challenge involving insertion of devices.

There is no comprehensive study on the prevalence of adverse events or errors in hemodialysis, and the available data are heterogeneous and based on different methodologies.

The Pennsylvania Patient Safety Authority analyzed all reports of incidents involving hemodialysis administration submitted through the Authority's reporting system during a one-year period [17]. Among 526 reports submitted, 5.5% resulted in harm to the patients. Medication errors were the most frequent events (29% of all reports) and among them, the greatest fraction involved dose omissions. Heparin errors were also common (3% of all events reported). Other events reported included failure to follow protocol, procedure complications, falls, equipment failures, and clotting. There were 32 reports of needle infiltration (blood infiltration into the surrounding tissue due to accidental piercing of the back wall of the graft or fistula during insertion of the needle) and an equal number of needle disconnections, together representing 12% of all hemodialysis administration events submitted to the Authority.

Needle infiltration most commonly occurred during the needle insertion. Lee et al. [18] reported an annual rate of major fistula infiltration leading to further intervention of 5.2%. Venous needle dislodgement is a rare but potentially serious event in hemodialysis [19]. A survey among nephrology nurses revealed that 77% of nurses had seen at least one venous needle dislodgement in the past 5 years [20]. Every second of the participating nurses reported to be concerned about venous needle dislodgement often or very often. The American Nephrology Nurses Association for instance provides valuable material for education of staff and patients about risk factors and prevention of venous needle dislodgment (https://www.annanurse.org/resources/venous-needle-dislodgement).

Holley [21] conducted a study of adverse events and medical errors in four hemodialysis units. Incident data are based on reports by the units' clinical directors. Among nearly 65,000 dialysis treatments, 88 errors occurred (1 event/733 treatments). Infiltration of the hemodialysis access, clotting of the dialysis circuit and omitted medications were common problems. In a surveillance study of dialysis patients in Gran Canaria (Spain), the incidence rate of adverse events was 8.6/100 patient-months [22]. The rate was higher among patients with arteriovenous fistula (9.1/100 patient-months) compared to patients with permanent catheter (2.9/100 patient-months). The preventability of the events is unknown.

As has been outlined above, important information about safety hazards can also be obtained from professionals (physicians and nurses) and patients (fig. 2). Garrick et al. [23] report about the results from a survey among ESRD patients

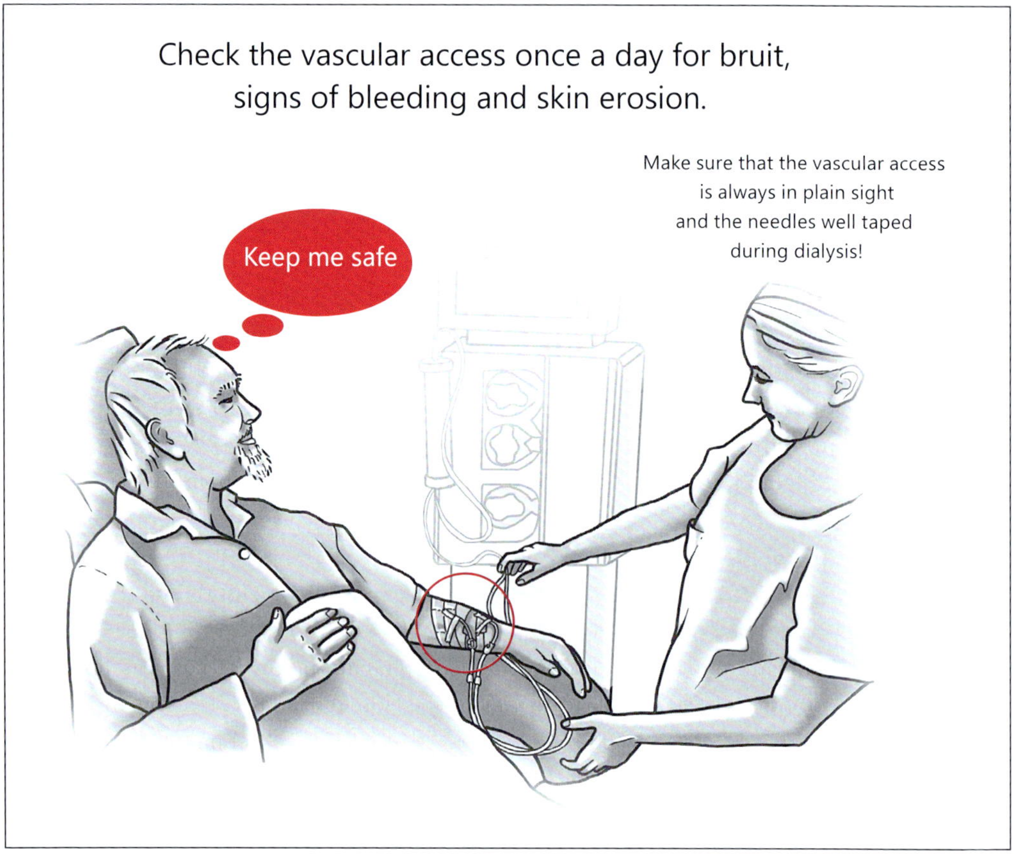

Fig. 2. Education posters for staff and patients may help to improve patient safety.

and professionals commissioned by the US Renal Physicians Association. In this survey study, 49% of patients reported to be worried about safety at least sometimes. 5% of patients reported falls at the dialysis center in the past 3 months. Almost half of patients indicated that the nurses or technicians inserting the needles for their dialysis treatments experience problems and 30% of patients indicated that staff tried more than twice to insert needles before getting assistance. Five specific threats to patient safety were identified from the survey among nurses and physicians: setting up an incorrect dialyzing solution prior to a dialysis session; patient falls following dialysis; medication omissions; staff failures to adhere to procedures (e.g. failure to take blood pressure), and staff noncompliance with hand disinfection or glove usage before touching a patient's access site. 55% of surveyed professionals attributed errors to staff failing to adhere to procedures.

Harel et al. [24] took a different yet highly important perspective in their study. They assessed how safe chronic dialysis patients are in hospital when admitted to surgical services, e.g. after fracture. They used retrospective chart review of patients receiving chronic hemodialysis and screened for safety lapses using a set of four predefined indicators. They detected 96 lapses in 38 patients. Failure to order an appropriate 'renal diet' was the most common problem, followed by inappropriate analgesic order, inappropriate intravenous fluid administration, and inappropriate antibiotic dosing. One adverse event directly attributable to these process errors was identified (volume overload). The authors also analyzed whether the problem was detected during hospitalization, by whom, and how long it took to be remediated. The majority of errors were detected by the consulting nephrology service. Inappropriate analgesia orders were only detected in 27% of cases during hospitalization. It took on average 2.5 days to detect that patients received the wrong diet. This study emphasizes that ESRD patients suffer risks not only associated with hemodialysis treatment, but also in the context of other, unrelated treatments. Obviously, general surgical units are often not sufficiently prepared to care for ESRD patients in their everyday routines.

Improving Systems – Improving Patient Safety

Recent research has demonstrated that sustainable improvements in patient safety are achievable. Well-recognized examples are a multifaceted intervention to reduce the incidence of catheter-related bloodstream infections and a surgical checklist to decrease adverse events and mortality in the operating room (OR) [25, 26]. The surgical safety checklist has proved effective in a broad range of surgical patient populations. In addition, the Pennsylvania Patient Safety Authority makes three specific recommendations for procedures involving the insertion of a device to prevent confusion during vascular access surgery [16]:

(1) The specific device should be mentioned on the schedule, the consent, and the surgeon's preoperative evaluation of the patient. This information should be checked for its presence and agreement with all the documents in the preoperative verification.
(2) The specific device should be mentioned during the time-out.
(3) The specific device should be called out when delivered onto the operative field.

Based on adverse event studies and reports, a number of specific risk reduction strategies for dialysis units have been recommended recently [17, 23]. These include for example:

- Independent double checks of i.v. heparin doses and infusions before dispensing
- Involvement of patients in their hemodialysis care and engagement to speak up if they note errors, observe rule violations
- Establishment of a policy to assess all hemodialysis patients for their risk of falling
- Monitoring and evaluation of infiltration problems that occurred to determine whether adjustments to cannulation techniques are necessary
- Systematic assessment of patients' risk for a serious venous needle dislodgement incident [20]
- Instruction of patients to keep all needle and blood line connections from being covered with blankets or other items so that staff can monitor the connections.

In the following chapters of this volume, experts present successful approaches and strategies to improve patient safety in vascular access patients. For example, Davidson et al. [pp. 97–106] discuss how team training and checklists can be used to improve safety in the OR, and Shemesh et al. [234–250] report about the important role of the hemodialysis patient in creating and maintaining safety.

From an organizational perspective, we suggest that every hemodialysis unit sets up an inclusive, interdisciplinary 'safety team' to assess and monitor risks at their specific environment. As a start of this safety team, patients and staff could be surveyed about risks, past incidents, violations of procedures and protocols and their perceptions of safety. Staff could be asked to report events to the hospital's critical incident reporting system. If such a system is not available, staff could complete a report form for every incident they observed (e.g. confusions or 'close calls'/near misses in the OR, missed medication dose, infection, clotting, fall, etc.) for a 4-week period. We also find it important that vascular access surgeons and hemodialysis clinicians and nurses have the opportunity to discuss their experiences of safety of care. This communication is often very restricted, irregular, and patient safety may be considerably improved if each involved specialty knows about the others' experiences, activities and concerns. Based on the individual unit's risk assessment, priorities for improvement can be set. The safety team could also serve as a connection to other units in the hospital which treat ESRD patients (e.g. general surgery) to ensure that safe care is provided outside the hemodialysis unit.

The following chapters provide valuable examples of important aspects of safe care for the vascular access patient. Many of the successful interventions focus on the performance of individuals. However, improvements at the systems level such as design of rooms, equipment and materials and work flow are often much more promising and effective, in particular in the prevention of lapses and slips, but have much too long been ignored. For example, rather than relying on staff education about proper hand disinfection practices, design of wards, patient rooms and devices can be designed to make failure much less likely [27, 28]. Similarly, instead of relying on the education of staff to be aware of line misconnections, research is underway to design and test material that does not allow dangerous misconnections [29]. Hopefully, such efforts will benefit the safety of care of vascular access patients in the future.

Disclosure Statement

The author has no conflict of interest to declare.

References

1 Institute of Medicine: To Err Is Human. Building a Safer Health System. Washington, National Academy Press, 1999.

2 Chedoe I, Molendijk H, Hospes W, Van den Heuvel ER, Taxis K: The effect of a multifaceted educational intervention on medication preparation and administration errors in neonatal intensive care. Arch Dis Child Fetal Neonatal Ed 2012;97:F449–F455.

3 Taxis K, Barber N: Incidence and severity of intravenous drug errors in a German hospital. Eur J Clin Pharmacol 2004;59:815–817.

4 Zegers M, de Bruijne MC, Wagner C, Hoonhout LHF, Waaijman R, Smits M, et al: Adverse events and potentially preventable deaths in Dutch hospitals: results of a retrospective patient record review study. Qual Saf Health Care 2009;18:297–302.

5 de Vries EN, Ramrattan MA, Smorenburg SM, Gouma DJ, Boermeester MA: The incidence and nature of in-hospital adverse events: a systematic review. Qual Saf Health Care 2008;17:216–223.

6 Soop M, Fryksmark U, Koster M, Haglund B: The incidence of adverse events in Swedish hospitals: a retrospective medical record review study. Int J Qual Health Care 2009;21: 285–291.

7 Tartaglia R, Albolino S, Bellandi T, Bianchini E, Biggeri A, Fabbro G, et al: Adverse events and preventable consequences: retrospective study in five large Italian hospitals. Epidemiol Prev 2012;36:151–161.

8 Aranaz-Andres JM, Aibar-Remon C, Vitaller-Burillo J, Requena-Puche J, Terol-Garcia E, Kelley E, et al: Impact and preventability of adverse events in Spanish public hospitals: results of the Spanish National Study of Adverse Events (ENEAS). Int J Qual Health Care 2009;21:408–414.

9 Hauck K, Zhao X: How dangerous is a day in hospital? A model of adverse events and length of stay for medical inpatients. Med Care 2011;49:1068–1075.

10 Landrigan CP, Parry GJ, Bones CB, Hackbarth AD, Goldmann DA, Sharek PJ: Temporal trends in rates of patient harm resulting from medical care. N Engl J Med 2010;363: 2124–2134.

11 Schwappach DLB: Risk factors for patient-reported medical errors in eleven countries. Health Expect 2014;17:321–331.

12 Schwappach DLB: Frequency of patient-reported infections among sicker adults in high-income countries: an international perspective. Am J Infect Control 2013;41:174–176.

13 Schwappach DLB, Wernli M: Chemotherapy patients' perceptions of drug administration safety. J Clin Oncol 2010;28:2896–2901.
14 Schwappach DLB, Wernli M: Am I (un)safe here? Chemotherapy patients' perspectives towards engaging in their safety. Qual Saf Health Care 2010;19:e9.
15 Van Den Bos J, Rustagi K, Gray T, Halford M, Ziemkiewicz E, Shreve J: The $17.1 billion problem: the annual cost of measurable medical errors. Health Aff 2011;30:596–603.
16 Pennsylvania Patient Safety Authority: Quarterly update on the preventing wrong-site surgery project. PA Patient Saf Advis 2010;7:108–110.
17 Pennsylvania Patient Safety Authority: Hemodialysis administration: strategies to ensure safe patient care. PA Patient Saf Advis 2010;7:87–96.
18 Lee T, Barker J, Allon M: Needle infiltration of arteriovenous fistulae in hemodialysis: risk factors and consequences. Am J Kidney Dis 2006;47:1020–1026.
19 Van Waeleghem JP, Chamney M, Lindley EJ, Pancirova J: Venous needle dislodgement: how to minimise the risks. J Ren Care 2008;34:163–168.
20 Axley B, Speranza-Reid J, Williams H: Venous needle dislodgement in patients on hemodialysis. Nephrol Nurs J 2012;39:435–445.
21 Holley JL: A descriptive report of errors and adverse events in chronic hemodialysis units. Nephrol News Issues 2006;20:57–63.
22 Quori A, Baamonde-Laborda E, Garcia-Canton C, Lago-Alonso MM, Toledo-Gonzalez A, Monzon-Jimenez E, et al: Surveillance for infections and other adverse events in dialysis patients in southern Gran Canaria. Nefrologia 2011;31:457–463.
23 Garrick R, Kliger A, Stefanchik B: Patient and facility safety in hemodialysis: opportunities and strategies to develop a culture of safety. Clin J Am Soc Nephrol 2012;7:680–688.
24 Harel Z, Wald R, Liu JJ, Bell CM: Lapses in safety in end-stage renal disease patients admitted to surgical services. Hemodial Int 2012;16:286–293.
25 Pronovost P, Needham D, Berenholtz S, Sinopoli D, Chu H, Cosgrove S, et al: An intervention to decrease catheter-related bloodstream infections in the ICU. N Engl J Med 2006;355:2725–2732.
26 Haynes AB, Weiser TG, Berry WR, Lipsitz SR, Breizat AH, Dellinger EP, et al: A surgical safety checklist to reduce morbidity and mortality in a global population. N Engl J Med 2009;360:491–499.
27 Birnbach DJ, Nevo I, Scheinman SR, Fitzpatrick M, Shekhter I, Lombard JL: Patient safety begins with proper planning: a quantitative method to improve hospital design. Qual Saf Health Care 2010;19:462–465.
28 Anderson O, Davey G, West J: Make It Better. Designing out Medical Error. London, Helen Hamlyn Centre, Royal College of Art, 2011.
29 Cook TM: Non-Luer connectors: are we nearly there yet? Anaesthesia 2012;67:784–792.

David Schwappach, MD, MPH
Swiss Patient Safety Foundation
Asylstrasse 77
CH–8032 Zürich (Switzerland)
E-Mail schwappach@patientensicherheit.ch

Widmer MK, Malik J (eds): Patient Safety in Dialysis Access.
Contrib Nephrol. Basel, Karger, 2015, vol 184, pp 13–23
DOI: 10.1159/000365498

Patients with Chronic Kidney Disease: Safety Aspects in the Preoperative Management

Marko Malovrh

Department of Nephrology, University Medical Center Ljubljana, Ljubljana, Slovenia

Abstract

Chronic kidney disease (CKD) is a major public health problem worldwide. Early detection and treatment of CKD can often prevent or delay some of the negative outcomes of CKD. This chapter shows how treatment of hypertension, proteinuria and metabolic disorders slow down the deterioration of renal function. Irrespective of the mode of renal replacement therapy, maintaining the veins in the upper extremities is of vital importance. Below are suggestions on how to protect blood vessels of the upper limbs and when to start preparing for the construction of vascular access. In this chapter, it is also shown how necessary it is to conduct a clinical evaluation of the blood vessels, which is required before the start of vascular access management. The methodology of noninvasive evaluation of vessels by duplex sonography is also presented. This method is very useful, especially if the vessels are not clinically visible, as well as the information concerning the morphological and functional properties of blood vessels.

Recommendations to Improve Patient Safety

- For patients with chronic kidney disease (CKD), overall recommendations are to delay progression of both kidney disease and its complications. Treatment of hypertension, proteinuria, dyslipidemia, calcium-phosphate regulation and anemia are the key elements.
- Patients with progressive CKD, especially when they require renal replacement therapy, have to have an education program which should include

modification of lifestyle, medication management, selection of treatment modality and instructions for vein preservation and for vascular access.
- Before vascular access surgery, physical and noninvasive examination by duplex ultrasonography of vessels is mandatory.

Chronic Kidney Disease

Chronic kidney disease (CKD) is a major public health problem worldwide. Kidney failure is becoming increasingly common and is associated with poor health outcomes and high medical expenditures. CKD is kidney damage for 3 or more months, as defined by structural or functional abnormalities of the kidney, with or without decreased glomerular filtration rate (GFR), manifested by pathologic abnormalities or markers of kidney damage, including abnormalities in the composition of the blood or urine or abnormalities in imaging tests or GFR <60 ml/min/1.73 m^2 for 3 months or more, with or without kidney damage. The classification of CKD stages is shown in table 1 [1].

Decreased kidney function is associated with complications of all organ systems. The major outcomes of CKD, regardless of the specific diagnosis (i.e. type of kidney disease), include progression to kidney failure, complications from decreased kidney function, and development of cardiovascular disease. Increasing evidence shows that early detection and treatment often can prevent or delay some of these adverse outcomes. Referral to a nephrologist depends on practice patterns, which are not uniform across health care system or geographic regions, even within countries. Most cases of nonprogressive CKD can be managed without referral to the nephrologist. One indication that is common to most guidelines is patients with severely decreased GFR (estimated GFR, eGFR, <30 ml/min/1.73 m^2). There are fewer consensuses about referral for patients with higher eGFR. Nephrologists can assist primary care physicians and other specialists in the diagnosis and care of patients at all stages of CKD. This includes determination of the cause of CKD, recommendations for specific therapy, suggestions for treatments to slow progression in patients who have not responded to conventional therapies, identification and treatment for kidney disease-related complications and preparation for renal replacement therapy [2].

Patients with CKD should be evaluated to determine the following:
- Specific diagnosis (type of kidney disease)
- Comorbid conditions
- Disease severity (assessed by the level of kidney function)
- Complications (related to the level of kidney function)

Table 1. Classification of CKD stages

Stage	Description	GFR, ml/min/1.73 m^2
1	Kidney damage with normal or increased GFR	≥90
2	Kidney damage with mildly decreased GFR	60–89
3	Moderately decreased GFR	30–59
4	Severely decreased GFR	15–29
5	Kidney failure	<15 (or dialysis)

- Risk for loss of kidney function
- Risk for development of cardiovascular disease

Treatment of patients with CKD includes the following:

- Therapy based on the specific diagnosis
- Evaluation and management of co morbid conditions
- Measures to:
  - slow loss of kidney function
  - prevent and treat cardiovascular disease
  - prevent and treat complications of decreased kidney function
- Preparation for kidney failure and kidney replacement therapy
- Replacement of kidney function by dialysis or transplantation if signs and symptoms of uremia are present

Medical Management of Patients with CKD

Progression of CKD toward end-stage renal disease (ESRD) is common in CKD patients, and once significant impairment of renal function has occurred, it tends to progress irrespective of the underlying kidney disorder. There is clear evidence from clinical studies that hypertension and proteinuria are key players in the pathophysiology of CKD progression in humans.

Hypertension is an independent risk factor for renal failure progression. Aggressive blood pressure reduction has always been shown to protect the kidney from further damage. The use of antihypertensive agents with antiproteinuric properties is also important but does not supersede the need to reach goal blood pressure. Antagonists of the renin-angiotensin system, such as ACE inhibitors and, more recently, angiotensin II type I receptor blockers have become pharmacotherapeutics of first choice. They significantly reduce blood pressure as well as urinary protein excretion and have an excellent safety profile. In adults with diabetic or nondiabetic kidney disease, several randomized trials demonstrate a more effective reduction of proteinuria, usually by 30–40%, by ACE inhibitors compared with placebo and/or other antihypertensive agents. Because hypertension is a multifactorial disorder, monotherapy is often not effective in lowering blood pressure or reducing proteinuria to the target range. Target blood pressure should be <130/80 or <125/75 mm Hg at more than 1 g/day/ 1.73 m^2 of proteinuria. It is generally recommended to administer these drugs, after confirming tolerability in a short run-in period, at their highest approved doses [4, 5].

Proteinuria is also a powerful independent risk factor for ESRD and overall mortality and is certainly predictive of the renal prognosis in adults with diabetic and nondiabetic kidney disorders. Reduction of proteinuria is associated with a slowing of GFR loss in the long term. Protein restriction may slow the progression of CKD, although the optimal level of protein intake has not been determined. The goal of any antiproteinuric treatment is to reduce proteinuria as much as possible, ideally to <300 $mg/m^2/day$. Renin-angiotensin system antagonists preserve kidney function, not only by lowering blood pressure but also through antiproteinuric and antifibrotic properties [6].

A wide range of disorders may develop as a consequence of the loss of renal function. These include disorders of fluid and electrolyte balance, such as volume overload, hyperkalemia, metabolic acidosis, and hyperphosphatemia, as well as abnormalities related to hormonal or systemic dysfunction, such as anorexia, nausea, vomiting, fatigue, hypertension, anemia, malnutrition, hyperlipidemia, and bone disease.

Dyslipidemia is common in patients with renal disease. Lipid-lowering medical treatment is commonly prescribed in adults with CKD based on the evident benefit of this approach for primary and secondary prevention of cardiovascular disease in the general adult population. Statin therapy is effective in reducing cardiovascular morbidity and mortality in adults with moderate to severe CKD although not in patients with ESRD. With respect to renoprotection, experimental evidence suggests that statins may retard renal disease progression not only by their lipid-lowering but also by lipid-independent pleiotropic effects [7].

There is an increasing tendency to retain hydrogen ions among patients with CKD. This can lead to a progressive metabolic acidosis with the serum bicarbonate concentration tending to stabilize between 12 and 20 mEq/l. Metabolic acidosis may be treated with bicarbonate supplementation. Bicarbonate supplementation requires careful monitoring of volume status because bicarbonate is administered with sodium [8].

Disorders of the calcium-phosphate metabolism are additional risk factors for renal disease progression. Several factors related to disturbed calcium-phosphorus metabolism, such as hyperphosphatemia, hyperparathyroidism, lack of active vitamin D, and possibly the phosphaturic hormone FGF23, may be considered to be – at least to a minor extent – involved in the progression of renal dysfunction. Dietary phosphate restriction, oral phosphate binders, vitamin D analogues, calcium supplementation and/or calcimimetics may limit the development of secondary hyperparathyroidism in patients with CKD [9].

Anemia is also an independent risk factor for progression of chronic renal failure. The anemia of CKD is, in most patients, normocytic and normochromic, and is due primarily to reduced production of erythropoietin (EPO) by the kidney (a presumed reflection of the reduction in functioning renal mass), low iron stores and shortened red cell survival. In 40%, it could be corrected by iron replacement. Early initiation of EPO therapy in patients with CKD and mild to moderate anemia significantly slowed down the progression of renal disease and delayed the need for renal replacement therapy. The target level of hemoglobin is 110 g/l [10].

Identifying Patients with CKD for Replacement Therapy and Vein Preservation

It is important to identify patients who may eventually require renal replacement therapy since adequate preparation can decrease morbidity and perhaps mortality. Early identification enables dialysis to be initiated at the optimal time with a functioning chronic access. The placement and adequate maturation of arteriovenous fistula (AVF) before the initiation of hemodialysis therapy requires timely patient education and counselling, selection of the preferred renal replacement modality, selection of an access type and location, and creation of the access at least several weeks to months in advance of its expected need. An early constructed AV fistula could also have a beneficial effect on the rapidity of worsening kidney failure. Reasons for this could be increased heart preload and consequently increased afterload or decreased peripheral resistance with increased renal perfusion. A simpler reason could be that patients after AV fistula construction become aware that situation is serious and they start to follow the therapy more accurately [11].

In patients with CKD, preservation of the integrity of peripheral and central veins is of vital importance for future hemodialysis access. Avoid i.v. infusion or vein puncture in the forearm and upper arm veins at both arms whenever possible. Insertion of venous access devices carries the risk to injure the veins and thereby incite phlebitis, sclerosis, stenosis or thrombosis and has to be avoided. Whenever a central venous catheter is needed, catheterization of the internal jugular or femoral vein is always preferred. Use of subclavian vein should be

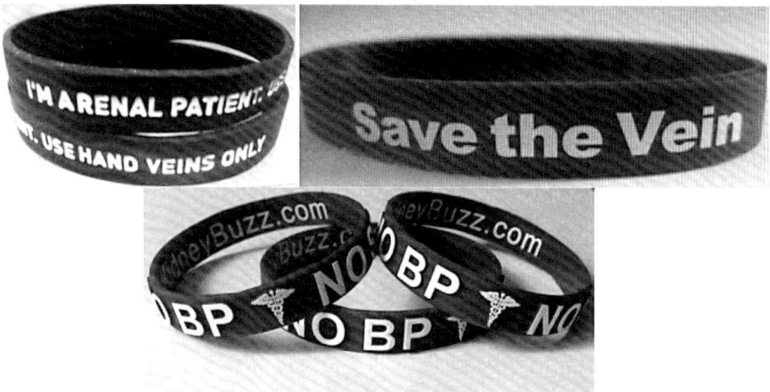
I'M A RENAL PATIENT
USE HAND VEINS ONLY
Save the Vein
KidneyBuzz.com
NO BP

Fig. 1. Different types of bracelets prevent the use of the best veins by health care professionals.

avoided because of frequent central vein stenosis later. An approach should be adopted in which education and vein protection begins in stage 3 CKD and planning for dialysis access takes place in stage 4 CKD. Besides other measures, use of the *'save the vein'* bracelet or similar could be very helpful (fig. 1). The patient's vessels should be examined early in the course of chronic renal failure and indicated to the patient so that he/she can prevent use of the best veins by health care professionals. The critical issue of vein preservation is not resolved once hemodialysis patients have a functional vascular access. Any hemodialysis vascular access is at risk of failure, and therefore protecting veins for future fistula creation remains an important part of the dialysis patient's health care. The same applies to ESRD patients with alternative forms of renal replacement therapy, including peritoneal dialysis or renal transplantation [12–14].

Evaluation of the Patient before Surgery for Vascular Access Construction

Careful clinical evaluation is mandatory before starting management of vascular access. Medical history and concomitant diseases have a strong impact on the choice of possible access site. One of the most important predictors of successful AVF development is the ability of the arterial and venous vessels to dilate under the influence of increased shear stress-vessel remodeling. The preoperative physical examination of the patients' forearm venous and arterial vessels includes inspection of the vein with a tourniquet in order to induce venous congestion, and of the quality of the arterial pulse including an Allen test. In heavily calcified arteries, the creation of an AVF is dangerous because there will be no adaptive flow-mediated dilatation. In complex cases, particularly in patients

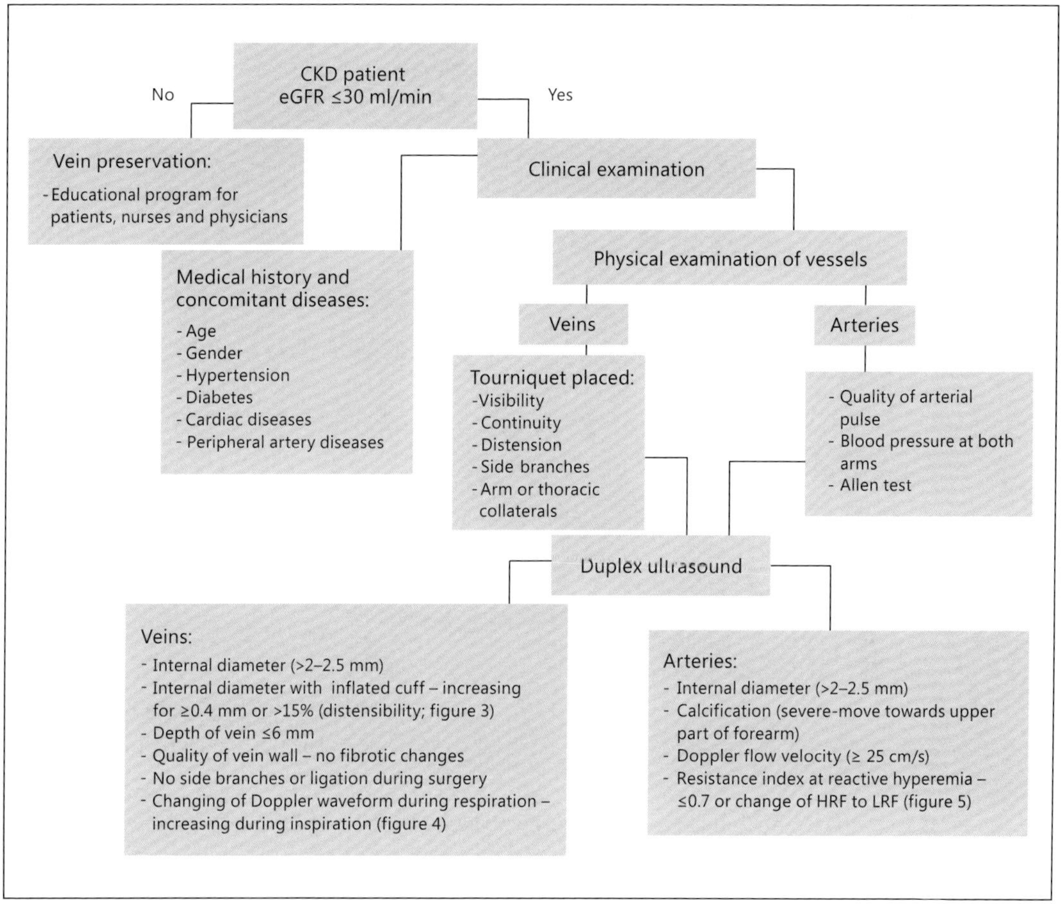

Fig. 2. Approach to the patient with CKD in need of a vascular access. HRF = High-resistance flow; LRF = low-resistance flow.

with a history of previous failed fistulae, prior vein cannulation, or in obese patients vein mapping using duplex ultrasonography, is a good and valuable tool. Also, in patients who previously had chronic cannulations of the subclavian or jugular veins, the central veins should be evaluated by duplex ultrasonography or phlebography to exclude any underlying stenosis or occlusion. It is suggested that duplex imaging should be used routinely to evaluate all patients prior to the creation of an AVF because there is a good correlation between the preoperative determination and perioperative findings (fig. 2) [15–17]. Routine preoperative sonographic vein mapping results in an increase in patients with suitable veins. Many patients were found to have large-caliber veins that were simply too deep to be visualized. The predictive value of the vein diameter for successful AVF is

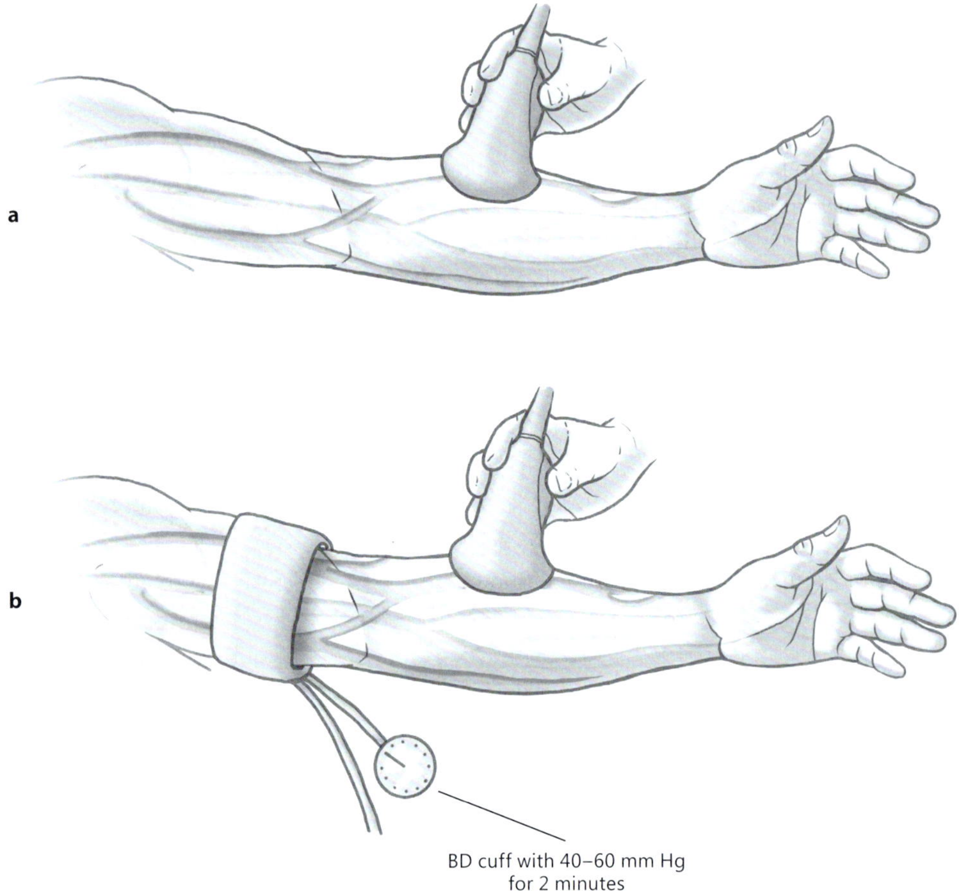

Fig. 3. Evaluation of vein distensibility. **a** Step 1: measurement of the inner vein diameter (IVD) without pressure (A). **b** Step 2: measurement of the IVD after 2 min of mild cuff pressure (B). Increase in IVD (%) = (B × 100/A) – 100.

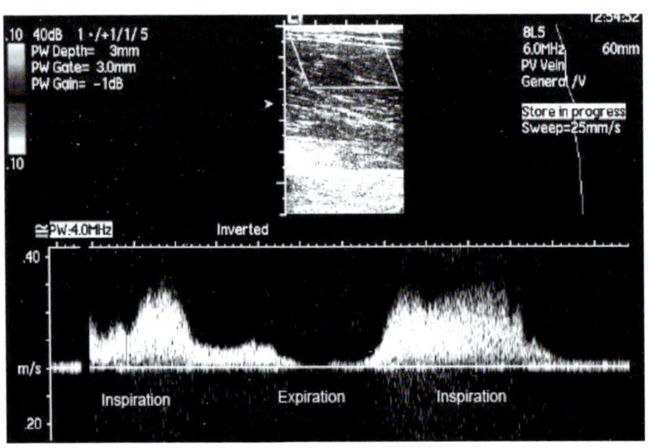

Fig. 4. Normal Doppler vein flow during respiration.

still to be established. Vein diameters <1.6 mm have been associated with AVF failure, while good patency rates were obtained in patients with AVF that were created on the basis of a selection of veins: diameter of cephalic vein at the wrist ≥2–2.5 mm or upper arm veins ≥3 mm. After AVF construction, the 'fistula vein' under the influence of increased blood flow and intravenous pressure is dilated. This ability of the vein could be determined before surgery by measuring the increase in the vein's inner diameter (IVD) after proximal vein compression. A blood pressure cuff should be placed around the upper arm as proximally as possible and inflated at 40–60 mm Hg for at least 2 min (fig. 3) [16, 18]. Based on this increase, it is possible to anticipate the increase in vein diameter at different intervals after construction and predict the time of AV fistula maturation. To determine if there is any disturbance in venous outflow, the continuity of the shape of the Doppler vein signal (DVS) and respiratory filling is used. At deep breath, the venous flow is increased because of low resistance to venous flow. If there is venous outflow disturbance (stenosis), DVS is not changed (fig. 4). Preoperative internal diameter of the feeding artery (IDA) is crucial for successful AVF construction. Most of the literature data suggest an IDA of 2.0–2.5 mm. Increased artery intima media thickness (IMT) is known to be a risk factor of early AVF failure. High-resolution ultrasonography is a simple and effective tool in measuring artery IMT. Besides morphological evaluation, the functional characteristics of the arteries could be evaluated by duplex ultrasonography, too. The feeding arteries dilate during access maturation. Consequently, it is obvious that not only the initial diameter, but also arterial compliance, affects access outcome.

The distensibility of the arterial wall can be assessed preoperatively by evaluating the Doppler waveform in the artery during reactive hyperemia (RH), induced by reopening a fist that was clenched for 2 min. The high-resistance triphasic Doppler ultrasound signal with clenched fist (regular signal of peripheral arteries) changes to a low-resistance biphasic waveform after releasing the fist, and the resistance index (RI) at RH can be calculated using the formula: (peak systolic velocity – peak diastolic velocity)/peak systolic velocity (fig. 5). The RI of <0.7 or even changing of high-resistance flow to low-resistance flow in the potential feeding artery after opening of the fist indicates that arterial blood flow will increase sufficiently, so that the chance of successful creation of an AV fistula exists. This maneuver is especially helpful in planning the location of the initial operation, i.e. selecting the wrist/forearm or elbow region. The preoperative duplex ultrasonography criteria for good outcome after AVF creation are: arterial luminal diameter >2.0 mm, venous luminal diameter (without use of tourniquet) >2.0 mm, and arterial RI <0.7 at RH [16, 17, 19].

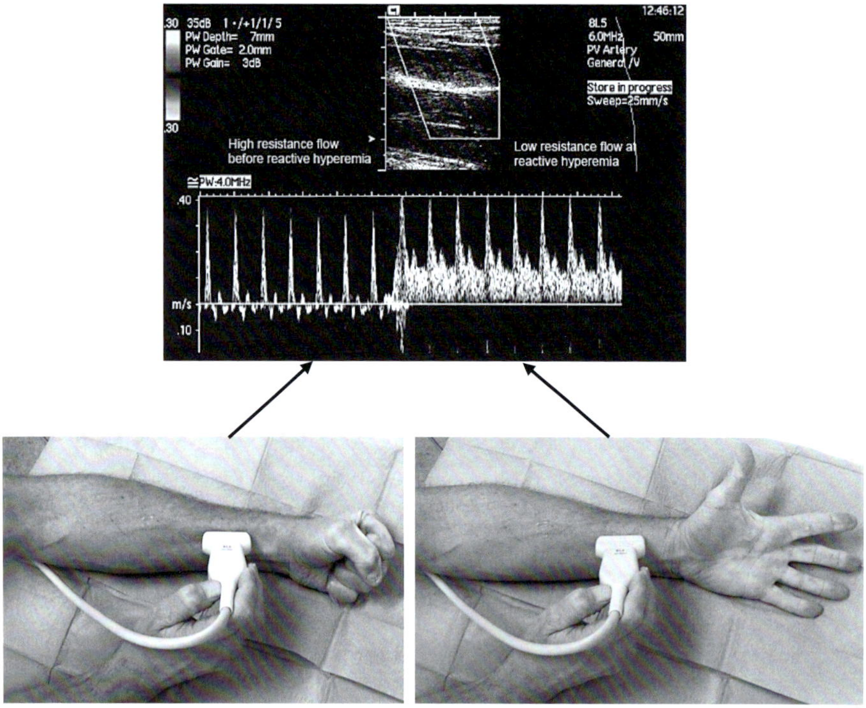

Fig. 5. Distensibility as a functional quality of the artery: changing of the arterial Doppler waveform at RH after opening of the fist clenched for 2 min.

Disclosure Statement

The author has no conflict of interest to declare.

References

1 K/DOQI clinical practice guidelines for chronic kidney disease: evaluation, classification, and stratification. Am J Kidney Dis 2002;39(suppl 1):S1–S266.

2 Bayliss EA, Bhardwaja B, Ross C, Beck A, Lanese DM: Multidisciplinary team care may slow the rate of decline in renal function. Clin J Am Soc Nephrol 2011;6:704–710.

3 Levin A, Hemmelgarn B, Culleton B, et al: Guidelines for management of chronic kidney disease. CMAJ 2008;179:1154–1162.

4 Rakugi H, Ogihara T, Umemoto S, et al: Combination therapy for hypertension in patients with CKD: a subanalysis of the combination therapy of hypertension to prevent cardiovascular events trial. Hypertens Res 2013;36:947–958.

5 Agarwal R, Andersen MJ: Prognostic importance of ambulatory blood pressure recordings in patients with chronic kidney disease. Kidney Int 2006;69:1175–1180.

6 Stevens PE, Levin A; Kidney Disease: Improving Global Outcomes Chronic Kidney Disease Guideline Development Work Group Members: Evaluation and management of chronic kidney disease: synopsis of the kidney disease: improving global outcomes 2012 clinical practice guideline. Ann Intern Med 2013;158:825–830.
7 Kwan BC, Kronenberg F, Beddhu S, et al: Lipoprotein metabolism and lipid management in chronic kidney disease. J Am Soc Nephrol 2007;18:1246–1261.
8 Kraut JA, Kurtz I: Metabolic acidosis of CKD: diagnosis, clinical characteristics, and treatment. Am J Kidney Dis 2005;45:978–993.
9 KDIGO clinical practice guidelines for the diagnosis, evaluation, prevention, and treatment of chronic kidney disease-mineral and bone disorder (CKD-MBD). Kidney Int 2009; 76(suppl 113):S1–S130.
10 Kazmi WH, Kausz AT, Khan S, et al: Anemia: an early complication of chronic renal insufficiency. Am J Kidney Dis 2001;38:803–812.
11 Jeong JU, Kim HK, Cho YP, Kwon TW, Kom SB: Arteriovenous access creation defer chronic hemodialysis initiation. Clin Nephrol 2011;75:113–119.
12 Malovrh M: Approach to patients with end-stage renal disease in need of arteriovenous fistula. Nephrol Dial Transplant 2003;18 (suppl 5):v50–v52.
13 Premru V: Preservation of veins in predialysis patients and early referral. Blood Purif 2002;20:2.
14 Hoggard J, Saad T, Schon D, et al: Guidelines for venous access in patients with chronic kidney disease. A Position Statement from the American Society of Diagnostic and Interventional Nephrology, Clinical Practice Committee and the Association for Vascular Access. Semin Dial 2008;21:186–191.
15 Ferring M, Claridge M, Smith SA, Wilmink T: Routine preoperative vascular ultrasound improves patency and use of arteriovenous fistulas for hemodialysis: a randomized trial. Clin J Am Soc Nephrol 2010;5:2236–2244.
16 Malovrh M: Native arteriovenous fistula: preoperative evaluation. Am J Kidney Dis 2002; 39:1218–1225.
17 Malovrh M: Non-invasive evaluation of vessels by duplex sonography prior to construction of arteriovenous fistulas for haemodialysis. Nephrol Dial Transplant 1998;13: 125–129.
18 Jemcov TK: Morphologic and functional vessels characteristics assessed by ultrasonography for prediction of radiocephalic fistula maturation. J Vasc Access 2013;14:356–363.
19 Ferring M, Henderson J, Wilmink T, Smith S: Vascular ultrasound for the pre-operative evaluation prior to arteriovenous fistula formation for haemodialysis: review of the evidence. Nephrol Dial Transplant 2008;23: 1809–1815.

Marko Malovrh, MD, PhD
Department of Nephrology
University Medical Center Ljubljana
Zaloška 7, SL–1525 Ljubljana (Slovenia)
E-Mail marko.malovrh@gmail.com

Widmer MK, Malik J (eds): Patient Safety in Dialysis Access.
Contrib Nephrol. Basel, Karger, 2015, vol 184, pp 24–50
DOI: 10.1159/000365821

What Every Doctor Should Know about Drug Safety in Patients with Chronic Kidney Disease

Maria Paparella[a] • Valentina Martina[b] • Maria Antonietta Rizzo[b] • Maurizio Gallieni[a, c]

[a] Nephrology and Dialysis Unit, Ospedale San Carlo Borromeo, [b] Graduate School of Nephrology, and [c] Department of Biomedical and Clinical Sciences 'L. Sacco' (DIBIC), University of Milan, Milan, Italy

Abstract

Drug safety is a very relevant issue when dealing with patients with chronic kidney disease (CKD) who need vascular access procedures and interventions. Drug dosage adjustments are needed for patients with acute or chronic kidney disease. In CKD patients, the estimated glomerular filtration rate is used to guide dose adjustments. Determining the influence of renal replacement therapies on drug dosage adjustment is also very important. Safety issues for the following drugs used for situations related to vascular access are reported: anticoagulants and antiplatelet agents, antibiotics, antimicrobials for catheter lock therapy, thrombolytics, local anesthetics, and painkillers. General principles of the interactions of drugs in CKD are also reported.

Recommendations to Improve Patient Safety

- The assessment of kidney function with estimated glomerular filtration rate (eGFR) using CKD-Epidemiology Collaboration (CKD-EPI) and Modification of Diet in Renal Disease (MDRD) formulas is key for correct and safe drug prescribing.
- Dosing adjustments are generally required when eGFR is below 60 ml/min/1.73 m^2.
- When choosing drugs for use in chronic kidney disease (CKD) patients, consider pharmacokinetics (PK) and pharmacodynamics (PD) characteristics for the best efficacy/safety profile.

- Drug interactions in CKD patients are more frequent for the large number of prescribed drugs and for the altered PK.
- Avoid (or use with extreme caution) drugs that have not been proved effective and safe in CKD.

Background

Introduction to the Use of Drugs in Chronic Kidney Disease Patients: Assessment of Kidney Function

Dialysis access procedures, from central venous catheter insertion to arteriovenous fistula and grafts placement, are performed in patients with different degrees of renal insufficiency, including patients with acute kidney injury (AKI) and chronic kidney disease (CKD) in different stages. AKI and CKD can change the pharmacokinetics (PK) and the pharmacodynamics (PD) of many drugs [1]. Moreover, drug removal by intermittent and continuous renal replacement therapies determines the need for evaluating drug transport across biological (the peritoneum) and artificial membranes. Identifying drugs for which individualization of the treatment regimen will be necessary and consequently adjusting drug dosage regimens is important to avoid overdosage and toxicity of the drugs and/or their metabolites in renally impaired patients. Therefore, prior to treating patients with CKD, one must define kidney function (fig. 1).

Which Is the Most Accurate and Reliable Index to Assess Kidney Function for Drug Dosing, Thus Improving Drug Safety?

Determination of GFR based on the administration of exogenous substances is not practical for routine individual drug dose calculations. Therefore, urinary clearance of inulin (the gold standard) is rarely performed except for research purposes. Moreover, determination of GFR using an endogenous substance (creatinine), based on the urinary clearance of creatinine derived from a 24-hour urine collection is of limited clinical value because of frequent urine collection errors and analytical interferences with the serum or urine creatinine assays as the result of concomitant diseases and drug therapies. Therefore, estimated glomerular filtration rate (eGFR) obtained in clinical practice from the measurement of endogenous substances such as serum creatinine (Scr) and then combined with patient factors is the most commonly used measure to define kidney function [2]. eGFR can be measured in several different ways (table 1). However, in those clinical

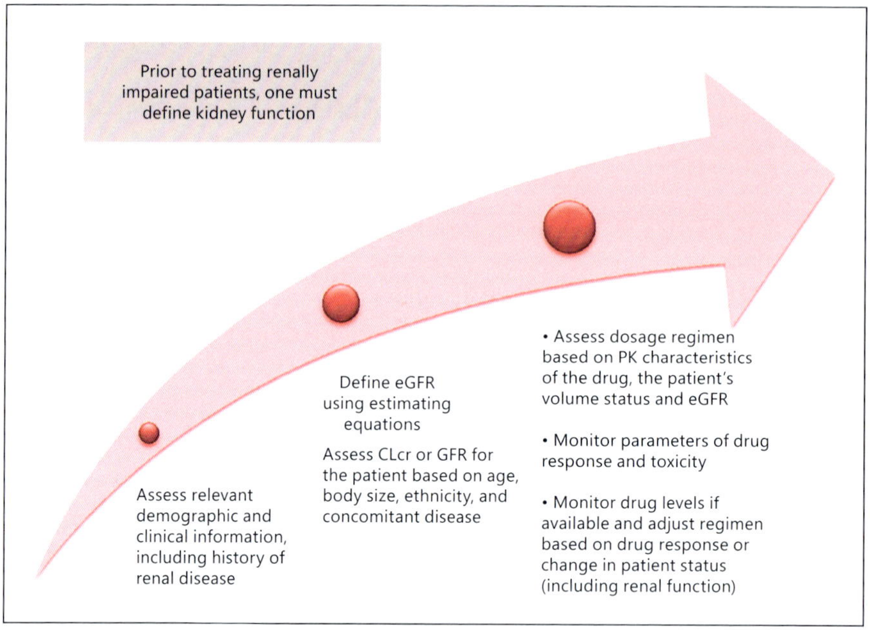

Fig. 1. Clinical algorithm for drug prescribing in CKD patients. CLcr = Urinary clearance of creatinine.

Table 1. List of the most common formulas for eGFR used for guiding drug dosage adjustment (see www.mdrd.com)

Cockcroft and Gault [6]	
MDRD-four variables [4]	(Modification of Diet in Renal Disease)
CKD-EPI [3, 5]	(Chronic Kidney Disease-Epidemiology Collaboration)

situations and for those drugs with a narrow therapeutic index for which dosing individualization is required, where any creatinine-based estimation equation is not likely to provide a good estimate of GFR, measured creatinine clearance or measured GFR using exogenous markers should be considered.

Which eGFR Equation Should Be Used for Assessment GFR as the Guide to Drug Dosage Regimens?

Several considerations regarding methods to estimate eGFR may guide us to choose the best option:

- Estimating equations are more accurate than measured creatinine clearance, given the errors in urine collection [3].
- Variability in Scr assays is a major source of bias, leading to differences in reported Scr values among laboratories as well as within laboratories over time. Use of isotope dilution mass spectroscopy (IDMS), a method to standardize creatinine assays, leads to less variation in eGFR and theoretically more consistent drug dosing recommendations across institutions and clinical settings. The MDRD Study [4] and CKD-Epidemiology Collaboration (CKD-EPI) [3, 5] equations should be preferentially used with IDMS-standardized creatinine.
- Keep in mind that in addition to the effect of GFR, Scr may be influenced by differences in muscle mass, diet and tubular secretion. Estimating equations capture the average differences in the rate of creatinine generation due to age, sex, race, and weight, but they do not capture all factors. Therefore, some individuals will have substantially different values of Scr than expected and eGFR will be higher or lower than the true GFR.
- In the past, before the availability of standardized approaches, variations of the Scr assays affected PK/PD drug studies. This may still determine difficulties in interpretation of product label drug dosing recommendations. However, it is not conceivable repeating all of the PK studies with standardized creatinine: considering that the MDRD equation has a similar performance at lower levels of GFR, where drug dose adjustment is frequent, it is still reasonable to use drug dosing adjustments suggested in the product labeling.
- The Cockcroft and Gault (CG) equation [6] has been shown to overestimate GFR with the use of standardized creatinine assays. The CG equation is reported in units not adjusted for body surface area (BSA), which is appropriate for drug dosage adjustment. However, it is worth noting that the CG equation considers the body weight in the mathematical approach.
- The Modification of Diet in Renal Disease (MDRD) equation was developed from an extensive sample of patients with known CKD, all of whom had a measured GFR <90 ml/min/1.73 m^2 [4]. This equation is now widely reported by clinical laboratories around the world whenever Scr is measured. Since the MDRD equation overestimates measured GFR in subjects with values >60 ml/min/1.73 m^2, values are only reported for GFR <60 ml/min/1.73 m^2 [3]. Use of IDMS-traceable creatinine values in the IDMS-MDRD Study equation results in a more accurate eGFR.
- The CKD-EPI equation, derived from studies including people with and without CKD, is more accurate than the MDRD equation, particularly at higher levels of GFR [5, 7].

- Formulas for eGFR are not accurate in individuals with extremes of body size or muscle mass, including the frail, elderly, critically ill, and subjects with unusual dietary habits. Kidney function is proportional to kidney size, which is proportional to BSA. BSA of 1.73 m^2 is the normal mean value for young adults. The eGFR ml/min/1.73 m^2 adjusted for BSA is necessary in patients whose body size is markedly different than average. If using eGFR in very large or very small patients, multiply the eGFR ml/min/1.73 m^2 by the BSA in order to obtain adjusted eGFR in units of ml/min.

In summary, it is very important to assess the GFR based on Scr levels. All the formulas considered in this chapter may give an acceptable estimate of GFR. The CKD-EPI equation appears to be preferable.

Drug Safety

Antimicrobial Drugs

Many antimicrobial agents are eliminated by the kidneys, and they require dosing adjustments in patients with CKD; however, several commonly used drugs do not require adjustments. Antibiotics should be used at the correct dose (see the section Drug Dosing in Patients with Renal Failure) to avoid undertreatment or, more commonly, drug toxicity.

Infectious complications are relevant causes of morbidity and mortality in hemodialysis patients [8, 9]. Of particular concern, vascular access has emerged as a major risk factor for infection and bacteremia [10]. Furthermore, the majority of these bacteremias are caused by staphylococci, associated with high rates of mortality (8–25%), recurrence (14.5–44%), and serious metastatic complications (14.5–44%) [11, 12]. When the source of fever is suspected to be vascular access (catheter or graft) related, antimicrobial therapy must reliably cover Gram-positive species (including methicillin-sensitive *Staphylococcus aureus*) since these organisms account for about two thirds of HD access-related bacteremias. Enterococci and Gram-negative organisms account for the majority of the remaining bacteremias, and antimicrobial therapy should target these organisms as well [12]. It has become common practice to treat the febrile HD patient empirically with a combination of parenteral vancomycin plus gentamycin or vancomycin plus a third generation cephalosporin [12]. With the emergence of vancomycin-resistant enterococci, the empiric use of vancomycin in the febrile patient on HD has been challenged: CDC published guidelines for the prudent use of vancomycin in an attempt to prevent the spread of vancomycin resistance [13]. In accordance with these guidelines, empiric treatment with vancomycin is appropriate in patients with β-lactam allergy or when serious infections with β-lactam-resistant Gram-positive bacteria are likely [12]. Continuing treatment, however, depends on culture results.

The appropriate management of catheter-related infections has become a major challenge for physicians, and the initial empiric antibiotic therapy should take into consideration the frequency of the bacterial isolates in such settings. Staphylococcal species are the most prevalent (60–100%) bacterial isolates in HD patients with catheter-related bacteremia [14, 15]; in some patients, both Gram-positive and Gram-negative organisms have been isolated from the bloodstream, indicating mixed bacteremia [16, 17]. These data mandate that empiric antibiotic therapy should target both Gram-positive and Gram-negative organisms.

For infections with documented sensitivity to cefazolin in anuric HD patients, intravenous postdialysis dosing of cefazolin is both safe and effective. Moreover, empiric treatment of non-life-threatening infections with cefazolin alone or in combination with gentamicin may be appropriate in HD patients pending culture results [18, 19].

Exit site infections are common and are recognized by redness, exudation and crusting. Topical agents applied to catheter exit site, such as povidone iodine, mupirocin, bacitracin zinc and polymixin B sulphate ointments have been proven effective [20, 21]. Oral rifampin or nasal mupirocin ointment reduced the incidence of *S. aureus* bacteremia [22].

Patient safety issues regarding the use of antibiotics are largely debated [23]. The WHO suggests that prescribing antibiotics without regard for the patient's underlying condition and whether antibiotics will help the patient, or administering multiple drugs without attention to the potential for adverse drug reactions, all have the potential for harm and patient injury. When considering CKD patients with end-stage renal disease, it should be kept in mind that if we want to avoid safety issues, use of the right antibiotic at the right dose is the ultimate goal.

Catheter Lock Therapy

Catheter-related bacteremia is the most relevant CVC-related complication, which can lead to catheter removal because bacteria colonize the catheter and may be difficult to eradicate.

Antibiotic-lock therapy (ALT) is used in addition to systemic treatment for CVC-related infections. After filling both catheter lumens with a mix of antibiotic and anticoagulant at the end of dialysis (catheter locking), antibiotic concentrations inside the catheter reach very high levels, much higher than the concentration reached during conventional treatment. The catheter lock can remain in place for many hours when the catheter is not in use, and it may limit biofilm formation. ALT is particularly important in central venous catheter-related infection of intraluminal origin, especially in patients with coagulase-negative staphylococci infections.

Published guidelines on the management of catheter-related infections are in favor of the use of ALT for the treatment of catheter-related infections [24]. The in vitro stability of antibiotic-heparin combinations in CVCs was studied by Vercaigne et al. [25]. While ciprofloxacin produced immediate precipitation with heparin, cefazolin, vancomycin and ceftazidime at 10 mg/ml and gentamycin at 5 mg/ml were successfully incubated with heparin (5,000 U/ml) for 72 h in the central venous catheter lumen. Although free antibiotic in CVC solution was reduced, the final concentration was still sufficient for an effective antibiotic-heparin lock [25]. Good evidence is available to support ALT in the prevention of catheter-related bacteremia in patients on hemodialysis [26, 27]. However, others have reported that the use of ALT may be limited due to antibiotic toxicity and the appearance of antibiotic-resistant microbial isolates [28, 29].

Sodium citrate locks are effective for prophylaxis against catheter-related infections [30], although increased rates of catheter thrombosis have been reported [31].

Catheter-related bloodstream infections are reduced by interdialytic locking with taurolidine, a nontoxic antimicrobial agent. Although the use of a formulation of 1.35% taurolidine in 4% citrate, compared to 5,000 U/ml heparin, was associated with a greater need for thrombolysis to maintain catheter patency [32], the addition of 500 U/ml heparin to taurolidine-citrate solution avoided the need for thrombolysis without increasing bacteremia, with catheter patency comparable to heparin 5,000 U/ml [33]. A taurolidine-citrate (4%)-urokinase (25,000 U) lock solution is now available.

Locking of catheters with ethanol is a promising technique: the agent is bactericidal, has low toxicity, is unlikely to produce resistant organisms, is able to disinfect organisms in biofilms and is cheap; ethanol is bactericidal by protein denaturation and is active against a wide variety of organism including Gram-positive bacteria, Gram-negative bacteria and fungi. A study has been designed comparing ethanol lock (70%) once a week versus standard heparin lock [34], but it recruited a limited number of patients and could not demonstrate a benefit of ethanol [35].

In patients with vascular access, the probability of dialysis access-related infection is considerably less for patients with native arteriovenous fistulae than for those with synthetic grafts [36]. Postoperative wound infection as well as poor aseptic technique at dialysis may cause infection of the fistula; silent infection in old nonfunctional clotted prosthetic arteriovenous grafts has been recognized as a frequent cause of bacteremia and morbidity among HD patients [12]. Patient safety, with the aim of avoiding infectious complications, should always be considered, even in the absence of a catheter.

Thrombolytics

Catheter thrombosis is another relevant problem for patients dialyzed with a CVC, leading to the use of thrombolytic therapy. Urokinase is used in Europe, and recombinant tissue plasminogen activator in the US for prevention and treatment of thrombosis.

Locking of the catheter with urokinase (5,000 IU instilled to each lumen for 30 min) may be used to open occluded CVCs [37], but in some patients is ineffective and is suggested in those patients who have contraindications to systemic urokinase. High-dose intradialytic urokinase (250,000 IU infused into the venous chamber over 3 h) is safe and effective in almost all instances of nonpositional malfunction of hemodialysis catheters without signs of sepsis; contraindications to high-dose systemic urokinase are rare in stable hemodialysis outpatients [38]. However, it is not indicated in patients with recent trauma or surgery.

The recombinant tissue plasminogen activator alteplase has recently been shown to be an effective alternative for restoring line patency [39]. In addition, a recent randomized trial demonstrated that the use of alteplase instead of heparin once weekly, as compared with the use of heparin three times a week, as a locking solution for central venous catheters significantly reduced the incidence of catheter malfunction and bacteremia [40]. It is also significantly more expensive than heparin and urokinase, but it can reduce the costs of unblocking or replacing clotted CVCs [41].

Analgesics

In CKD patients, analgesic drugs are difficult to handle, and pain is often undertreated as renal failure modifies the PK and PD of analgesics. In addition, most analgesics and their active metabolites are distributed in different tissues and their distribution volume is frequently altered in renal failure. Therefore, it is possible to observe side effects even at low doses of analgesics. In addition, many patients with CKD follow complex polypharmacy therapies for which there is a high risk of drug interactions.

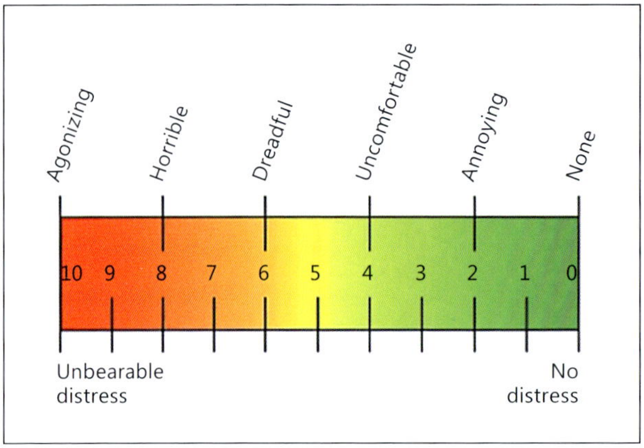

Fig. 2. Example of a VAS, where 0 is no pain and 10 is agonizing pain. Pain is a subjective sensation, and patients can adequately express the level of pain they are feeling and the level of pain they consider acceptable using the VAS.

Before starting treatment of pain, it is always necessary to understand its cause. In the general population, different drugs are available for the treatment of acute and chronic pain: peripherally acting analgesics (paracetamol and non-steroidal anti-inflammatory drugs, NSAIDs), centrally acting analgesics (opioids), clonidine, adjuvants (anticonvulsants, antidepressants, ketamine), peripheral neuronal blocking. NSAIDs are known for their renal toxicity and they should be avoided in renal failure. In addition, local anesthetics are generally used for control of surgery-related acute pain prevention and treatment.

Somatic pain responds well to NSAIDs and narcotics. Visceral pain, deep and poorly localized, caused by irritation of the serous or distension or ischemic tissue (for example pain associated with nephrolithiasis or pancreatitis) responds better to narcotics. In some cases, however, the narcotics themselves can exacerbate the problem (for example in case of bile duct obstruction). Neuropathic pain is characterized by excruciating burning pain, and is frequently associated with hypersensitivity. It may be more responsive to anticonvulsants and antidepressants than to opioids.

The knowledge of formulations, PK, potency and duration of analgesics is required for optimal analgesic therapy practice.

For a good treatment plan, one must first establish visual-analogue scale pain intensity (fig. 2), which is broadly classified as follows: mild pain (visual analogue scale, VAS, 1–4), moderate pain (VAS 5–6), and severe pain (VAS 7–10).

Barakzoy and Moss [42] validated in patients with renal failure the three-step scale of the World Health Organization for the treatment of pain, achieving ad-

Table 2. General principles for the treatment of chronic pain in CKD patients

Pain level	Recommended analgesic	Safety issues
Mild pain: VAS 1–3	Paracetamol (±adjuvant) is the nonnarcotic agent of choice NSAID are not indicated (topical gels may be used in small amounts)	Paracetamol: at high doses (over 4 g/day), liver toxicity is possible, especially in patients with chronic liver disease (viral or alcohol related) NSAID: increased risk of gastrointestinal bleeding; oliguria/anuria due to sodium and water retention; hyperkalemia; worsening of renal function
Moderate pain: VAS 4–6	Tramadol (with dose adjustment according to residual renal function)	Side effects are similar to those observed with opioids: constipation; nausea; central nervous system depression; seizures (in conditions with lower seizure threshold) May precipitate excess serotonin activity (serotonin syndrome), when patients are concomitantly treated with serotonergic drugs
Severe pain: VAS 7–10	Fentanyl (mostly cleared by the liver; inactive metabolites) Buprenorphine (with dose adjustment according to residual renal function; mostly cleared by the liver; inactive metabolites) Methadone (mostly cleared by the liver; inactive metabolites)	Safe for treatments over short periods; all may accumulate in the long term Reassess the need and dose of opioids every 24–48 h Use caution in opioid-naïve patients (monitor for central nervous system and respiratory effects) Fentanyl and methadone are highly protein bound and not dialyzable Constipation; nausea; central nervous system depression; seizures (in conditions with lower seizure threshold) May precipitate excess serotonin activity (serotonin syndrome), when patients are concomitantly treated with serotonergic drugs

equate analgesia in 96% of patients. However, this scheme is not applicable to acute pain for the long kinetics of tramadol, methadone and fentanyl; for the treatment of acute pain, rapid action and easy handling therapy is necessary. With this understanding, the general principles for the treatment of chronic pain in CKD are summarized in table 2, while in table 3 a treatment algorithm is proposed for acute pain [42, 43].

Analgesic drugs can be administered intravenously or orally. It is a doctor's duty to prevent the onset of severe pain by early administration of an analgesic rather than waiting until the patient has severe pain. The goal is the absence of pain, but also the limitation of side effects.

Table 3. Treatment of acute pain in CKD patients

Severity of pain	CKD EPI 50–10 ml/min[1]	CKD EPI <10 ml/min or dialysis[2]
Mild pain	paracetamol 1 g × 4; tramadol 100 mg may be added	paracetamol 1 g × 3; tramadol 50 mg may be added
Moderate pain	paracetamol 1 g × 4 + tramadol 100 mg × 2; buprenorphine 0.15 mg may be added	paracetamol 1 g × 3 + tramadol 50 mg × 2; buprenorphine 0.15 mg may be added
Severe pain[3]	buprenorphine 0.3 mg × 2 + paracetamol 1 g × 4; buprenorphine (3rd dose)	buprenorphine 0.3 mg × 2 + paracetamol 1 g × 3; buprenorphine (3rd dose)

[1] An eGFR of 50–10 ml/min calculated with the CKD-EPI formula usually corresponds to an Scr level between 1.5 and 5 mg/dl for males and between 1.25 and 4 mg/dl for females.
[2] An eGFR <10 ml/min or dialysis calculated with the CKD-EPI formula usually corresponds to an Scr level >5 mg/dl for males and >4 mg/dl for females.
[3] The combination oxycodone/naloxone is an opioid analgesic which may also be used for severe pain in CKD patients. Oxycodone is responsible for the pain-relieving effects, while naloxone reduces opioid-induced constipation.

Anesthetics

The anesthetist treating CKD patients is confronted with a number of clinical challenges related to altered drug handling, the production and accumulation of active metabolites and difficulties with vascular access and fluid balance [44]. CKD is a risk factor for serious postoperative complications, such as acute renal failure and cardiovascular complications, which are associated with an increased morbidity and mortality [45].

Dose adjustments are not usually necessary until GFR falls below 50 ml/min. CKD may influence both the PK and the PD of a drug [44].

Local anesthetics have two plasma protein-binding sites: a high-affinity and low-capacity site, and a low-affinity high-capacity site on albumin; the albumin-binding site becomes increasingly important as the plasma concentration of the local anesthetic increases. Metabolic acidosis increases the percentage of unbound drug, and this effect is more pronounced with bupivacaine [46].

Local anesthetics, such as lidocaine, are metabolized in the liver and excreted by the kidneys. Acute or chronic deterioration of renal function can lead to their inadequate clearance. Use of local anesthetics is not contraindicated in CKD patients with eGFR <50 ml/min, but dosages should be kept to a minimum and the interval between injections adequately extended.

Local anesthesia and regional blocks, commonly used in vascular access surgery, may affect vein diameter and fistula blood flow rates, which are important predictors of fistula failure. Regional block anesthesia (brachial plexus block) is associated with vasodilation in both the cephalic and basilic veins and with increased fistula blood flow.

Intravenous Anesthetic Agents

- Propofol PK are unaltered by established renal failure; the time interval between cessation of a propofol infusion and eye opening is significantly shorter in renal failure patients than controls, although blood propofol concentrations are not significantly different on waking [47].
- Thiopental has an increased volume of distribution and reduced plasma protein binding in renal failure, and the brain is exposed to a higher free drug concentration, so the rate of administration should be reduced [48].

Potent Inhalation Agents

- Methoxyflurane anesthesia may determine elevated serum inorganic fluoride levels and polyuric renal failure (serum fluoride levels >50 μmol/dl were associated with an increased risk of renal damage) [49].
- Enflurane: case reports of renal failure after enflurane anesthesia suggest that it is best avoided in patients with renal dysfunction [50].
- Desflurane and isoflurane are not associated with renal toxicity and appear safe to use in patients with CKD [51].

Anticoagulants and Platelet Aggregation Inhibitors

The prevalence of atrial fibrillation (AF) in end-stage renal disease is high, with an increased risk of stroke among these patients with AF compared with the AF population without severe renal impairment. Many trials have shown the clinical benefit of oral anticoagulation therapy for primary and secondary prevention of stroke in patients with AF. However, current stroke risk stratification schemes are based on studies that have deliberately excluded patients with severe renal impairment. Indeed, there are no large randomized controlled trials assessing the real risk/benefit of full intensity anticoagulation in patients with severe renal impairment. In addition, rates of major bleeding episodes in anticoagulated hemodialysis patients with AF are high [52].

Using data from the international Dialysis Outcomes and Practice Patterns Study (DOPPS) studying patients with AF, Wizemann et al. [53] found that warfarin use was associated with an overall significantly higher stroke risk due to an increased risk of bleeding, particularly in those over 75 years of age. This study shows that AF is common and associated with elevated risk of adverse clinical outcomes, and this risk is even higher among elderly patients prescribed warfarin. The effectiveness and safety of warfarin in hemodialysis patients require additional investigation [53].

Many physicians prescribe anticoagulants and antiplatelet medications to prevent thromboembolic events and access thrombosis in dialysis patients despite limited evidence of their efficacy in this population. Chan et al. [54] concluded that warfarin, aspirin, or clopidogrel prescription is associated with higher mortality among hemodialysis patients [54].

Recently, several novel oral anticoagulants (NOACs; rivaroxaban, dabigatran, apixaban) have been tested in large trials involving patients with AF and venous thromboembolism (VTE). All of these new anticoagulants are partially eliminated by renal clearance. In CKD patients, therefore, the half-lives of these novel anticoagulants may be prolonged, resulting in enhanced antithrombotic activity. On the other hand, there might be a higher risk of bleeding in CKD patients with these compounds.

The ROCKET-AF study [55] tested the efficacy and safety of rivaroxaban, a novel factor Xa inhibitor, in 14,264 patients with nonvalvular AF and additional stroke risk factors compared with standard warfarin therapy aiming at an international normalized ratio (INR) of 2.0–3.0. Rivaroxaban is predominantly metabolized by the liver, but approximately one third of the drug is cleared by the kidneys. The ROCKET-AF trial excluded patients with an eGFR <30 ml/min, whereas the daily dose of rivaroxaban was reduced from 20 to 15 mg in patients with an eGFR of 30–49 ml/min based on available PD data and PK modelling [55].

In the setting of chronic nonvalvular AF or venous thromboembolism, a recent systematic review of 8 randomized controlled trials among patients with CKD who received NOACs compared with those who received vitamin K antagonists (VKAs) identified no difference in the risk of stroke and systemic thromboembolism, recurrent thromboembolism or thromboembolism-related death, or bleeding. CKD was defined as a creatinine clearance between 30 and 50 ml/min [56]. Collectively, the NOACs have demonstrated efficacy and safety similar to those of the VKAs in patients with moderate CKD (CrCl 30–50 ml/min); however, trials evaluating the effect of these agents on important clinical outcomes in patients with more severe CKD, including patients undergoing dialysis, are lacking [56].

When planning vascular access interventions, one important safety aspect is the management of already established anticoagulant and antiplatelet treatments. Oral anticoagulation should be substituted with unfractionated heparin, which can be easily monitored with activated partial thromboplastin time and stopped the day before surgery. Low-molecular-weight heparins, on the other hand, pose an increased risk of bleeding because they accumulate in patients with CKD, unless their activity is monitored by the anti-factor Xa assay, which currently is not widely available.

Patients with CKD, including dialysis patients, are often prescribed platelet aggregation inhibitors. However, safety with antiplatelet therapy is a major concern in patients with renal impairment because they are at increased risk of bleeding compared with the general population for the concurrent uremia-related platelet dysfunction [57]. Therefore, understanding strategies of antiplatelet management in patients with CKD is of key importance. The most commonly used agents are ticlopidine, clopidogrel, and aspirin, which sometimes are combined.

A systematic review identified 16 studies including 40,676 patients, and found an increased bleeding risk for hemodialysis patients treated with combination antiplatelet therapy, while there are mixed results for studies using a single antiplatelet agent [58]. The study also suggested that antiplatelet agents appear to be effective in preventing shunt and central venous catheter thrombosis, but not for preventing thrombosis of arteriovenous grafts. Considering risks and benefits, the usefulness of antiplatelet agents for the prevention of access thrombosis in dialysis patients remains poorly defined. Individual risk stratification taking into account the increased risk of bleeding should be considered before initiating antiplatelet agents, especially in combination therapy [58].

Ongoing treatment with antiplatelet agents is generally stopped before planned vascular access surgery because they might increase the bleeding and the overall surgical risk in CKD patients. A recent retrospective study in renal transplantation, however, highlighted that these drugs are associated with a low risk of bleeding during renal transplantation, and their use does not seem to be a contraindication for renal transplant surgery [59]. The same might be true for vascular access surgery, especially when considering risks in patients needing urgent interventions for vascular access dysfunction.

Martinez Salazar et al. [60] reported no bleeding complications after 53 tunneled hemodialysis catheter procedures performed in dialysis patients on clopidogrel therapy, indicating that cardiologic indications to continue clopidogrel after cardiac procedures can be followed with low risks of complications during dialysis catheter procedures.

After vascular access surgery, benefits and risks of antithrombotic medications should be considered. The aim of such treatment is increasing the access duration, but its suitability for needling is also an important outcome to be considered.

Antiplatelet agents represent a logical strategy to prevent vascular access failure. Clopidogrel activity has been studied in patients with renal function impairment [61], although no data are reported in the drug prescribing information. Dose adjustment in patients with severe renal failure (GFR 5–15 ml/min) and moderate renal impairment (GFR 30–60 ml/min) does not appear to be required [61].

Clopidogrel has been evaluated for prevention of AV fistula nonmaturation [62] in a multicenter randomized clinical trial. Patients received either clopidogrel or placebo for 6 weeks after surgery. Although the frequency of access thrombosis within 6 weeks was significantly lower in patients receiving clopidogrel (12.2 vs. 19.5%), AV fistula nonmaturation was similar (and surprisingly very high) in both groups (61.8 vs. 59.5%). Antithrombotics for prevention of stenosis or thrombosis of AV grafts have also been evaluated with randomized trials. Neither warfarin nor aspirin plus clopidogrel prevented AV graft thrombosis, but unfortunately they increased the risk of bleeding complications [63, 64]. Dipyridamole plus aspirin produced a modest, although significant, prolongation of primary unassisted AV graft survival [65].

Interestingly, long-term fish oil ingestion (four 1-gram capsules/day) in patients with new hemodialysis grafts decreased by 22% (although statistically nonsignificant) the proportion of grafts with loss of native patency within 12 months [66]. In addition, fish oil improved some relevant secondary outcomes such as graft patency (RR 0.58), rates of thrombosis (RR 0.50), and angioplasty (RR 0.59). Unexpected benefits on cardiovascular events were also observed: improved cardiovascular event-free survival (hazard ratio, 0.43) and lower mean systolic blood pressure, indicating a favorable risk/benefit ratio for this pharmacological approach [66].

Systemic anticoagulation for the prevention of dialysis catheter thrombosis is controversial for its inherent risk-benefit issues: while it may improve catheter survival, it can also increase the risk of side effects, such as bleeding and cardiovascular calcifications due to inhibition of vitamin K-dependent proteins such as MGP (Matrix Gla protein) [67, 68].

Warfarin at the mini-dose of 1 mg/day was not effective in preventing thrombus formation with hemodialysis catheters, although catheter survival improved in patients with an INR greater than 1.00 [69]. A retrospective study found a significantly reduced thrombosis rate of tunneled catheters using anticoagulation at therapeutic levels [70]. Similar results were reported in patients anticoagulated after treatment with urokinase for thrombosis [71] and in patients at high risk for thrombosis with the maintenance of target INR in the range of 1.5–2.0 [72]. Twardowski [73] proposed a stepwise anticoagulation strategy in which the warfarin dose, started at 1 mg/day, is titrated upwards until thrombotic episodes resolve.

Thus, anticoagulation appears to be effective in preventing catheter thrombosis, but the available evidence is based on retrospective and noncontrolled studies, where the risks of bleeding, vascular calcification and bone side effects were not assessed. This raises a relevant safety issue, and in the absence of controlled prospective studies confirming the overall benefits of anticoagulation use, its general use cannot be currently recommended [74].

Interactions of Drugs: General Principles

CKD patients are affected by many comorbidities that require multiple pharmacological treatments. One of the factors that can modify the response to drugs is the concurrent administration of other drugs. This phenomenon is defined as drug interaction. Drug interactions may lead to adverse effects and occasionally to fatal outcomes [75]. Adverse effects due to drug interactions are often predictable from previous reports and careful knowledge of pharmacologic principles, but many clinicians have a low awareness of these possible adverse events.

Drug interaction is a condition of pharmacological incompatibilities, in which a drug affects the activity of another drug when they are administered together (drug-drug interaction, DDI); moreover, this reaction may also happen between drug and food, or between drug and medical plants.

Potential DDIs have been frequently reported, but only few studies have been conducted on actual interactions. Some data are available about drug interactions among elderly patients hospitalized for drug toxicity [76]. In a recent review [77], differences between actual and potential DDIs were outlined: the incidence of actual DDIs resulted lower than that of potential DDIs; important adverse effects occur only in the presence of specific risk factors, such as age or genetic polymorphisms.

There are several mechanisms by which drugs may interact; they can be classified as PK, PD, or combined interactions [78, 79]. Drug action can be synergistic (when the drug's effect is increased), antagonistic (when the drug's effect is decreased), or it may produce new effects. Drug interactions depend on both patient-specific factors (intrinsic drug clearance, genetics, gender, concurrent diseases, diet), and drug-specific factors (dose, route of administration, drug formulation, and the sequence of drug administration).

PD Interactions

PD interactions can occur through pharmacological receptors or signal transductor mechanisms [79]. The drugs may or may not act on the same receptor to produce pharmacological effects. When drugs with similar pharmacologic effects are concurrently administered, an additive or synergistic response is usually seen.

If the drugs act on the same receptor, they in turn can be:

- Pure agonists, binding to the receptor's main locus and causing a similar effect.
- Partial agonists, binding to one of the receptor's secondary loci, causing the same effect, but with a lower intensity in contrast to the principle drug.
- Antagonists, binding the receptor's main locus but with an opposite effect to that of the main drug. If they compete with the main drug to bind with the receptor, they are defined as competitive antagonists; but, when the antagonist irreversibly binds to the receptor and it is not released until the receptor is saturated, it is called uncompetitive antagonist.

PK Interactions

Different basic PK parameters must be considered for obtaining a careful drug management [78]. The most important are clearance, distribution volume, amount bound in plasma, half-life. Clearance is the measure of capacity to eliminate the drug, while volume of distribution is the measure of the apparent body space available to contain the drug. Moreover, half-life represents the time required to reduce the amount of drug in the body by one half during elimination and attain 50% of steady state. Finally, the renal eliminated fraction of a drug is the key to predict its PK.

PK interactions may modify drug concentrations by interfering with different mechanisms such as absorption, distribution, metabolism, and excretion of the drug [78].

Absorption is strictly related to gastric pH, drug solubility or gastrointestinal motility, while distribution is influenced by competition of plasma protein binding, displacement from tissue-binding sites, or alterations in local tissue barriers.

Metabolism is regulated by metabolizing enzymes, which are typically activated through nuclear receptors. It primarily occurs in liver tissue and small intestine, followed by other sides, such as plasma, lung and kidney. The most important of this enzymatic system is the system of cytochrome P450 isozymes. A result of interactions between endogenous or exogenous factors on enzymatic systems may stimulate the function of the enzyme (enzyme induction) or inhibit it (enzyme inhibition) [80]. The final action is a modification in drug metabolism.

Table 4. Potential effects of kidney failure on drug PK

Absorption
Diabetic or uremic gastroparesis may alter gastrointestinal transit time and modify drug absorption
A drug able to alter gastric pH (e.g. antacids ad phosphate binders) can reduce the absorption of other drugs
Gastrointestinal tract edema caused by congestive heart failure or nephrotic syndrome can slow drug absorption
Distribution
Edema or ascites may increase the distribution volume for protein-bound and water-soluble drugs
Uremia can alter plasma protein binding, affecting acidic drugs
Hypoalbuminemia and altered plasma protein binding increase free or unbound concentrations of drugs
Tissue protein drug binding is reduced in uremic states
Metabolism
Renal failure may affect liver function, increasing or decreasing hepatic bio-transformations
Excretion
Reduced excretion and prolonged half-life; renal failure may alter glomerular filtration, tubular secretion, reabsorption

Finally, the excretion interactions principally depend on renal function. Drugs are removed from the plasma by the kidney with different mechanisms: passive filtration, reabsorption and active secretion. Filtration depends on urine pH, so that renal excretion of certain drugs that are weak acids or weak bases may be influenced by other drugs that affect urinary pH (for example, drugs acting as weak bases are more easily excreted with acid urine pH; the inverse it is true for weak acids). Finally, secretion is a process based on saturability of the transported molecule and competition between substrates. P-glycoprotein, organic anion and cation transporters are involved in active tubular secretion of some drugs, and inhibition of these transporters can reduce renal elimination of the drugs, causing an increase in their serum levels [81].

Considering the key role of the kidneys in drug metabolism and excretion, kidney failure obviously modifies drug PK (table 4).

Drug Dosing in Patients with Renal Failure

The standard dose of a drug derives from studies in healthy volunteers and patients with normal capacity to metabolize and eliminate drugs [78]. However, the effective dose may be different from patient to patient. Pathologic conditions

Table 5. Drug dosage individualization in patients with CKD

eGFR should be calculated for evaluating the stage of CKD and drug dosing purposes
Dosing adjustments are generally required when GFR falls below 50 ml/min/1.73 m^2
The impact of interactions of all drugs commonly used in CKD patients (e.g. phosphate binders) should be evaluated
The volume of distribution (VD) of many drugs is increased in patients with moderate to severe CKD as well as in those with pre-existing CKD who develop AKI; the increase in VD may be the result of decreased protein binding or fluid overload; obese CKD and AKI patients and those with large variations in serum protein levels should have their drug dosage individualized
Dosing changes can involve dose reduction, increasing the interval between doses or both
Loading doses may be required if a drug has a long half-life and there is a need to rapidly achieve the desired steady-state concentrations or if the VD of a drug is significantly increased
Maintenance dose: most commonly, prolonging the dosing interval but maintaining the same dose will result in the achievement of similar peak and trough concentrations as well as area under the curve and thus may be preferred
A more accurate drug dosage adjustment is recommended for agents that have a narrow therapeutic index; when available, measurement of therapeutic drug levels may optimize therapeutic regimens; hypoalbuminemia may influence the interpretation of drug concentrations

(heart, liver or renal failure) may demand dosage adjustment in individual patients because they modify specific PK parameters of the drugs.

For the predominant role of the kidneys in drug metabolism and excretion, patients affected by renal failure require an adjustment of dosing for substances cleared and metabolized by the kidney. The principles for drug dosage individualization in CKD patients are summarized in table 5.

Dose adjustment is based on a combination of PK and PD effects, determining the relationship between the concentration of a drug and its final effect on organs [82]. In case of a marked reduction of glomerular filtration, certain drugs should no longer be given, either because they may further damage the kidneys or because they are insufficiently eliminated and will accumulate, causing adverse events.

Dosages of drugs cleared by kidney should be adjusted according to creatinine clearance or GFR calculated using online or electronic calculators [83], as previously outlined.

A careful assessment of renal function is necessary before starting a drug. It is necessary to evaluate if a drug should be administrated or not, and/or if a dosing adjustment is required according to GFR.

Attention in the use of antibiotics is particularly important. Patients with fluid overload may require a larger loading dose, in contrast to dehydrated patients. Patients with renal insufficiency generally need a higher starting dose, and then the maintenance dose is adjusted according to renal function, depending on drug half-life. The starting dose is important for both types of antibiotic, those whose effect is concentration dependent and those whose effect is time dependent. For adjusting the maintenance dosage in patients affected by kidney failure, it is possible to reduce the dose or to increase the intervals between doses, keeping the dose size normal. In clinical practice, a combination of the two methods is often useful. Finally, in patients requiring dialysis, many drugs are given at the end of the dialysis session, minimizing removal during dialysis. As a clinical alternative, it is often useful to search for drugs that are similar to the principal drugs but not metabolized by the kidney [83].

Detailed dosing recommendations for individual drugs are available in specific textbooks [84, 85]. Nevertheless, although guidelines are available, indications and regimens must be always individualized according to patient response and serum drug concentrations.

Problematic Drugs in CKD

Many drugs are commonly administered in CKD and dialysis patients. Here, we focus our attention on drugs required for management of vascular access: antimicrobials, anticoagulants, analgesics and anesthetics. PK parameters may be modified in kidney failure and dosing adjustment based on GFR may be required, especially for antimicrobials (table 6). Again, we want to emphasize that patients affected by renal failure are at high risk of adverse events induced by NSAIDs [86]. The most frequent are acute kidney failure, nephritic/nephrotic syndrome, papillary necrosis. In patients with preexisting renal damage, the use of NSAIDs can lead to permanent renal damage. The risk of renal damage is increased if NSAIDs are administrated together with ace inhibitors, in dehydrated conditions and for prolonged time. They should be avoided in renal failure.

Measurement of Therapeutic Drug Levels

Measuring drug concentrations is one way to optimize therapeutic regimens and account for changes between individuals. Therapeutic drug monitoring mainly involves antibiotics (i.e. vancomycin, gentamicin), immunosuppressives (cyclosporine), anti-seizure drugs (carbamazepine, phenytoin and valproic acid), mood stabilizers (lithium), and antipsychotics.

Table 6. PK parameters for selected drugs used in CKD/dialysis patients and dosing adjustment according to GFR

Drug	Urinary excretion, %	Bound to plasma proteins, %	Volume of distribution, l/kg	Half-life normal/ESRD, h	Dose for normal renal function	Dosing adjustment for eGFR	
						30–15 ml/min (CKD IV)	<15 ml/min (CKD V)
Antiplatelet and anticoagulant drugs							
Acetylsalicylic acid (aspirin) for prophylaxis of thrombosis	5–80% (highly variable: increases with increased urinary pH)	80–90	0.1–0.2	2 (salicylate)/unchanged	75–325 mg q24 h	75–325 mg q24 h	not recommended[a]
Warfarin	3	99	0.15	34–45/unchanged	2–10 mg[b]	100%	10%
Ticlopidine	2	98	no data	12/no data (single dose) 24–33/no data (repeat dosing)	250 mg q12 h	100%	100%
Clopidogrel	50	98	no data	6–8/no data	75 mg q24 h	100%	100%
Heparin	–	90	0.06–0.1	0.3–2/unchanged	50–75 IU/kg per day	100%	100%[c]
Low-molecular-weight heparin	–	no data	0.06–0.13	22.6/4–10	30–40 mg q12 h[d]	100%	50%[d]
Pain medications/analgesics							
Paracetamol (acetaminophen)	3	20–30	1–2	2/2	500–1,000 mg q4 h	500–1,000 mg q6 h[e]	500–1,000 mg q8 h[e]
Tramadol	95	20	2–3	5–7/11 (range up to 20 h)	50–100 mg q12–4 h depending on severity of pain	50–100 mg q12 h[f]	50 mg q12 h[f]
Buprenorphine	30 (inactive metabolites)	96	2.8	37/unchanged	0.3 mg q6 h (initial dose)	0.15–0.3 mg q12 h	0.15–0.3 mg q12 h
Fentanyl	10	84	3–4	i.v.: 6/no data sublingual: 6.6/no data transdermal: 20–27/no data	sublingual: 100 μg (initial dose) transdermal: 25 μg/h (initial dose)	75%	50%
Codeine	>90	7	3–4	2.5–3.5/no data	30–60 mg q4–6 h	avoid[g]	avoid[g]

Table 6 (continued)

Drug	Urinary excretion, %	Bound to plasma proteins, %	Volume of distribution, l/kg	Half-life normal/ESRD, h	Dose for normal renal function	Dosing adjustment for eGFR	
						30–15 ml/min (CKD IV)	<15 ml/min (CKD V)
Methadone	highly variable (reduced with increased urinary pH)	85–90	1–8	30/unchanged	2.5–10 mg q8–12 h	75%[g]	50%[g]
Morphine	8%	20–30	3.5	1–4/unchanged	20–25 mg q4 h	avoid[g]	avoid[g]
Antimicrobial drugs							
Gentamicin	76	10	0.23–0.28	1.8–3/20–60	1.7 mg/kg q8 h	100% q12–24 h	100% q48 h
Ciprofloxacin	65	40	2.5	3–6/6–9	500–750 mg q12 h	50–75%	50%
Levofloxacin	60–80	24–38	1.1–1.5	4–8/76	250–750 mg q24 h	250–750 mg q24–48 h[h]	250–500 mg q48 h[h]
Vancomycin	80	30	0.4–1.1	4–6/200–250	1 g q12 h	1 g q24–96 h	1 g q4–7 days[i]
Amoxicillin	50–70	15–25	0.26	0.9–2.3/5–20	250–500 mg q8 h	250–500 mg q8–12 h	250–500 mg q24 h
Ampicillin	30–90	20	0.17–0.31	0.8–1.5/7–20	250 mg to 2 g 6 h	250 mg to 2 g q6–12 h	250 mg to 2 g q12–24 h
Cefazolin	90	80	0.13–0.22	2/40–70	0.25–2 g q6 h	100% q12 h	50% q24–48 h
Ceftazidime	60–80	5–24	0.18–0.31	1.2/13–25	1–2 g q8 h	1–2 g q12–24 h	1–2 g q24–48 h
Ceftriaxone	30	90	0.12–0.18	7–9/12–24	0.25–2 g q12–24 h	100%	100%
Meropenem	70	2	0.35	1.1/6–10	1–2 g q8 h	100% q12 h	100% q24 h
Imipenem	70	13–21	0.17–0.3	1/4	0.2 mg to 1 g q6 h	50%[j]	25%[j]
Local anesthetics							
Lidocaine 0.5 – 1%	<10	70	1.1	1.8/5.0	5–300 mg (1–60 ml)	75%	75%

Modified from Holford [78], Berns and Aronoff [84], and Gilbert et al. [85].
[a] Nephrotoxic at high doses (a potential GFR reduction when renal blood flux is supported by prostaglandins); dose of 100 mg when administrated as antiplatelet action. [b] According to INR, reduced binding to plasma protein in CKD. [c] Increased risk of bleeding – measure activated partial thromboplastin time. [d] 1 mg = 100 IU; monitored by anti-Xa factor activity; reduced elimination in renal failure. Avoid in renal failure if anti-Xa factor activity cannot be monitored. [e] Safe in CKD. [f] 100 mg extended-release tablets should not be used. [g] Opioid use causes adverse events in CKD patients. [h] Loading dose 500 mg. [i] Measure serum levels. [j] Administered together with cilastatin to prevent nephrotoxicity.

Therapeutic drug monitoring requires availability of rapid, specific, and reliable assays and known correlations of drug concentration to therapeutic and adverse outcomes. Hypoalbuminemia may influence the interpretation of drug concentrations as the total drug concentration may be reduced even when the active unbound drug concentration is not. Unbound drug concentrations are often not clinically available, and therefore clinicians must empirically consider the impact of hypoalbuminemia in their interpretation of measured total drug concentrations.

Conclusions

Safety of pharmacologic therapy in CKD patients is a major concern. Therefore, understanding strategies of drug management in this patient population is of key importance. The lack of studies performed specifically in patients with impaired renal function, particularly those with AKI or end-stage renal disease, who are generally excluded from many large-scale clinical trials, often leads to either no recommendation on the most appropriate pharmacologic treatment regimen or to opinion-based indications. Overall, the choice and combination of drugs prescribed to CKD patients should be balanced against the individual risk of adverse events. More data from large-scale clinical trials including CKD patients or even better from dedicated studies in patients with CKD are warranted in order to define the most effective and safe drugs for CKD patients.

Disclosure Statement

The authors have no conflicts of interest to declare.

References

1 Matzke GR, Comstock T: Influence of renal disease and dialysis on pharmacokinetics; in Evans W, Schentag J, Burton M (eds): Applied Pharmacokinetics: Principles of Therapeutic Drug Monitoring, ed 4. Baltimore, Lippincott, Williams & Wilkins, 2005, pp 187–212.

2 Kasiske B, Keane W: Laboratory assessment in kidney disease: clearance, urinalysis, and renal biopsy; in Brenner B (ed): Brenner and Rector's The Kidney, ed 6. Philadelphia, WB Saunders, 2000, pp 1129–1170.

3 Levey AS, Stevens LA: Estimating GFR using the epidemiology collaboration (CKD-EPI) creatinine equation: more accurate GFR estimates, lower CKD prevalence estimates, and better risk predictions. Am J Kidney Dis 2010;55:622–627.
4 Levey AS, Bosch JP, Lewis JB, Greene T, Rogers N, Roth D: A more accurate method to estimate glomerular filtration rate from serum creatinine: a new prediction equation. Modification of Diet in Renal Disease Study Group. Ann Intern Med 1999;130:461–470.
5 Levey AS, Stevens LA, Schmid CH, et al: A new equation to estimate glomerular filtration rate. Ann Intern Med 2009;150:604–612.
6 Cockcroft DW, Gault MH: Prediction of creatinine clearance from serum creatinine. Nephron 1976;16:31–41.
7 Stevens LA, Schmid CH, Zhang Y, et al: Development and validation of GFR-estimating equations using diabetes, transplant and weight. Nephrol Dial Transplant 2009;25: 449–457.
8 Di Iorio BR, Bellizzi V, Cillo N, et al: Vascular access for hemodialysis: the impact on morbidity and mortality. J Nephrol 2004;17: 19–25.
9 United States Renal Data System. Causes of death. Am J Kidney Dis 1997;30(suppl 1): S107–S117.
10 Bloembergen WE, Port FK: Epidemiological perspective on infections in chronic dialysis patients. Adv Ren Replace Ther 1996;3:201–217.
11 Powe NR, Jaar B, Furth SL, Hermann J, Briggs W: Septicemia in dialysis patients: incidence, risk factors, and prognosis. Kidney Int 1999;55:1081–1090.
12 Nassar GM, Ayus JC: Infectious complications of the hemodialysis access. Kidney Int 2001;60:1–13.
13 Centers for Disease Control and Prevention: Recommendations for preventing the spread of vancomycin resistance: recommendations of the Hospital Infection Control Practices Advisory Committee (HICPAC). MMWR 1995;44:1–13.
14 Nielsen J, Ladefoged SD, Kolmos HJ: Dialysis catheter-related septicaemia – focus on *Staphylococcus aureus* septicaemia. Nephrol Dial Transplant 1998;13:2847–2852.
15 Dobkin JF, Miller MH, Steigbigel NH: Septicemia in patients on chronic hemodialysis. Ann Intern Med 1978;88:28–33.
16 Beathard GA: Management of bacteremia associated with tunneled-cuffed hemodialysis catheters. J Am Soc Nephrol 1999;10:1045–1049.
17 Saad TF: Bacteremia associated with tunneled, cuffed hemodialysis catheters. Am J Kidney Dis 1999;34:1114–1124.
18 Fogel MA, Nussbaum PB, Feintzeig ID, Hunt WA, Gavin JP, Kim RC: Cefazolin in chronic hemodialysis patients: a safe, effective alternative to vancomycin. Am J Kidney Dis 1998; 32:401–409.
19 Marx MA, Frye RF, Matzke GR, Golper TA: Cefazolin as empiric therapy in hemodialysis-related infections: efficacy and blood concentrations. Am J Kidney Dis 1998;32:410–414.
20 Fong IW: Prevention of haemodialysis and peritoneal dialysis catheter related infection by topical povidone-iodine. Postgrad Med J 1993;69(suppl 3):S15–S17.
21 Johnson DW, MacGinley R, Kay TD, Hawley CM, Campbell SB, Isbel NM, Hollett P: A randomized controlled trial of topical exit site mupirocin application in patients with tunnelled, cuffed haemodialysis catheters. Nephrol Dial Transplant 2002;17:1802–1807.
22 Yu VL, Goetz A, Wagener M, Smith PB, Rihs JD, Hanchett J, Zuravleff JJ: *Staphylococcus aureus* nasal carriage and infection in patients on hemodialysis. Efficacy of antibiotic prophylaxis. N Engl J Med 1986;315:91–96.
23 World Health Organization: WHO patient safety curriculum guide for medical schools. Topic 1. What is patient safety. Geneva, WHO, 2009.
24 Mermel LA, Farr BM, Sherertz RJ, et al: Guidelines for the management of intravascular catheter-related infections. J Intraven Nurs 2001;24:180–205.
25 Vercaigne LM, Sitar DS, Penner SB, Bernstein K, Wang GQ, Burczynski FJ: Antibiotic-heparin lock: in vitro antibiotic stability combined with heparin in a central venous catheter. Pharmacotherapy 2000;20:394–399.
26 Kim SH, Song KI, Chang JW, Prevention of uncuffed hemodialysis catheter-related bacteremia using an antibiotic lock technique: a prospective, randomized clinical trial. Kidney Int 2006;69:161–164.
27 Capdevila JA, Gavaldà J, Fortea J, et al: Lack of antimicrobial activity of sodium heparin for treating experimental catheter-related infection due to *Staphylococcus aureus* using the antibiotic-lock technique. Clin Microbiol Infect 2001;7:206–212.

28 Abbas SA, Haloob IA, Taylor SL, et al: Effect of antimicrobial locks for tunneled hemodialysis catheters on bloodstream infection and bacterial resistance: a quality improvement report. Am J Kidney Dis 2009;53:492–502.
29 Dogra GK, Herson H, Hutchison B: Prevention of tunneled hemodialysis catheter-related infections using catheter-restricted filling with gentamicin and citrate: a randomized controlled study. J Am Soc Nephrol 2002;13: 2133–2139.
30 Yahav D, Rozen-Zvi B, Gafter-Gvili A, Leibovici L, Gafter U, Paul M: Antimicrobial lock solutions for the prevention of infections associated with intravascular catheters in patients undergoing hemodialysis: systematic review and meta-analysis of randomized, controlled trials. Clin Infect Dis 2008;47:83–93.
31 Power A, Duncan N, Singh SK, et al: Sodium citrate versus heparin catheter locks for cuffed central venous catheters: a single-center randomized controlled trial. Am J Kidney Dis 2009;53:1034–1041.
32 Solomon LR, Cheesbrough JS, Ebah L, et al: A randomized double-blind controlled trial of taurolidine-citrate catheter locks for the prevention of bacteremia in patients treated with hemodialysis. Am J Kidney Dis 2010;55: 1060–1068.
33 Solomon LR, Cheesbrough JS, Bhargava R, Mitsides N, Heap M, Green G, Diggle P: Observational study of need for thrombolytic therapy and incidence of bacteremia using taurolidine-citrate-heparin, taurolidine-citrate and heparin catheter locks in patients treated with hemodialysis. Semin Dial 2012; 25:233–238.
34 Broom JK, O'Shea S, Govindarajulu S, et al: Rationale and design of the HEALTHY-CATH trial: a randomised controlled trial of Heparin versus EthAnol Lock THerapY for the prevention of Catheter Associated infecTion in Haemodialysis patients. BMC Nephrol 2009;10:23.
35 Broom JK, Krishnasamy R, Hawley CM, Playford EG, Johnson DW: A randomised controlled trial of Heparin versus EthAnol Lock THerapY for the prevention of Catheter Associated infecTion in Haemodialysis patients – the HEALTHY-CATH trial. BMC Nephrol 2012;13:146.
36 Bonomo RA, Rice D, Whalen C, Linn D, Eckstein E, Shlaes DM: Risk factors associated with permanent access-site infections in chronic hemodialysis patients. Infect Control Hosp Epidemiol 1997;18:757–761.
37 Schwab SJ, Buller GL, McCann RL, Bollinger RR, Stickel DL: Prospective evaluation of a Dacron cuffed hemodialysis catheter for prolonged use. Am J Kidney Dis 1988;11:166–169.
38 Twardowski ZJ: The clotted central vein catheter for haemodialysis. Nephrol Dial Transplant 1998;13:2203–2206.
39 Bamgbola OF, del Rio M, Kaskel FJ, Flynn JT: Recombinant tissue plasminogen activator infusion for hemodialysis catheter clearance. Pediatr Nephrol 2005;20:989–993.
40 Hemmelgarn BR, Moist LM, Lok CE, et al: Prevention of dialysis catheter malfunction with recombinant tissue plasminogen activator. N Engl J Med 2011;364:303–312.
41 Gittins NS, Hunter-Blair YL, Matthews JN, Coulthard MG: Comparison of alteplase and heparin in maintaining the patency of paediatric central venous haemodialysis lines: a randomised controlled trial. Arch Dis Child 2007;92:499–501.
42 Barakzoy AS, Moss AH: Efficacy of the world health organization analgesic ladder to treat pain in end-stage renal disease. J Am Soc Nephrol 2006;17:3198–3203.
43 Glick N, Davison SN: Managing chronic pain in advanced chronic kidney disease. US Nephrol 2011;6:21–28.
44 Craig RG, Hunter JM: Recent developments in the perioperative management of adult patients with chronic kidney disease. Br J Anaesth 2008;101:296–310.
45 Novis BK, Roizen MF, Aronson S, Thisted RA: Association of preoperative risk factors with postoperative acute renal failure. Anesth Analg 1994;78:143–149.
46 Nancarrow C, Runciman WB, Mather LE, Upton RN, Plummer JL: The influence of acidosis on the distribution of lidocaine and bupivacaine into the myocardium and brain of the sheep. Anesth Analg 1987;66:925–935.
47 Ickx B, Cockshott ID, Barvais L, et al: Propofol infusion for induction and maintenance of anaesthesia in patients with end-stage renal disease. Br J Anaesth 1998;81:854–860.
48 Sear JW: Drug handling in renal impairment. Curr Anaesth Crit Care 1992;3:133–139.

49 Cousins MJ, Mazze RI, Kosek JC, Hitt BA, Love FV: The etiology of methoxyflurane nephrotoxicity. J Pharmacol Exp Ther 1974;190:530–541.
50 Eichhorn JH, Hedley-Whyte J, Steinman TI, Kaufmann JM, Laasbert LH: Renal failure following enflurane anesthesia. Anesthesiology 1976;45:557–560.
51 Litz RJ, Hübler M, Lorenz W, Meier VK, Albrecht DM: Renal responses to desflurane and isoflurane in patients with renal insufficiency. Anesthesiology 2002;97:1133–1136.
52 Marinigh R, Lane DA, Lip GY: Severe renal impairment and stroke prevention in atrial fibrillation: implications for thromboprophylaxis and bleeding risk. J Am Coll Cardiol 2011;57:1339–1348.
53 Wizemann V, Tong L, Satayathum S, et al: Atrial fibrillation in hemodialysis patients: clinical features and associations with anticoagulant therapy. Kidney Int 2010;77:1098–1106.
54 Chan KE, Lazarus JM, Thadhani R, Hakim RM: Anticoagulant and antiplatelet usage associates with mortality among hemodialysis patients. J Am Soc Nephrol 2009;20:872–881.
55 Goodman SG, Wojdyla DM, Piccini JP, et al: Factors associated with major bleeding events: insights from the ROCKET AF trial (rivaroxaban once-daily oral direct factor Xa inhibition compared with vitamin K antagonism for prevention of stroke and embolism trial in atrial fibrillation). J Am Coll Cardiol 2014;63:891–900.
56 Harel Z, Sholzberg M, Shah PS, et al: Comparisons between novel oral anticoagulants and vitamin K antagonists in patients with CKD. J Am Soc Nephrol 2014;25:431–442.
57 Capodanno D, Angiolillo DJ: Antithrombotic therapy in patients with chronic kidney disease. Circulation 2012;125:2649–2661.
58 Hiremath S, Holden RM, Fergusson D, Zimmerman DL: Antiplatelet medications in hemodialysis patients: a systematic review of bleeding rates. Clin J Am Soc Nephrol 2009;4:1347–1355.
59 Benahmed A, Kianda M, Ghisda L, et al: Ticlopidine and clopidogrel, sometimes combined with aspirin, only minimally increase the surgical risk in renal transplantation: a case-control study. Nephrol Dial Transplant 2014;29:463–466.
60 Martinez Salazar GM, Tan CS, Spearman K, Wicky S, Wu S: Safety of percutaneous tunneled hemodialysis catheter procedures in patients receiving concurrent clopidogrel therapy. J Vasc Access 2014;15:33–37.
61 Deray G, Bagnis C, Brouard R, et al: Clopidogrel activities in patients with renal function impairment. Clin Drug Investig 1998;16:319–328.
62 Dember LM, Beck GJ, Allon M, et al: Effect of clopidogrel on early failure of arteriovenous fistulas for hemodialysis: a randomized controlled trial. JAMA 2008;299:2164–2171.
63 Crowther MA, Clase CM, Margetts PJ, et al: Low-intensity warfarin is ineffective for the prevention of PTFE graft failure in patients on hemodialysis: a randomized controlled trial. J Am Soc Nephrol 2002;13:2331–2337.
64 Kaufman JS, O'Connor TZ, Zhang JH, et al: Veterans Affairs Cooperative Study Group on Hemodialysis Access Graft Thrombosis: randomized controlled trial of clopidogrel plus aspirin to prevent hemodialysis access graft thrombosis. J Am Soc Nephrol 2003;14:2313–2321.
65 Dixon BS, Beck GJ, Vazquez MA, et al: Effect of dipyridamole plus aspirin on hemodialysis graft patency. N Engl J Med 2009;360:2191–2201.
66 Lok CE, Moist LM, Hemmelgarn BR, et al: Effect of fish oil supplementation on graft patency and cardiovascular events among patients with new synthetic arteriovenous hemodialysis grafts: a randomized controlled trial. JAMA 2012;307:1809–1816.
67 Fusaro M, Crepaldi G, Maggi S, et al: Bleeding, vertebral fractures and vascular calcifications in patients treated with warfarin: hope for lower risks with alternative therapies. Curr Vasc Pharmacol 2011;9:763–769.
68 Fusaro M, Tripepi G, Noale M, et al: Prevalence of vertebral fractures, vascular calcifications, and mortality in warfarin treated hemodialysis patients. Curr Vasc Pharmacol 2013, Epub ahead of print.
69 Mokrzycki MH, Jean-Jerome K, Rush H, Zdunek MP, Rosenberg SO: A randomized trial of minidose warfarin for the prevention of late malfunction in tunneled, cuffed hemodialysis catheters. Kidney Int 2001;59:1935–1942.
70 Lee O, Raque JD, Lee LJ, et al: Retrospective assessment of risk factors to predict tunneled hemodialysis catheter outcome. J Vasc Interv Radiol 2004;15:457–461.

71 Webb A, Abdalla M, Russell GI: A protocol of urokinase infusion and warfarin for the management of the thrombosed haemodialysis catheter. Nephrol Dial Transplant 2001; 16:2075–2078.
72 Zellweger M, Bouchard J, Raymond-Carrier S, Laforest-Renald A, Quérin S, Madore F: Systemic anticoagulation and prevention of hemodialysis catheter malfunction. ASAIO J 2005;51:360–365.
73 Twardowski ZJ: Stepwise anticoagulation with warfarin for prevention of intravenous catheter thrombosis. Hemodial Int 2000;4: 37–41.
74 Beathard GA: Thrombosis Associated with Chronic Hemodialysis Vascular Access: Catheters. UpToDate Topic 1906, version 3.0. 2014.
75 Manley HJ, Drayer DK, Muther RS: Medication-related problem type and appearance rate in ambulatory hemodialysis patients. BMC Nephrol 2003;4:10.
76 Juurlink DN, Mamdani M, Kopp A, Laupacis A, Redelmeier DA: Drug-drug interactions among elderly patients hospitalized for drug toxicity. JAMA 2003;289:1652–1658.
77 Magro L, Moretti U, Leone R: Epidemiology and characteristics of adverse drug reactions caused by drug-drug interactions. Expert Opin Drug Saf 2012;11:83–94.
78 Holford HG: Pharmacokinetics and pharmacodynamics: rational dosing and the time course of drug action; in Katzung BG, Masters SB, Trevor AJ (eds): Basic and Clinical Pharmacology, ed 12. New York, McGraw-Hill, 2011, chapter 3, pp 37–51.
79 Horn JR: Important drug interactions and their mechanisms; in Katzung BG, Masters SB, Trevor AJ (eds): Basic and Clinical Pharmacology, ed 12. New York, McGraw-Hill, 2011, chapter 66, pp 1149–1162.
80 Danielson P: The cytochrome P450 superfamily: biochemistry, evolution and drug metabolism in humans. Curr Drug Metab 2002; 3:561–597.
81 Kappel J, Calissi P: Nephrology. 3. Safe drug prescribing for patients with renal insufficiency. Can Med Assoc J 2002;166:473–477.
82 Hartmann B, Czock D, Keller Munar F: Drug therapy in patients with chronic renal failure. Dtsch Arztebl Int 2010;107:647–656.
83 Munar MY, Singh H: Drug dosing adjustments in patients with chronic kidney disease. Am Fam Physician 2007;75:1487–1496.
84 Berns JS, Aronoff GR: Drug Prescribing in Renal Failure. Dosing Guidelines for Adults, ed 4. Philadelphia, American College of Physicians, 1999.
85 Gilbert DN, Moellering RC Jr, Eliopoulos GM, Chambers HF, Saag MS (eds): The Sanford Guide to Antimicrobial Therapy 2014, ed 44. Sperryville, Antimicrobial Therapy, 2014.
86 Bennett WM, Henrich WL, Stoff JS: The renal effects of nonsteroidal anti-inflammatory drugs: summary and recommendations. Am J Kidney Dis 1996;28(suppl 1):S56–S62.

Maurizio Gallieni, MD
Nephrology and Dialysis Unit, Ospedale San Carlo Borromeo
via Pio II, 3
IT–20153 Milan (Italy)
E-Mail maurizio.gallieni@fastwebnet.it

Widmer MK, Malik J (eds): Patient Safety in Dialysis Access.
Contrib Nephrol. Basel, Karger, 2015, vol 184, pp 51–58
DOI: 10.1159/000365822

Patient Safety in Vascular Access Patients on Hemodialysis: Contrast Agents and Renal Function

Bruno Vogt

Department of Nephrology, Hypertension and Clinical Pharmacology, Inselspital, Bern University Hospital, Bern, Switzerland

Abstract

Patient safety is a major concern in medical practice. Today, the health care system is faced with a growing number of patients at increased risk with serious conditions, older patients, and multimorbidity and kidney disease. In these patients, not only the correct diagnostic but also the time to get the correct diagnosis and the strategy of treatment are of great importance. For this reason, the numbers of imaging, interventional radiological procedures and the administration of potentially nephrotoxic agents are increasing. Preventive strategies for contrast-induced side effects, especially contrast-induced renal failure, are of 'real life' importance.

Recommendations to Improve Patient Safety

- Always follow rule one: Does the indication for the planned examination stand up?
- Always follow rule two: What is the exact question to be answered by the test?
- Always follow rule three: Can the question be answered by a less invasive and/or less dangerous procedure/test?
- Always follow rule one once again: Is the test indicated?

Introduction

Radiology is an integral component in the evaluation of the kidney. For decades, the primary imaging of the urinary tract has been excretion radiography following intravenous administration of iodinated contrast media (CM). This technique is called intravenous urography or pyelography, or excretory urography. In the last 30 years, we have witnessed an extraordinary development of the renal imaging technique. Ultrasounds, with or without ultrasound CM, computed tomography (CT) with or without iodinated CM, magnetic resonance imaging (MRI), with or without gadolinium-containing CM, are used with increased frequency. The aim is to compensate for the limitations of intravenous pyelography, to limit radiation exposure, and to limit CM side effects. In the same context, a reappraisal of scintigraphic methods using radioactive tracer is observed, including positron-based techniques. And to compensate for potential side effects of CM, and to get more information from MRI, new techniques are developed. These MRI techniques are resumed in the term functional MRI, including diffusion MRI, BOLD-MRI (blood oxygen level determination MRI), or new angiography MRI methods without the use of CM.

This chapter will outline the problems of CM, the iodinated for radiography and the gadolinium based for MRI, when treating patients with impaired renal function.

Contrast Media

We are in an excellent situation today that we have intravenous CM for radiography containing iodine, CM with gadolinium for MRI, and gas-containing bubbles used as CM for ultrasound examinations. This chapter will focus on iodinated and on gadolinium-containing CM, but not on the recently developed ultrasound CM. However, these new ultrasound based techniques might well replace some of the conventional techniques with CT or MRI in the future.

Iodinated CM

These contrast agents continue to have a role in many imaging techniques. A tri-iodinated benzene ring forms the chemical basis for all intravascular contrast agents for x-ray examinations. Mortality is increased in patients with acute renal failure following exposure to CM [1–3]. For this reason, strategies to reduce nephrotoxicity have been developed. The toxicity of the CM has been reduced

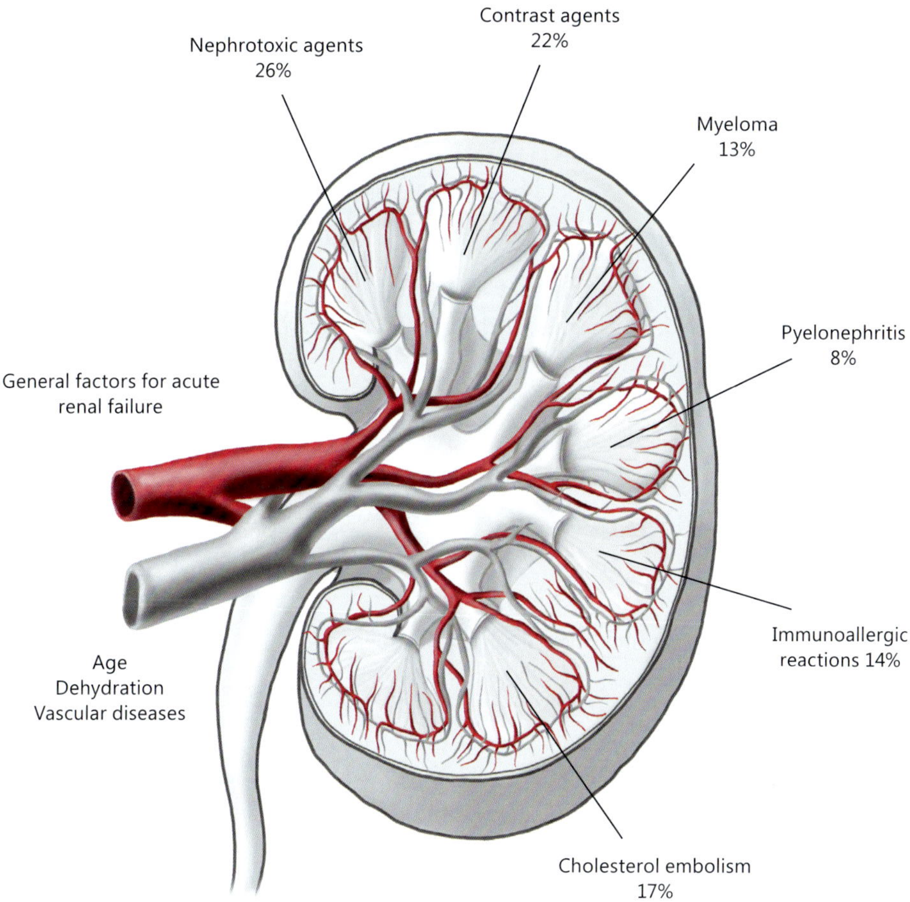

Fig. 1. Acute kidney injury in noncritically ill patients admitted to a tertiary care academic center in medical and surgical services (after Meier et al. [3]).

by developing low- and iso-osmolar agents, and by better identification and preparation of patients with high risk for contrast-induced nephropathy (fig. 1). Despite optimal preparation in a tertiary hospital, contrast nephropathy is still a major factor for renal failure. However, one has to be aware that a clear separation between CM nephropathy and cholesterol embolism is not possible, and mixed clinical pictures can exist. This has to be clear in mind today with increasing numbers of intravascular interventions.

Historically, contrast agents used to have very high osmolality. This was due to the high iodine content for increasing the contrast capacity. These agents had almost 5 times higher osmolality than normal plasma. This chemical characteristic contributes to the excellence of contrast imaging, but the high osmolality

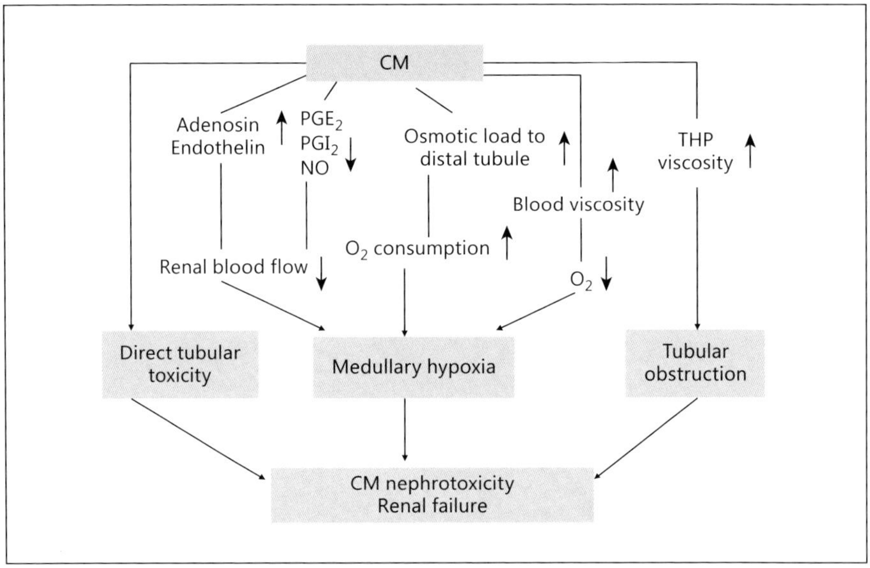

Fig. 2. Different mechanisms of renal toxicity of iodinated CM. THP = Tamm-Horsfall glycoprotein.

contributes to the toxicity. Furthermore, in the old times patients were dehydrated to get fine renal contrast images, a practice that contributed to renal failure after exposure, especially in myeloma patients: 'Since the *dehydration* utilized in the preparation of patients for intravenous pyelography will tend to optimize the circumstances for precipitation of the abnormal urine proteins, it would seem reasonable to suggest that patients with myeloma should not be prepared for this examination by *dehydration*' [4]. New iodinated contrast agents have been developed with the aim to give the same image quality but less toxicity.

It is important to realize that the so-called low-osmolar CM do not have lower osmolality than plasma, but twice the plasma osmolality. Indeed, the term low-osmolality refers to the old CM, i.e. they are lower than the old CM that were around 1,200 mosm/l, and the low-osmolar CM are around 600 mosm/l. Iso-osmolar refers to the plasma, and means that these CM are comparable to plasma osmolality, i.e. around 300 mosm/l.

The high osmolality of CM explains another important feature of these agents. They are osmotic active and act similar to osmotic diuretics such as mannitol. After administration, an increased diuresis is observed. This observation supports the necessity to perform hydration of the patient not only before, but also after administration of CM to balance the CM-induced diuresis. The histological lesions in the kidney are of the same type as the lesions observed after administration of mannitol or other agents inducing osmotic diuresis.

Medullary oxygenation decreases when iodinated CM is administrated (fig. 2). This has been shown first in animals and later in human after exposure to intravenous CM [5]. There is an important difference between rodent models and human; indeed, the human kidney is more sensitive to iodinated intravenous CM responding immediately with decreased medullary oxygenation. Strategies to minimize nephrotoxicity of CM such as the antioxidant N-acetylcysteine might have an effect through this mechanism. Interestingly, dark Swiss chocolate might increase renal medullary oxygenation in human [6]. The role in preventing CM nephropathy has not been studied.

Two other factors have to be mentioned that affect renal medullary oxygen content. First with age, the renal medullary oxygenation decreases, which might increase the risk in elderly patients [7]. Second, the use of nonsteroidal anti-inflammatory drugs decreases the kidney response to hydration and might well contribute to CM-induced nephropathy by this mechanism [8].

Iodinated CM in Patients with Impaired Renal Function

Before administration of CM, the indication of the test should be controlled and replaced by another examination without CM if possible.

If CM will be administrated in a patient with CKD or acute renal failure, low-osmolality CM should be used [9]. Correct hydration is essential. Because the CM acts as an osmotic diuretic, hydration after CM administration is as important as hydration before CM administration. For more than a decade, the classic scheme of Solomon and collaborators was highly recommended [10]. The procedure included hydration with a 0.45% NaCl i.v. solution 1 ml/kg body weight over 12 h before and 12 h after the administration of CM. The 0.45% solution has been replaced by 0.9% NaCl after the study was published, and recently bicarbonate solutions are used in a similar way [11]. This is generally accepted but the hydration might be a problem in heart failure patients. New techniques are investigated for this purpose, a promising one is the use of controlled intense hydration by a feedback loop using urinary output through the so called RenalGuard System [12]. Basically, this system matches automatically the intravenous replacement solutions to the urinary flow allowing to achieve very high urinary volumes up to 1,000 ml per hour. Today, this method is not yet entered in routine clinical practice.

The role of concomitant medication is not clear due to the lack of good clinical studies [9]. It is recommended to stop nonsteroidal anti-inflammatory drugs, metformin for the risk of lactic acidosis with decreasing renal function, and diuretics. Usually, diuretics used for long-term treatment of hypertension and inhibitors of the renin-angiotensin system should not be discontinued.

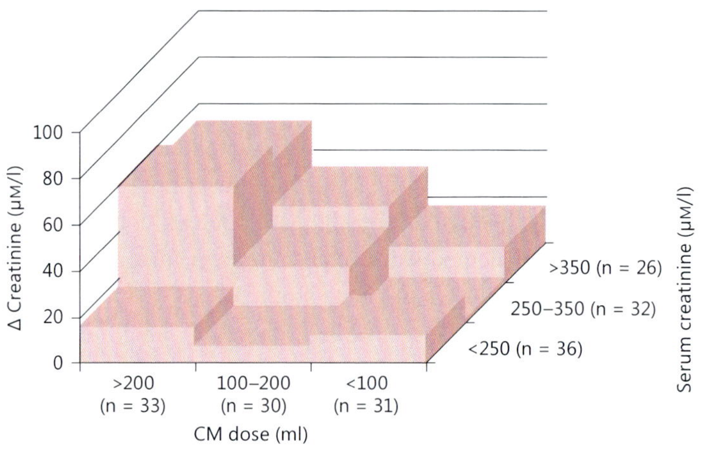

Fig. 3. Change in serum creatinine at day 6 after CM exposure as a function of baseline serum creatinine and amount of CM administered [13].

It is important to use the lower necessary amount of CM. Figure 3 shows a post hoc analysis of a study conducted by Vogt and coworkers demonstrating that 6 days after exposure to CM in patients with renal impairment, high dose of CM and high initial creatinine have the worst outcome. In the same study, hemodialysis therapy immediately after CM exposure had no beneficial effect. Indeed, hemodialysis access complications can be harmful for the patient [13]. However, hemodialysis after CM exposure might be necessary for therapy of volume overload and patients with advanced CKD. According to one study, there might be a role of hemodialysis after CM exposure in patients with severe advanced CKD of GFR <15 ml/min [14]. But that is a subject of controversy and is not clinical practice in most centers [15].

Gadolinium and Nephrogenic Systemic Fibrosis

Nephrogenic systemic fibrosis (NSF) occurs in patients with advanced CKD or acute renal failure, most commonly following exposure to gadolinium-based contrast agents. NSF is associated with increased morbidity and mortality [16, 17]. Despite the claim of some investigators that the association of NSF with gadolinium-based MRI is putative, the reality was different. The incidence of NSF has decreased dramatically following increasing clinician awareness and application of guidelines to avoid gadolinium-based CM in advanced CKD and in end-stage renal disease.

This appears to be the only effective means of decreasing NSF incidence. Retrospectively, NSF seems to be linked directly to the unstable form of gadolinium in the linear and nonionic form. The type of gadolinium chelate affects its thermodynamic and therapeutic properties. Cyclic forms of gadolinium CM seem to be safer, and following the guidelines are given in at-risk patients with a clear indication and no alternative possibility of procedure. Indeed, this is a rare event, and basically gadolinium-based CM can be avoided in patients with severe CKD (eGFR <30 ml/min), and in end-stage renal disease. Increasing clinician awareness of the danger and potentially lethal effect of specific gadolinium-based CD in advanced renal failure should help avoid them all in these conditions. If no other possibility exists, gadolinium-based CM with known low risk should be used exclusively [16, 17].

The clinical picture is devastating. One third of the patients will die, and one third will be disabled permanently! Typically, fibrosis of the skin develops, but the face remains unaffected. With developing disease, the skin gets so fibrotic that the movement of limbs gets difficult to impossible. The understanding of the pathogenic mechanisms and treatment of NSF remains unknown.

In summary, in all patients the lowest dose of gadolinium-based CM should be administered, name and dose always recorded, readministration avoided several weeks after the first administration, and CM should not or with utmost care be given in patients with advanced renal failure. The exact gadolinium-based CM should be selected following the guidelines. Nevertheless, considering the new techniques of functional MRI and the development of CT techniques with less exposure to radiation and CM, and having seen several patients die from NSF, the authors think that gadolinium-based CM should not be used in patients with a GFR below 30 ml/min!

Conclusions

What research project should be done to overcome the problems in relation to CM and nephrotoxicity? Such research programs should have two aims: First, define the optimal strategy for intravenous solutions for optimal hydration and protection, i.e. the kind of solution used, the amount and the time before and after CM administration. Second, research should focus on the indication of specific imaging methods and the added value of CM in regard of sensitivity, specificity and clinical decision making.

Disclosure Statement

The author has no conflict of interest to declare.

References

1 Levy EM, Viscoli CM, Ralph I, Horwitz RI: The effect of acute renal failure on mortality. A cohort analysis. JAMA 1996;275:1489–1494.

2 Kohli SH, Bhaskaran MC, Muthukumar T, Thennarasu K, Sud K, Jha V, Gupta KL, Sakhuja V: Treatment-related acute renal failure in the elderly: a hospital-based prospective study. Nephrol Dial Transplant 2000;15:212–217.

3 Meier P, Bonfils RM, Vogt B, Burnand B, Burnier M: Referral patterns and outcomes in non-critically ill patients with hospital-acquired acute kidney injury. Clin J Am Soc Nephrol 2011;6:2215–2225.

4 Lasser EC, Lang JH, Zaeadski ZA: Contrast media: myeloma protein precipitates in urography. JAMA 1966;198:273–275.

5 Hofmann L, Simon-Zoula S, Nowak A, Giger A, Vock P, C Boesch C, Frey FJ, Vogt B: BOLD-MRI for the assessment of renal oxygenation in humans: acute effect of nephrotoxic xenobiotics. Kidney Int 2006;70:144–150.

6 Pruijm M, Hofmann L, Charollais-Thoenig J, Forni V, Maillard M, Coristine A, Stuber M, Burnier M, Vogt B: Effect of dark chocolate on renal tissue oxygenation as measured by BOLD-MRI in healthy volunteers. Clin Nephrol 2013;80:211–217.

7 Simon-Zoula SC, Hofmann L, Giger A, Vogt B, Vock P, Frey FJ, Boesch C: Non-invasive monitoring of renal oxygenation using BOLD-MRI: a reproducibility study. NMR Biomed 2006;19:84–89.

8 Tumkur SM, Vu AT, Li LP, L Pierchala, Prasad PV: Evaluation of intra-renal oxygenation during water diuresis: a time-resolved study using BOLD MRI. Kidney Int 2006;70:139–143.

9 Solomon R, Deray G, Consensus Panel for CIN: How to prevent contrast-induced nephropathy and manage risk patients: practical recommendations. Kidney Int 2006;69:S51–S53.

10 Solomon R, Werner C, Mann D, D'Elia J, Silva P: Effects of saline, mannitol, and furosemide on acute decreases in renal function induced by radiocontrast agents. N Engl J Med 1994;331:1416–1420.

11 Mueller C, Buerkle G, Buettner HJ, Petersen J, Perruchoud AP, Eriksson U, Marsch S, Roskamm H: Prevention of contrast media-associated nephropathy randomized comparison of 2 hydration regimens in 1,620 patients undergoing coronary angioplasty. Arch Intern Med 2002;162:329–336.

12 Briguori C, Visconti G, Focaccio A, Airoldi F, Valgimigli M, Sangiorgi GM, Golia B, Ricciardelli B, Condorelli G; REMEDIAL II Investigators: Renal Insufficiency After Contrast Media Administration Trial II (REMEDIAL II). Renal Guard System in High-Risk Patients for Contrast-Induced Acute Kidney Injury. Circulation 2011;124:1260–1269.

13 Vogt B, Ferrari P, Schönholzer C, Marti H-P, Mohaupt M, Wiederkehr M, Cereghetti C, Serra A, Huynh-Do U, Uehlinger DE, Frey FJ: Prophylactic hemodialysis after radiocontrast media in patients with renal insufficiency is potentially harmful. Am J Med 2001;111:692–698.

14 Lee P-T, Chou K-J, Liu C-P, Mar G-Y, Chen C-L, Hsu C-Y, Fang H-C, Chung H-M: Renal protection for coronary angiography in advanced renal failure patients by prophylactic hemodialysis: a randomized controlled trial. J Am Coll Cardiol 2007;50:1015–1020.

15 Uehlinger DE: Prophylactic use of hemodialysis to prevent radiocontrast-induced nephropathy: the discussion is open again! J Am Coll Cardiol 2008;51:1047–1048.

16 Daftari Besheli LD, Aran S, Shaqdan K, Kay J, Abujudeh H: Current status of nephrogenic systemic fibrosis (review). Clin Radiol 2014;69:661–668.

17 Agarwal R, Brunelli SM, Williams K, Mitchell MD, Feldman HI, Umscheid CA: Gadolinium-based contrast agents and nephrogenic systemic fibrosis: a systematic review and meta-analysis. Nephrol Dial Transplant 2009;24:856–863.

Bruno Vogt, MD
Department of Nephrology, Hypertension and
Clinical Pharmacology, Inselspital, Bern University Hospital
Freiburgstrasse 10, CH–3010 Bern (Switzerland)
E-Mail bruno.vogt@insel.ch

Widmer MK, Malik J (eds): Patient Safety in Dialysis Access.
Contrib Nephrol. Basel, Karger, 2015, vol 184, pp 59–74
DOI: 10.1159/000365823

Contrast Agents and Ionization with Respect to Safety for Patients and Doctors

Hendrik von Tengg-Kobligk[a–c] · Levent Kara[a] · Thorsten Klink[a] · Elham Khanicheh[a] · Johannes T. Heverhagen[a] · Ingrid B. Böhm[a]

[a]Department of Diagnostic, Interventional and Pediatric Radiology, Inselspital, Bern University Hospital, Bern, Switzerland; [b]Department of Diagnostic and Interventional Radiology, University Hospital Heidelberg, Heidelberg, Germany; [c]Department of Radiology, Wright Medical Center of Innovation, Ohio State University, Columbus, Ohio, USA

Abstract

In hemodialysis patients, radiographic imaging with iodinated contrast medium (ICM) application plays a central role in the diagnosis and/or follow-up of disease-related conditions. Therefore, safety aspects concerning ICM administration and radiation exposure have a great impact on this group of patients. Current hardware and software improvements including the design and synthesis of modern contrast compounds allow the use of very small amounts of ICM in concert with low radiation exposure. Undesirable ICM side effects are divided into type A (predictable reactions such as heat feeling, headache, and contrast-induced acute kidney injury, for example) and type B (nonpredictable or hypersensitivity) reactions; this chapter deals with the latter. The first onset cannot be prevented. To prevent hypersensitivity upon reexposure of ICM, an allergological workup is recommended. If this is not possible and ICM is necessary, the patient should receive a premedication (H1 antihistamine with or without corticosteroids). Current imaging hardware and software improvements (e.g. such as additional filtration of the X-ray beam) allow the use of very small amount of ICM and small X-ray doses. Proper communication among the team involved in the treatment of a patient may allow to apply imaging protocols and efficient imaging strategies limiting radiation exposure to a minimum. Practical recommendations will guide the reader how to use radiation and ICM efficiently to improve both patient and staff safety.

Recommendations to Improve Safety for Both the Patient and the Radiological Staff

- Careful assessment of the patient's history including actual condition, actual medication, previous interventions, previous radiological procedures, and previous tolerability of ionic contrast media (ICM).
- Avoid both frequent contrast-enhanced and native image-guided examinations.
- If the application of ICM is necessary, use the lowest dose possible (approximately 5 ml of a nonionic ICM such as iopromide, for example).
- Use a low frame rate (e.g. 3 pulses/s) and a small field of view to achieve a minimum radiation exposure for both patients and staff – according to the ALARA (as low as reasonably achievable) principle.
- Patients with a history of ICM hypersensitivity have an increased risk to react again after reexposure. Therefore, these patients should be closely diagnosed. If this is not possible, native radiological X-ray examinations or ultrasound examinations are recommended. If ICM is necessary, a premedication should be given, and one should be aware that this procedure does not absolutely protect from hypersensitivity reactions.

Overview of Iodinated Contrast Media

There is a huge amount of literature describing the spectrum of and differences between commercially available iodinated contrast media (ICM) [1, 2]. The initial group of ionic, high-osmolar ICM has been nearly completely replaced by low- and iso-osmolar nonionic ICM that generally have a better safety profile than the former ones. Therefore, this book chapter does not further discuss ionic, high-osmolar ICM.

Currently, all available nonionic ICM (fig. 1) either have low osmolality or iso-osmolality (i.e. <859 mosm/kg H_2O) [1, 3].

Adverse Reactions

Like drug-induced reactions in general, the broad spectrum of ICM-induced adverse events in particular can be divided into type A and type B reactions [4, 5]. The first category is defined as predictable reactions that are dose-dependent side effects induced by the pharmacological compound(s). Heat feeling, vomiting, emesis, headache, renal complaints, and thyrotoxic events are ICM-related

Nonionic ICM	Generic name	Iodine concentration (mg I/l)	Osmolality (mOsm/kg water)
Low osmolar	Iobitridol	300/350	695/915
	Iohexol	300/350	672/844
	Iomeprol	300/400	521/726
	Iopamidol	300/370	616/796
	Iopentol	300	640/818
	Iopromide	300/370	607/774
	Ioversol	320/350	702/792
	Ioxilan	300/350	585/695
Iso-osmolar	Iodixanol	270/320	290

Fig. 1. Currently available and safe ICM.

type A reactions. On the other hand, type B reactions are not predictable. These are hypersensitivity reactions that can be further categorized as either allergic or nonallergic reactions [6].

Contrast-Induced Acute Kidney Injury

One should be aware that all ICM including all nonionic compounds are nephrotoxic substances. Therefore, they have the potential to induce contrast-induced acute kidney injury (AKI) also called contrast-induced nephropathy (CIN).

To date, the results from studies comparing low- and iso-osmolar ICM in terms of safety outcomes and specifically the incidence of CIN in patients with preexisting renal dysfunction have been inconclusive. Early studies showed the lower incidence of CIN in patients with renal dysfunction after administration of iso-osmolar ICM compared to low-osmolar ICM [7, 8], whereas subsequent trials failed to prove the advantage of iso-osmolar over low-osmolar ICM in the development of CIN [9, 10].

Patients with impaired renal function (i.e. all patients undergoing hemodialysis) are at risk to acquire CIN compared to patients with normal renal function [11].

Hypersensitivity to ICM

Most hypersensitivity reactions to ICM occur immediately, and may be either allergic or nonallergic [6]. The clinical features of both pathological conditions are identical, and comprise localized/generalized urticaria, angioedema, asthma bronchiale, tachycardia, and drop of blood pressure, for example. Both radiological in general and interventional teams in particular that are involved in ICM application should be aware of various reactions that may occur after ICM injection.

While mild reactions spontaneously disappear, moderate hypersensitivity needs adequate treatment. The observed symptoms should be individually treated (e.g. H1 antihistaminics are suitable for generalized urticaria). Severe hypersensitivity reactions manifest as anaphylactic shock and should be treated in collaboration with the hospital emergency team.

A regular training of the involved team may improve patient management and outcome [12].

Apart from immediate or so-called type I reactions, nonimmediate or so-called type IV reactions may occur after ICM administration. The latter allergy subgroup manifests either with maculopapular exanthema, fixed drug eruption or other very rare conditions such as Stevens-Johnson syndrome [13–15].

Prevalence of ICM Hypersensitivity

The prevalence or incidence rates of ICM-induced hypersensitivity show great variability in the literature [5–17]. The reason for this phenomenon is unclear. The study design/setting, the use of different ICM, different doses in different patient groups, and the experience of involved medical personnel may be responsible for this phenomenon. Furthermore, the definition of adverse events differs from paper to paper. While some authors report on prevalence rate of adverse ICM reactions in general, others focus on hypersensitivity reactions, and found prevalences of 0.7–3.1% [16, 18].

Most hypersensitivity reactions are mild. Severe reactions have been reported to occur in 0.02–0.04% [18, 19]. A recent retrospective study analyzed reactions in 84,928 patients after i.v. administration of nonionic ICM during CT: in total, 0.6% showed a hypersensitivity reaction [20]. Of 545 hypersensitivity reactions, 77% were mild, 21% moderate, and 2% severe [20].

Although the incidence of severe hypersensitivity reactions to intravascular administration of nonionic ICM is rather rare, the fact that more than 75 million times ICM are administered annually to patients worldwide [21] relates to a significant number of patients who may experience hypersensitivity to ICM.

Nonimmediate or delayed hypersensitivity reactions are T cell based [8] and occur several hours or even days after an ICM administration. The observed prevalence affects 1–3% of patients [22] and is mainly induced by nonionic iso-osmolar dimer ICM [16, 22]. These reactions are generally mild, and mainly involve the skin. Only very rarely, can they be life threatening [14, 23].

Risks for Hypersensitivity Reactions

Although a lot of risk factors have been described in the literature [12, 13], only few are of clinical relevance. Important risks are a history of ICM-induced hypersensitivity, especially moderate and severe manifestations, and acute severe allergy against other allergens (e.g. allergic asthma) [24].

In anxious patients, reactions may occur that mimic immediate hypersensitivity.

A relationship between ICM-induced hypersensitivity and iodine or seafood allergies does not exist [25, 26].

Treatment, Testing and Prevention of Hypersensitivity Reactions

Some recommendations regarding the treatment of type 1 reactions to ICM are summarized in table 1.

Unfortunately, currently an international standard regimen to prevent, minimize or avoid hypersensitivity reactions to ICM does not exist.

Patients with a history of ICM-induced hypersensitivity should be tested in vivo and in vitro with the culprit ICM, and additional ICM 4 up to 6 weeks after they displayed the hypersensitivity reaction [13, 26–28]. In addition, one should be aware that especially in patients undergoing radiological interventional procedures not only ICM but also a variety of other allergens (e.g. latex, heparins) may induce the observed hypersensitivity [29].

If testing is not possible, a premedication should be given. Unfortunately, currently there is no standard regimen, drugs given for premedication themselves can induce adverse drug reactions, and premedication does not guarantee absolute protection from hypersensitivity reaction after ICM reexposure [30].

Amongst numerous pretreatment regimes, almost all include histamine 1 (H1) antagonist to antagonize the effects of histamine, and some additionally use a corticosteroid to target the inflammatory response. Other regimens also include ephedrine for bronchodilation as well as cimetidine because of its antagonism at the H2 receptor. If the patients' history reveals a serious reaction to

Table 1. Recommended treatment of adverse reactions to ICM

Symptoms		Treatments
Mild	Pruritus and urticaria	Usually self-limited – no treatment
Moderate	Mild to moderate urticaria	Diphenhydramine (i.v., i.m., oral)
	Mild to moderate bronchospasm	Supplemental oxygen and inhaled β_2-agonist
	Severe bronchospasm	High-flow supplemental oxygen; inhaled β_2-agonist; epinephrine (s.c./i.v.), antihistamine (i.v.), corticosteroid (i.v.), diphenhydramine (i.v.)
	Facial and laryngeal edema	Intubation in the setting of airway compromise; high-flow supplemental oxygen; inhaled β_2-agonist; epinephrine (s.c./i.v.), antihistamine (i.v.), corticosteroid (i.v.), diphenhydramine (i.v.)
Severe	Hypotension with brady-/tachycardia	Elevate patient's lower extremities; high-flow supplemental oxygen; epinephrine (s.c./i.v.); i.v. fluid resuscitation
	Seizure	Turn patient to their side to prevent aspiration; high-flow supplemental oxygen; diazepam (i.v.)

ICM, different premedications do exist. Here are only two examples for premedication that can be applied before the next exam: (1) prednisone: 50 mg orally 12–20 h and 2 h or (2) methylprednisolone 62.5 mg i.v. 12 and 2 h.

H1 antagonists or H1 blockers and possibly H2 antihistaminics should be combined with the above-mentioned steroids, and should be given 30 min before ICM injection.

How to Minimize the Use of i.v. ICM during Radiological Procedures

Preinterventional Procedure

Awareness of the patient's past medical history regarding the current fistula is mandatory. If the patient had prior surgery, the interventionist should contact the surgeon or should request the report. The surgical report should provide information about surgery date, region of anastomosis, surgical technique or type of access, as well as vessels being used, details about the dysfunctional shunt, or any prior interventions.

Before starting the intervention, the team should examine the relevant region using duplex sonography, which does not require any ionizing radiation or any administration of ICM [31]. Duplex sonography allows to detect possible stenoses, occlusions with or without thrombus and aneurysms. Duplex sonography prior to interventional procedures can reduce the amount of ICM as well as radiation dose.

Patients with a known shunt problem need to be controlled quite frequently. In these cases, the imaging procedure can only be focused on the shunt, which saves time, radiation and volume of ICM.

To achieve optimal management of patients undergoing hemodialysis, the following recommendations are made:

(1) Interventionists should be familiar with anatomy and potential hazards:
- Anatomical variants
- Individual pathology
- Access strategy
- Visualization of the preintervention road map, e.g. based on CT angiography (CTA) or magnetic resonance angiography (MRA)
- Efficient use of the interventional unit (movement, zoom, shielding, etc.)
- Use of the road map acquired during first angiography

(2) Careful case planning including consideration of both potential complications and their adequate management.

Use of an ICM (200–400 mg I/ml) in a volume of 5–10 ml is possible (if image quality allows, use a 1:1 dilution with normal saline; see fig. 3 and 4). Since CIN is triggered by the amount of administered ICM, it is crucial, especially in patients with renal function impairment, to use as minimal contrast medium (CM) as reasonably possible. An amount of <10 g of iodine (approx. 25 ml ICM with a concentration of 370 mg I/ml) per examination should be aimed at for initial diagnosis. A recent study testing the compatibility of ICM with trisodium citrate, a catheter lock solution as a replacement of heparin, suggests that the catheter should be thoroughly flushed ex-vivo with saline if an ICM has been previously injected. Otherwise, the potential for precipitation is increased [32].

Check and report peripheral pulses after procedure. Document the interventional procedure including the used material. Dialysis after intervention depends on the patient's condition, levels of electrolytes particular potassium and dialysis schedule. In urgent cases, it is usually no problem to perform hemofiltration on the same day of intervention since hemodialysis has not been proven to be effective [33].

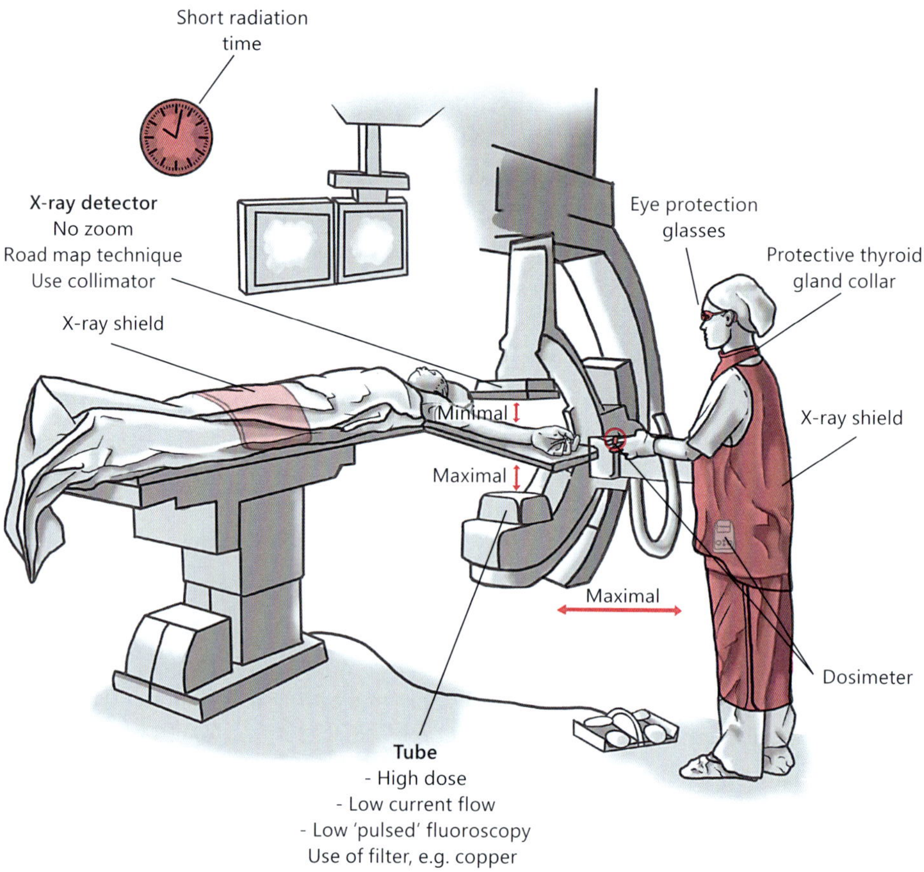

Fig. 2. Common protection setup to minimize ionization during intervention for patients and physicians.

Minimizing Ionization Risks: Techniques and Strategies

Radiation exposure of both patients and the staff should be closely monitored in order to minimize it (fig. 2). There are several techniques and options to realize the ALARA (as low as reasonable achievable) principle [34–36].

Optimized Radiation Doses to Patients

The surgeon influences the exposure of patients and thus must be trained in the application of proper radiologic techniques. A first step is presetting fluoroscopy and angiography parameters. The tube current time product (mAs) range and voltage (kV) determine X-ray energy and intensity. In patients, the exposed anatomic region has a major influence on the amount of the required radiation dose. Interventions in hemodialysis patients with surgically produced forearm shunts (e.g. Cimino AVF) require much lower doses compared to patients with abdominal interventions. Automatic exposure control measures the attenuation of tissue density during the fluoroscopy and immediately adapts the current settings for sufficient exposure. Therefore, it is important to keep possibly overlaying high-density materials (e.g. lead shields) out of the beam. Modern technology renders 'smart' X-ray beams with modified and patient-adapted energy spectra, beam shapes, and frequency. As a general rule, exposure is reduced by keeping the tube voltage as high and the tube current as low as possible.

The X-ray energy spectrum includes low-energy radiation that hits the patient but has not the energy to pass through. This radiation is not involved in image generation and harmful to skin and superficial tissue. Thus, X-ray filters are necessary. These X-ray filters consist of aluminum and copper, and absorb the unwanted low-energy fraction of the X-ray spectrum, thus minimizing superficial radiation injuries.

The X-ray generator can be set to produce the X-ray beam continuously or intermittently. The intermittent X-ray beam, used during 'pulsed' fluoroscopy, substantially reduces X-ray dose by applying a certain number of exposures per second (frame rate) instead of a continuous exposure. The number of exposures per second is usually chosen with regard to expected (hemo-)dynamics. Technically modern angiography tubes render frame rates of 0.5–30 per second. Major dose savings are achieved when very low pulse frequencies are chosen. Newest X-ray tubes also allow very short lengths of pulse itself (about 10 ms).

Collimator shutters (X-ray shades) are used to limit the exposed body area to the necessary minimum field size. Besides the dose-saving effects, it reduces image noise due to less scatter radiation. Magnification also increases radiation doses and should be used only when high-resolution images are required.

Radiation doses during fluoroscopy are optimized by maximizing the distance between the X-ray tube and the patient, and by minimizing the distance between the patient and the X-ray detector. Surgeons have to control exposure time (beam-on-time). Different projections reduce skin dose of smaller areas (fig. 3, 4).

Minimized Radiation Doses to Surgeons and Staff of Radiological Units

Both single radiation doses and number of radiation exposures should be kept to a minimum for surgeons and staff. For sufficient protection, operators and staff should be trained and supervised, and radiation doses should be controlled

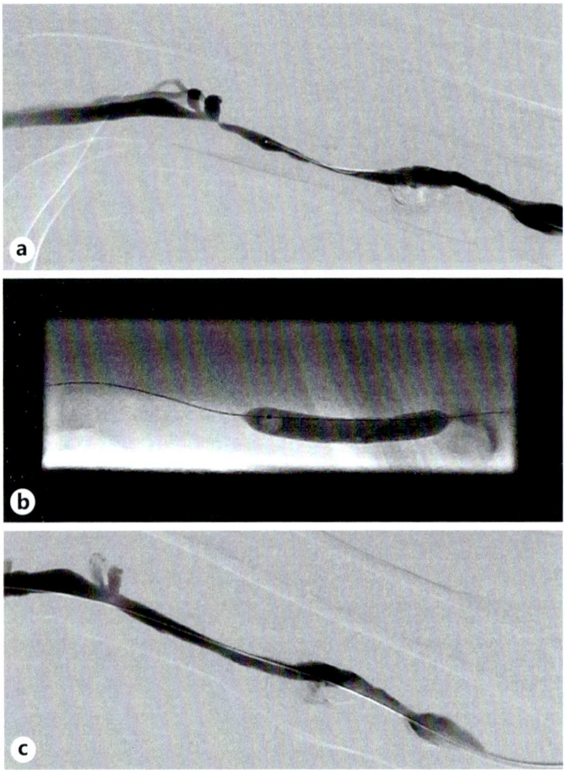

Fig. 3. Diagnostic DSA prior to intervention; image of fistula stenosis using 5 ml of contrast agent. **a** With a minimum amount of contrast agent, it is possible to use the 'road map' technique to localize stenosis prior to balloon angioplasty. **b** Balloon angioplasty without using i.v. contrast agent. The fluoro mode is focused with magnification at the balloon, and only a screen shot has been taken to save radiation dose and to document balloon performance. **c** Outcome after PTA.

and documented. One simple step for protection is to keep as much distance as possible to the X-ray source. All staff members that sojourn within the intervention suite should protect themselves using personal equipment and X-ray shields including lead aprons and lead thyroid collars. For weight reasons and flexibility, lead-rubber composite materials are used for protection wear, whereas the thickness and efficacy in radiation absorption are labelled in the form of the lead-equivalent value. The lead-equivalent value correlates with the thickness (mm) of a pure lead layer. Sufficient radiation protection is mostly achieved with a lead equivalent of 0.7 on the body side that is directed towards the X-ray source. Surgeons and other medical staff working in close relation to the radiation source should wear leaded glasses. Leaded gloves are effective hand protectors

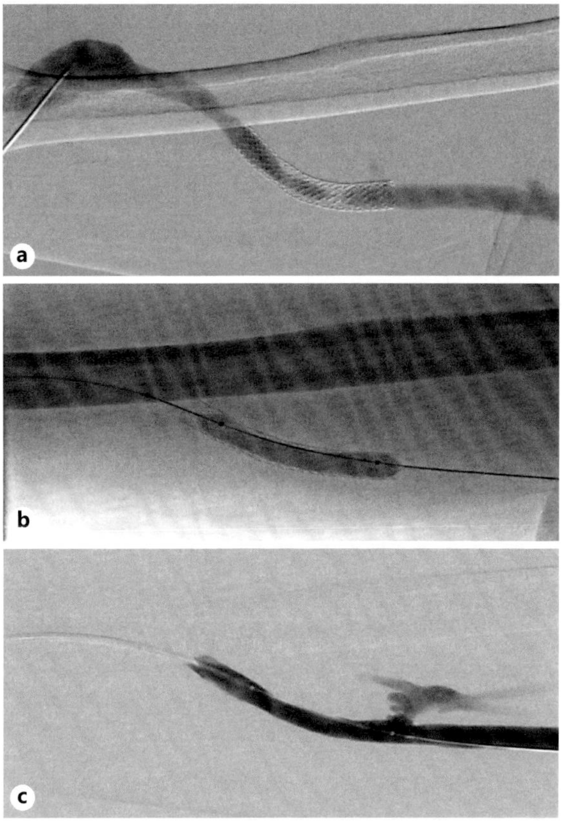

Fig. 4. Orientation in anatomical structures or guidance using foreign body markers for further procedures like PTA or stent placement may significantly reduce the amount of contrast agent for further procedures. **a** Diagnostic DSA prior to intervention, image of high-grade in-stent fistula stenosis using 5 ml of contrast agent. **b** In-stent PTA, no contrast agent necessary. **c** Outcome after in-stent PTA with a physiologic connection between a reopened artery and vein.

but may impair fine motor skills, and are often relinquished. To ensure effective hand protection, hands should be kept out of the active X-ray beam.

X-ray shields are very effective for radiation protection. Suitable shields are moveable, either using moveable frames with wheels and lead drapes or glass, or ceiling-mounted lead acrylic windows. Their use in routine practice may be difficult in certain positions due to individual patient and equipment setup, but they are highly effective when placed closely to the particular X-ray scatter source (patient).

Occupational radiation exposure to surgeons and medical/radiological staff is monitored by using personal dosimeter badges. These badges must be worn when working with radiation. They are best worn under the lead apron to assess the body exposure. They allow for personal risk estimation, and are exchanged on a monthly basis in many hospitals. Then, dosimetry records are reviewed and annually reported to prevent overexposure to staff. For operators and staff with a more excessive exposure further dosimetry devices are recommended. Another badge may be worn outside of the collar to document the radiation exposure of the eyes. Interventionists should wear their ring dosimeters on the hand that is closer to the X-ray beam. In the OR, these rings should be sterilized in alcohol before they can be placed on one finger of the hand covered with two gloves.

Contrast-enhanced (CE) MRA can acquire a static 3D vascular tree in submillimeter resolution. Time-resolved CE-MRA would be feasible but temporal resolution would be lower compared to conventional digital subtraction angiography (DSA), e.g. one 3-D MRA data set within a few seconds (<5 s) is possible [37]. Prior to surgery, high spatial resolution steady-state CE-MRA of the upper extremity using the contrast agent Ablavar® (gadofosveset trisodium, Lantheus Medical Imaging) may provide radiation-free submillimeter anatomy of arteries and veins of the upper extremity [38]. However, in Europe Ablavar is not available anymore, i.e. this method is not established for this indication and body region.

Alternative Imaging Methods in Patients with End-Stage Renal Disease

End-stage renal disease (ESRD) is defined as stage 5 of chronic kidney damage (CKD), i.e. there is very severely reduced kidney function (end stage or ESRF/ESRD) with less than 15% (eGFR <15 ml/min/1.73 m^2) [39]. On the other hand, ESRD includes patients treated by dialysis or transplantation, irrespective of the level of GFR [40].

Duplex sonography is the gold standard prior to surgery for ESRD patients. Other imaging modalities are all problematic or quite challenging in ESRD patients. A feasibility study by Bode et al. [41] showed that MRA can also be performed without external contrast agent, which could be promising for ESRD patients. However, image quality of the arteries and vessel to background ratios were lower using non-CE (NCE) MRA. In addition, currently no shunt intervention is being performed in the MR scanner in clinical routine.

In some clinical centers, CE-MRA is not an option anymore for ESRD patients due to the risk to develop nephrotic systemic fibrosis (NSF) [17], although the safety profile of MR contrast agents with respect to hypersensitivity reactions is very good [42].

Although the incidence of NSF has declined after 2006 [43], this adverse condition is still a problem in the context of gadolinium-based contrast agents

(GBCA), because of its unknown pathophysiology, its harmful character, and the lack of an effective treatment. Therefore, prophylaxis is of great impact. This means that all physicians who are involved in GBCA application should closely observe the FDA or other national guidelines. High doses of GBCA should be omitted in cases with eGFR $\leq$15 ml/min/1.73 m^2, and GBCA with lower thermodynamic stability such as gadodiamide, gadopentetate dimeglumine, and gadoversetamide are contraindicated in patients with eGFR $\leq$30 ml/min/1.73 m^2 [44, 45]. The European Society of Urogenital Radiology published a guideline on how to deal with ESRD patients and gadolinium-based CM for MRI [46]. For patients with a GFR <15 ml/min/1.73 m^2 (CKD stage 5), it is recommended to use the recommended CM with caution. If not available, only CM from the group 'lowest risk of NSF' should be administered i.v.: gadobutrol (Gadovist®, Bayer Healthcare), gadoterate meglumine (Dotarem®, Guerbet) or gadoteridol (ProHance®, Bracco). For more detailed information, see Heverhagen et al. [47].

CO_2 angiography of an antebrachial dialysis shunt is contraindicated due to the risk of cerebral gas emboli. Gadolinium-based intraarterial DSA used off-label is not being routinely performed as an alternative because higher volumes of GBCA are necessary, etc.

A relatively high radiation dose results if dynamic/multiphasic CTA is performed. The required volume of i.v. applied CM is typically higher than for intraarterial DSA. The achieved vessel contrast-to-noise ratio is lower using CTA. In summary, CTA is not considered as a real alternative imaging method.

Conclusion

Most patients under hemodialysis tolerate ICM given for CE shunt imaging very well. Only a small proportion of patients acquire type A or B reactions (hypersensitivity). Currently, there is no straightforward guideline for prevention of hypersensitivity reactions. But in patients with a history of ICM-induced hypersensitivity (especially moderate and severe forms), a careful individual management should be carried out in order to prevent similar reactions after ICM reexposure.

An image-guided, shunt-related intervention can be performed with small amounts of a nonionic ICM. Radiation dose can be substantially reduced with the latest technology and recommendations from experienced users.

Disclosure Statement

The authors have no conflicts of interest to declare.

References

1 Reimer P, Vosshenrich R: Contrast agents in radiology: current agents approved, recommendations, and safety aspects (in German). Radiologe 2013;53:153–164.
2 von Tengg-Kobligk HM, Mehndiratta A, Giesel FL: Contrast agents in radiology; in Miller C, Krasnow J, Schwartz LH (ed): Medical Imaging in Clinical Trials. London, Springer, 2014, pp 327–357.
3 Newmark JL, Mehra A, Singla AK: Radiocontrast media allergic reactions and interventional pain practice – a review. Pain Physician 2012;15:E665–E675.
4 Rawlins MD, Thompson W: Mechanisms of adverse drug reactions; in Davies DM (ed): Textbook of Adverse Drug Reaction. New York, Oxford University Press, 1991.
5 Böhm I, Heverhagen JT, Klose KJ: Classification of acute and delayed contrast media-induced reactions: proposal of a three-step system. Contrast Media Mol Imaging 2012;7:537–541.
6 Böhm I, Schild H: Contrast-media-induced hypersensitivity or allergic/allergic-like reactions? Suggestion for a more appropriate use of the nomenclature. Eur J Clin Pharmacol 2008;64:931–932; author reply 933–934.
7 Aspelin P, Aubry P, Fransson SG, Strasser R, Willenbrock R, Berg KJ: Nephrotoxic effects in high-risk patients undergoing angiography. N Engl J Med 2003;348:491–499.
8 Jo SH, Youn TJ, Koo BK, Park JS, Kang HJ, Cho YS, Chung WY, Joo GW, Chae IH, Choi DJ, Oh BH, Lee MM, Park YB, Kim HS: Renal toxicity evaluation and comparison between visipaque (iodixanol) and hexabrix (ioxaglate) in patients with renal insufficiency undergoing coronary angiography: the recover study: a randomized controlled trial. J Am Coll Cardiol 2006;48:924–930.
9 Rudnick MR, Davidson C, Laskey W, Stafford JL, Sherwin PF: Nephrotoxicity of iodixanol versus ioversol in patients with chronic kidney disease: the visipaque angiography/interventions with laboratory outcomes in renal insufficiency (VALOR) trial. Am Heart J 2008;156:776–782.
10 Laskey W, Aspelin P, Davidson C, Rudnick M, Aubry P, Kumar S, Gietzen F, Wiemer M: Nephrotoxicity of iodixanol versus iopamidol in patients with chronic kidney disease and diabetes mellitus undergoing coronary angiographic procedures. Am Heart J 2009;158:822–828 e823.
11 Widmark JM: Imaging-related medications: a class overview. Proc (Bayl Univ Med Cent) 2007;20:408–417.
12 Petscavage-Thomas JM, Kaneda H, Bruno MA: The value of training technologists for adverse reactions to contrast. Radiol Technol 2014;85:256–260.
13 Böhm I, Medina J, Prieto P, Block W, Schild HH: Fixed drug eruption induced by an iodinated non-ionic X-ray contrast medium: a practical approach to identify the causative agent and to prevent its recurrence. Eur Radiol 2007;17:485–489.
14 Laffitte E, Nenadov Beck M, Hofer M, Hohl D, Panizzon RG: Severe Stevens-Johnson syndrome induced by contrast medium iopentol (imagopaque). Br J Dermatol 2004;150:376–378.
15 Böhm I, Schild HH: A practical guide to diagnose lesser-known immediate and delayed contrast media-induced adverse cutaneous reactions. Eur Radiol 2006;16:1570–1579.
16 Schild HH, Kuhl CK, Hubner-Steiner U, Böhm I, Speck U: Adverse events after unenhanced and monomeric and dimeric contrast-enhanced CT: a prospective randomized controlled trial. Radiology 2006;240:56–64.
17 Katayama H, Yamaguchi K, Kozuka T, Takashima T, Seez P, Matsuura K: Adverse reactions to ionic and nonionic contrast media. A report from the Japanese committee on the safety of contrast media. Radiology 1990;175:621–628.
18 Katayama H: Survey of safety of clinical contrast media. Invest Radiol 1990;25(suppl 1):S7–S10.
19 Caro JJ, Trindade E, McGregor M: The risks of death and of severe nonfatal reactions with high- vs low-osmolality contrast media: a meta-analysis. AJR Am J Roentgenol 1991;156:825–832.

20 Wang CL, Cohan RH, Ellis JH, Caoili EM, Wang G, Francis IR: Frequency, outcome, and appropriateness of treatment of nonionic iodinated contrast media reactions. AJR Am J Roentgenol 2008;191:409–415.
21 Katzberg RW: 'Acute reactions to urographic contrast medium: incidence, clinical characteristics, and relationship to history of hypersensitivity states' – a commentary. AJR Am J Roentgenol 2008;190:1431–1432.
22 Hosoya T, Yamaguchi K, Akutsu T, Mitsuhashi Y, Kondo S, Sugai Y, Adachi M: Delayed adverse reactions to iodinated contrast media and their risk factors. Radiat Med 2000;18:39–45.
23 Torres MJ, Mayorga C, Cornejo-Garcia JA, Lopez S, Chaves P, Rondon C, Fernandez T, Blanca M: Monitoring non-immediate allergic reactions to iodine contrast media. Clin Exp Immunol 2008;152:233–238.
24 Boehm I: Contrast medium and patients at risk: asthma. Acta Radiol 2009;50:348.
25 Schabelman E, Witting M: The relationship of radiocontrast, iodine, and seafood allergies: a medical myth exposed. J Emerg Med 2010;39:701–707.
26 Boehm I: Iodinated contrast agents are not forbidden in patients with iodine allergy. Cardiovasc Intervent Radiol 2010;33:435–436; author reply 437.
27 Böhm I, Pfützner W, Klose KJ: Individual management permits contrast media enhanced CT examination without premedication (in German). Rofo 2012;184:1161–1162.
28 Böhm I, Speck U, Schild HH: Pilot study on basophil activation induced by contrast medium. Fundam Clin Pharmacol 2011;25:267–276.
29 Böhm I, Alfke H, Klose KJ: Hypersensitivity reactions and contrast medium injection: are they always related? Eur J Radiol 2011;80:368–372.
30 Tramer MR, von Elm E, Loubeyre P, Hauser C: Pharmacological prevention of serious anaphylactic reactions due to iodinated contrast media: systematic review. BMJ 2006;333:675.
31 Malovrh M: Non-invasive evaluation of vessels by duplex sonography prior to construction of arteriovenous fistulas for haemodialysis. Nephrol Dial Transplant 1998;13:125–129.
32 Delcour C, Bruninx G: Incompatibility of contrast medium and trisodium citrate. Cardiovasc Intervent Radiol 2013;36:237–238.
33 Ellis JH, Cohan RH: Prevention of contrast-induced nephropathy: an overview. Radiol Clin North Am 2009;47:801–811, v.
34 Vano E, Rosenstein M, Liniecki J, Rehani M, Martin CJ, Vetter RJ: Education and training in radiological protection for diagnostic and interventional procedures. Ann ICRP 2009;39.
35 Aichinger HDJ, Joite-Barfuss S, Säbel M: Radiation Exposure and Image Quality in X-Ray Diagnostic Radiology. Berlin, Springer, 2012.
36 Kaufmann JLM: Vascular and Interventional Radiology: The Requisites. St. Louis, Mosby, 2004, pp 31–82.
37 Winterer JT, Blanke P, Schaefer A, Pache G, Langer M, Markl M: Bilateral contrast-enhanced MR angiography of the hand: diagnostic image quality of accelerated MRI using echo sharing with interleaved stochastic trajectories (TWIST). Eur Radiol 2011;21:1026–1033.
38 Rohrl B, Kunz RP, Oberholzer K, Pitton MB, Neufang A, Dueber C, Kreitner KF: Gadofosveset-enhanced MR angiography of the pedal arteries in patients with diabetes mellitus and comparison with selective intraarterial DSA. Eur Radiol 2009;19:2993–3001.
39 The Renal Association: Stage 4–5 CKD. Petersfield, The Renal Association, 2014.
40 National Kidney Foundation: KDOQI Guidelines. New York, National Kidney Foundation, 2002.
41 Bode AS, Planken RN, Merkx MA, van der Sande FM, Geerts L, Tordoir JH, Leiner T: Feasibility of non-contrast-enhanced magnetic resonance angiography for imaging upper extremity vasculature prior to vascular access creation. Eur J Vasc Endovasc Surg 2012;43:88–94.
42 Kanal E, Barkovich AJ, Bell C, Borgstede JP, Bradley WG Jr, Froelich JW, Gimbel JR, Gosbee JW, Kuhni-Kaminski E, Larson PA, Lester JW Jr, Nyenhuis J, Schaefer DJ, Sebek EA, Weinreb J, Wilkoff BL, Woods TO, Lucey L, Hernandez D: ACR guidance document on MR safe practices: 2013. J Magn Reson Imaging 2013;37:501–530.

43 Becker S, Walter S, Witzke O, Wilde B, Hillen U, Napieralski D, Kreuter A, Altmeyer P, Schieren G, Daul A, Rump LC, Kribben A: The German registry for nephrogenic systemic fibrosis: findings from 23 patients. Clin Nephrol 2010;73:426–430.
44 FDA: Public health advisory – gadolinium-containing contrast agents for magnetic resonance imaging (MRI). Silver Spring, FDA, 2013.
45 FDA: New warnings required on use of gadolinium-based contrast agents enhanced screening recommended to detect kidney dysfunction. Silver Spring, FDA, 2013.
46 European Society of Urogenital Radiology: Guidelines on contrast media. Vienna, European Society of Urogenital Radiology, 2014.
47 Heverhagen JT, Krombach GA, Gizewski E: Application of extracellular gadolinium-based MRI contrast agents and the risk of nephrogenic systemic fibrosis. Rofo 2014;186: 661–669.

Hendrik von Tengg-Kobligk, MD
Diagnostic, Interventional and Pediatric Radiology (DIPR)
Inselspital, Bern University Hospital
Freiburgstrasse 10, CH–3010 Bern (Switzerland)
E-Mail hendrik.vonTengg@insel.ch

Widmer MK, Malik J (eds): Patient Safety in Dialysis Access.
Contrib Nephrol. Basel, Karger, 2015, vol 184, pp 75–86
DOI: 10.1159/000365499

Cardiac Safety in Vascular Access Surgery and Maintenance

Jan Malik[a] · Jaroslav Kudlicka[a] · Vladimir Tesar[b] · Ales Linhart[c]

[a]3rd Department of Internal Medicine, [b]Department of Nephrology, and [c]Second Department of Internal Medicine, General University Hospital Prague and First Faculty of Medicine, Charles University Prague, Prague, Czech Republic

Abstract

More than 50% of all end-stage renal disease (ESRD) patients die from cardiovascular complications. Among them, heart failure and pulmonary hypertension play a major role, and published studies document significantly higher mortality rates in patients with these two states. Arteriovenous fistulas (AVF) and arteriovenous grafts (AVG) are the preferred types of vascular access (VA). However, both AVF and AVG increase cardiac output and in turn could contribute to (the decompensation of) heart failure or pulmonary hypertension. No really safe access flow volume exists, and the ESRD patients' reactions to it vary considerably. We review the mechanisms involved in the cardiovascular consequences of increased cardiac output and available literary data. The link between access flow volume and increased mortality due to pulmonary hypertension or heart failure probably exists, but still has not been directly evidenced. Regular echocardiography is advisable especially in patients with symptoms or with high VA flow (>1,500 ml/min).

Recommendations to Improve Patient Safety

- Patients with vascular access (VA) should be checked for congestive heart failure and pulmonary hypertension prior to and after access creation.
- Echocardiography is advisable prior to VA creation. If the finding is pathological, consult a cardiologist.
- Any arteriovenous VA flow could be too high for a particular patient, but always exclude other causes, such as inappropriate dry weight setting.
- Asymptomatic patients with arteriovenous VA flow >1,500–2,000 ml/min could benefit from regular echocardiography (every 6 months).

Cardiovascular Morbidity in End-Stage Renal Disease Patients

The end-stage renal disease (ESRD) population is at a high risk of cardiovascular morbidity, and more than 50% of ESRD patients die from cardiovascular complications [1]. One of the typical features is accelerated atherosclerosis due to the higher prevalence of many risk factors in ESRD patients, such as arterial hypertension, diabetes mellitus and so-called uremic dyslipidemia. Moreover, several specific factors contribute to the process including higher activity of subclinical inflammation, increased level of ADMA (asymmetric di-methylarginine, an endogenous inhibitor of nitric oxide synthase) and others [2]. Atherosclerosis presents as coronary artery disease, cerebrovascular disease or peripheral vascular disease. Metabolic changes (parathormone and phosphate increase, vitamin D decrease, etc.) lead to arterial stiffening and medial calcifications ('arteriosclerosis'). Many ESRD patients suffer from left ventricular hypertrophy, which is associated with myocardial oxygen supply impairment, left ventricular diastolic dysfunction and increased mortality. Heart failure, another frequent condition, has a multifactorial origin and will be discussed together with pulmonary hypertension in detail below.

Heart Failure

Heart failure is present in up to 30% of new dialysis patients [3]. ESRD patients with heart failure have significantly shorter lifespan than patients without this condition. By definition, heart failure is a state when the heart is not able to maintain adequate perfusion of the target tissues and organs at rest or during exercise, or if it is able to do it only at the cost of higher filling pressures. The left-sided heart failure is mostly leading to shortness of breath, fatigue, and decreased exercise capacity. The right-sided heart failure is usually presenting with leg edemas and ascites. Many conditions could lead to heart failure. The most frequent of them is the left ventricular systolic dysfunction (as a result of myocardial infarction, dilated cardiomyopathy, myocarditis, etc.), described roughly by the ejection fraction, which is the relation of the stroke volume and end-diastolic volume (normal value >50%). Another cause of heart failure is left ventricular diastolic dysfunction, which corresponds to the impaired diastolic filling due to impaired relaxation and myocardial compliance. This so-called heart failure with preserved ejection fraction (HF-PEF) is encountered in patients with left ventricular hypertrophy or its disperse fibrotization. However, a newly emerging concept of HF-PEF suggests that in a substantial proportion of patients this condition is caused by increased stiffness of great arteries leading to

Table 1. Specific factors contributing to the development of heart failure in the ESRD population

Volume overload between dialysis sessions
Arterial hypertension (present in >80% of all patients)
Cardiovascular calcifications (valvular disease, higher arterial stiffness)
Anemia
Inflammation
Vascular access flow volume
Arrhythmias (caused by sympathetic activation and ionic changes)

an inappropriate afterload increase, which requires compensatory mechanisms leading to prolongation and alteration of myocardial relaxation. Further mechanisms of heart failure in ESRD patients include moderate to severe valve stenosis or regurgitation, arterial hypertension, arrhythmias, etc.

In ESRD patients, there are also other specific and significant factors contributing to the development of heart failure (table 1). These include volume overload between dialysis sessions, the amount of blood flowing through the arteriovenous shunt and anemia. Their role will be discussed in detail below.

Pulmonary Hypertension

Pulmonary hypertension is, by definition, a state when the mean pulmonary arterial pressure at rest is >25 mm Hg. Symptoms of pulmonary hypertension include shortness of breath, dizziness, fainting, leg swelling and others. A recent study found 38% prevalence of pulmonary hypertension among ESRD patients. This condition was associated with a >2-fold increase in all-cause mortality independent of other risk factors [4]. Another study found up to 56% prevalence of pulmonary hypertension in ESRD patients [5]. Many factors contribute to its development. They include volume overload, left ventricular failure, arterial hypertension, vascular access (VA) flow and the complex metabolic changes of ESRD [6].

The gold standard for the measurement of pulmonary arterial pressure is right-sided catheterization. However, this invasive procedure has a limited application in common clinical practice. Alternatively, the pulmonary artery pressure (mainly systolic) could be estimated by echocardiography. There is a large number of pulmonary hypertension signs on echo, but the most precise is the measurement of the peak tricuspid regurgitation gradient (if present). By adding the estimation of the central venous pressure, we could estimate the systolic right ventricular (and pulmonary arterial) pressure.

Hemodynamic Changes Associated with Vascular Access

Heart Failure

Physiologically, the blood flow through extremities is regulated mainly by the peripheral vascular resistance, that is by the tone (and diameter) of resistant arterioles. Under resting conditions, the flow is low (for example flow volume in the brachial artery is 60–150 ml/min [own unpubl. data]). However, during a muscle work, the flow increases several times. Arteriovenous fistulas (AVF) and arteriovenous grafts (AVG) used in ESRD patients bypass the resistance arterioles. The resulting access flow ('normal values' range between 600 and 1,500 ml/min) is 10–20 times higher than the normal values of the resting extremity; higher values are especially in the more proximal VA. Moreover, such values represent about 10–30% of resting cardiac output (CO; normal values range between 4 and 6 l/min in adults). If we compare all these values, there is no surprise that creation of VA could cause heart problems. The concept of effective CO, that is the real CO minus access flow, has been introduced [7]. Surprisingly, there are still only few experts believing that higher access flow is truly toxic for the heart and that it is associated with shorter lifespan of the dialysis patients.

The reason why AVF issues remain controversial is that our evidence of fistula-related deleterious cardiac changes is limited. In the literature, we have 3 groups of studies: (1) the effect of AVF in animal models; (2) the effect of AVF creation in humans, and (3) the effect of flow-reducing procedures or fistula closure.

Aortocaval fistula in rats is a frequently used model of (hyperkinetic) heart failure. The rats develop cardiomegaly and pulmonary hypertension, and die earlier than the animals without this fistula [8]. Different expression of as many as 66 proteins was found by this group in the hearts of AVF rats.

Human Studies of the Consequences of AVF Creation

Shortly after access creation, CO increases due to both left ventricular ejection fraction and heart rate increase [9]. These changes are probably driven by the decrease in systemic vascular resistance (caused by the arterial anastomosis of the VA) and by the increase of preload (venous return to the heart). Such changes could be considered rather physiological. However, within some weeks after access creation, Iwashima et al. [10] observed also an increase in the left ventricular diastolic diameter; the indices of diastolic left ventricle function worsened, and levels of natriuretic peptides increased. The rise of B-natriuretic peptide (BNP) correlated with the diastolic function (E/A ratio, which is early/atrial left ventricular filling). Similar findings were observed in our center in a group that had their first VA with the access flow volume of only 789 ± 361 ml/min 6 weeks after access creation [11]. Even treatment of access stenosis by the balloon angioplasty could lead to a pulmonary edema because of the sudden increase in access flow [12]. There are only very limited data of the medium- or long-term effect of access creation on the heart. In our study [11], 6 months after access creation, we observed a trend of BNP decrease despite somewhat higher access flow than at 6 weeks. In an interesting study by Movilli et al. [13], the patients were echocardiographically evaluated 6 months after fistula ligation due to long-term malfunction and conversion to a permanent catheter. Left ventricular mass decrease after access ligation was associated with an increase in ejection fraction.

Effects of Flow-Reducing Procedures or Fistula Closure

Hemodynamic changes occur even during short arteriovenous access compression, as was shown already in the early 1970s [14] – increase in systemic vascular resistance associated with the decreased CO due to slower heart rate. Chemla et al. [15] monitored the effect of surgical flow reduction by the distalization of the anastomosis technique in a group of patients having very high access flow (3,135 ± 692 ml/min, minimum 1,600 ml/min) and overt (hyperkinetic) heart failure with the mean CO of 8.0 l/min. After the procedure, the mean access flow dropped to 1,025 ml/min and the mean CO to 5.6 l/min. Similar findings were observed also by other authors [16, 17].

Pulmonary Hypertension

Normal resting pulmonary artery mean pressure (PAMP) is less than 25 mm Hg. This value is the sum of the left atrial pressure (LAP) and the pressure gradient needed to shift blood from the pulmonary arteries to the left atrium (fig. 1). The latter is called transpulmonary gradient (TPG). Therefore, TPG = PAMP – LAP. Pulmonary artery pressure depends on pulmonary vascular resistance (PVR) and also on the CO. The latter may change due to various reasons, in particular due to physical exercise. According to hemodynamic studies [18], physical exercise in healthy older people (especially >70 years) leads to an acute increase in PAMP more than in younger people. If CO doubles (e.g. from 5 to 10 l/min), PAMP and LAP rise approximately twice. This phenomenon is likely due to the worsened diastolic function of the left ventricle in the elderly. As we already mentioned, left ventricular diastolic dysfunction is frequently associated also with ESRD.

The hemodynamics of pulmonary circulation are best described by using the concept of PVR [PVR = TPG/CO or (PAMP – LAP)/CO]. From this equation, it is obvious that PVR is dependent on age (in parallel with PAMP). TPG increases with increasing CO in all age categories, but the differences are much smaller. Finally,

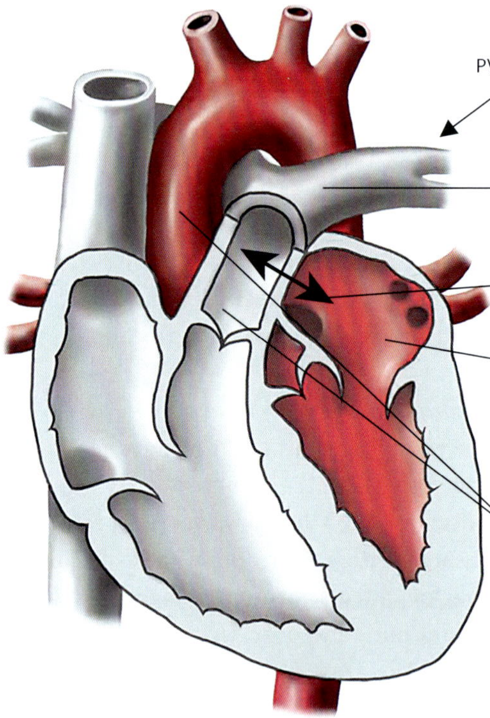

Fig. 1. Hemodynamics in normal patients and changes after VA creation. PAMP normal values <20–25 mm Hg; LAP <12 mm Hg; TPG <12 mm Hg; CO 4.0–6.0 l/min; PVR = TPG/CO or (PAMP – LAP)/CO.

another formulation of this equation (PAMP = CO/PVR + LAP) can explain how the AVF could influence the pulmonary artery pressure. CO is increased by the AVF (and also by anemia, volume retention etc.). Indeed, pulmonary hypertension was more frequent in a group with proximal VA (mean flow 2,500 ml/min) than in distal accesses in the study by Beigi et al. [19]. Case reports of severe pulmonary hypertension caused by large AVF and its reversal after fistula ligation have also been published [20]. This observation may be explained by secondary pulmonary vascular changes primarily induced by an increased CO. These may be responsible for the observation that in a group of 20 prospectively evaluated patients before and after fistula creation, pulmonary hypertension did not correlate with fistula flow [21].

Other Hemodynamic Consequences

According to case reports, other consequences of AVF flow include the risk of the benign intracranial hypertension as a result of the chronically elevated cen-

Table 2. Creation of AVF or AVG should probably be avoided in the following groups of patients

Patients with very short life expectancy (<3–6 months)
Patients with severe heart failure with systemic hypotension[1]
Patients with severe pulmonary hypertension[2]
Patients with the presence or high risk of hand ischemia
Patients having a coronary artery bypass with the use of the left internal mammary artery – restriction of the left-hand access

[1] Reversible causes, such as valvular or coronary arterial stenosis, should be excluded as well as inadequately low setting of the dry weight.
[2] Reversible causes should be excluded (especially pulmonary embolism).

tral venous pressure [22]. After the closure of a long-term AVF, a true aneurysm of the feeding artery could occur [23]. Hand growth retardation can develop in children on the side of the fistula [24]. Acute cardiorenal failure was attributed to high-flow fistula in a patient after kidney transplantation [25]. The explanation for these contradictory findings is in the multiple etiology of pulmonary hypertension in ESRD patients.

Safe Access Creation – Cardiological Examination prior to Surgery

Based on the potential cardiovascular adverse effects of AVF, it may seem that the best VA is a permanent catheter. However, patients with catheters have a higher mortality, especially due to infections [26]. The vast majority of patients tolerate AVF and AVG well. The choice between the latter two depends mostly on local factors, but the native fistula should be preferred.

The latter recommendations (table 2) mirror the authors' experience because the official guidelines do not cover this topic. A close cooperation of the nephrologist, vascular surgeon and cardiologist is advisable.

Cardiac Safety in Access Maintenance

Harmful hemodynamic consequences of the arteriovenous shunt described in this chapter are, fortunately, not very common. Moreover, although we know that heart failure and/or pulmonary hypertension are associated with significantly shorter lifespan of dialysis patients, there is up to now no evidence of a direct link between high access flow and increased mortality. Many patients tolerate access flow 2–3 l/min without symptoms, although the question for how long remains. Heart failure and pulmonary hypertension associated with higher access flow are usually reversible and disappear after flow reduction surgery. Therefore, the emerging questions are: (1) When is access flow too high? (2) Who and when should be examined for possible complications?

The answers to these questions cannot be simple. Numerically, access flow is considered high when it exceeds 1,500–2,000 ml/min [2]. Such values represent more than 30% of resting normal CO, so the patients could be at risk of heart failure and/or pulmonary hypertension. These patients are examined by echocardiography twice per year in our center, even if they have no symptoms. Left ventricular dilatation and/or decrease in its ejection fraction are the most common indications for flow-reducing surgery. Other authors recommend the relation of access flow to CO suggesting a cutoff value of 0.3 [27, 28]. Figure 2 summarizes the algorithm in the creation and maintenance of VA.

Since *any* access flow could be too high for a particular patient in his/her particular state, the clinical approach seems to be more practical and appropriate. Clinical symptoms of heart failure or pulmonary hypertension should lead to a careful examination of the patient, and the access flow should play only a minor role. Practically, it is important to keep in mind that both heart failure and pulmonary hypertension significantly depend on the patient's actual hydration status. The latter changes with hemodialysis and significant reduction of left ventricular size and mass occur after hemodialysis [29]. Furthermore, the correct setting of dry weight plays a fundamental role. Inadequately high dry weight setting frequently leads to shortness of breath and fatigue. In these patients, echocardiography often reveals signs of left ventricular systolic (and diastolic) dysfunction, valve regurgitation and pulmonary hypertension. Echocardiography should also estimate the actual central venous pressure (by the inferior vena cava diameter and the level of inspiratory collapse). An attempt to lower the patient's dry weight value should be done prior to further cardiological investigation! Other causes of heart failure, such as treatable arrhythmia, coronary artery disease, valvular disease, etc. should always be excluded.

Access Flow Measurement

Several methods are used for the VA flow volume measurement during hemodialysis [30]. Mostly, they are based on dilution techniques and are used for early detection of access stenosis. However, they are important also in terms of systemic hemodynamics. It should be especially kept in mind that the obtained

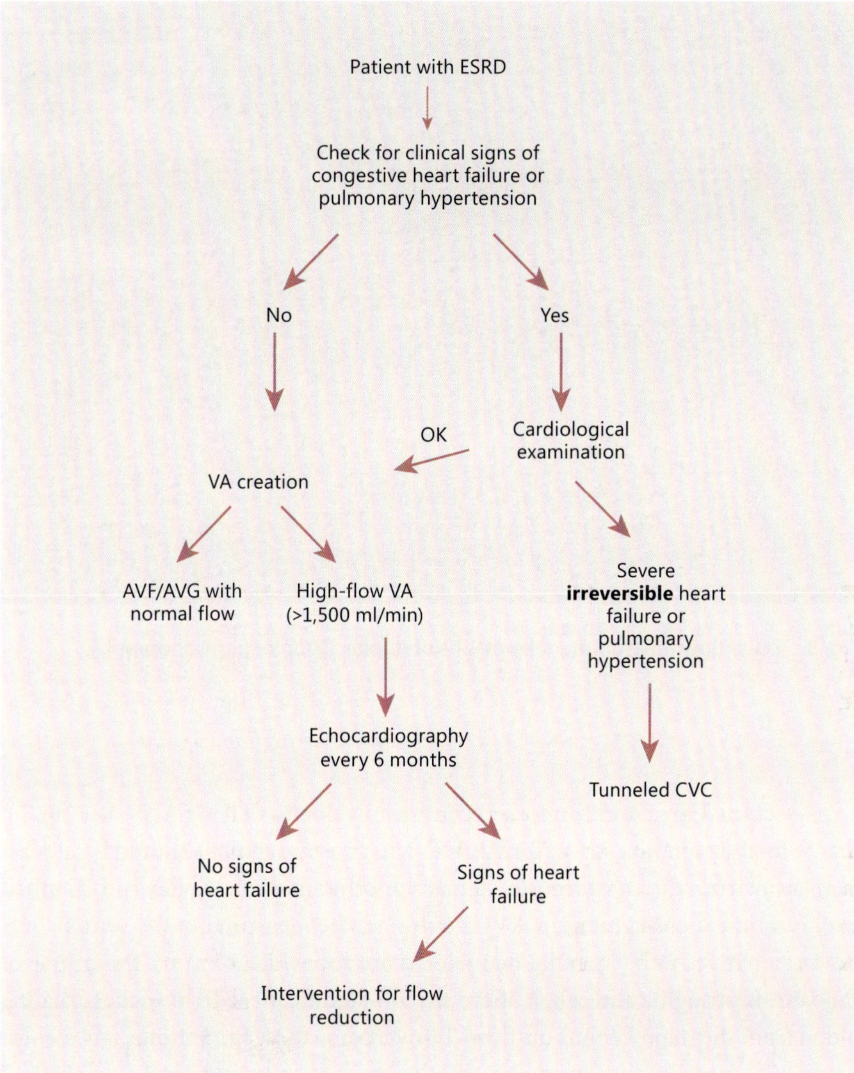

Fig. 2. Algorithm for patients with a (risk for) heart failure. CVC = Central venous catheter.

values vary, depending on actual hemodynamic status, hydration, blood pressure, cardiac rhythm, etc. Physiological access flow variation was observed in an interesting study – the mean coefficient of variation was as high as 23.3% [31].

During echocardiography or vascular sonography, the access flow can also be calculated using a linear high-frequency probe, as shown in figure 3.

The access flow should be measured in a straight vascular segment without excessive dilatation by the longitudinal section. It is based on multiplying the

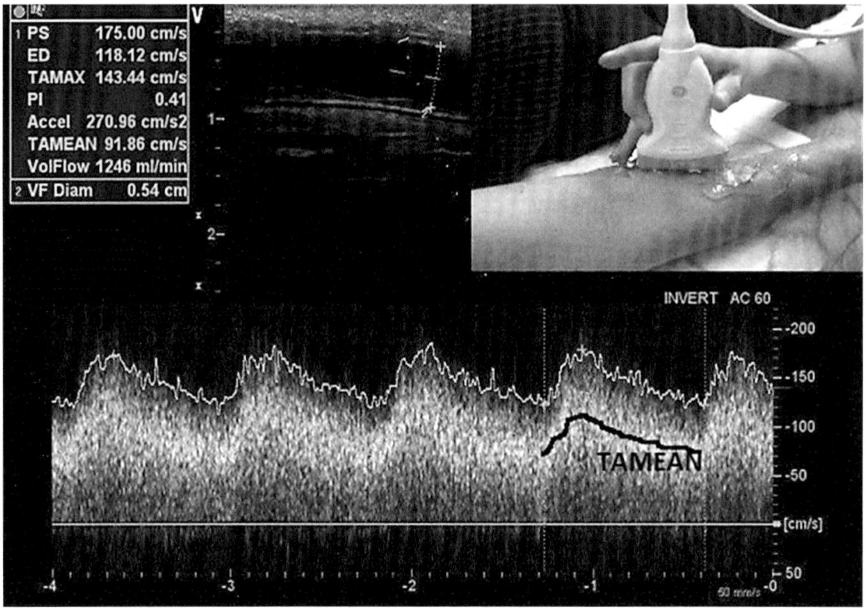

Fig. 3. Access flow measurement by means of duplex Doppler ultrasonography.

cross-sectional area and time-averaged mean velocity (TAMEAN – see fig. 3), that is by the equation $\pi r^2 \times$ TAMEAN. The chosen segment should be at least 5 cm away from the anastomosis, stenosis or other major irregularity. It is much easier to find such segment in AVGs. Flow can be measured in the venous outflow of a native AVF when the diameter is not too wide (<7 mm), the course of the vein is straight, and when there are no significant side branches stealing blood from the main venous outflow. To overcome these limitations, it is recommended to measure the flow volume in the brachial artery at least 5 cm proximal to the anastomosis, bearing in mind that less than 100 ml/min of blood flow is consumed by the tissues below the level of the anastomosis. We advise to measure the access flow in a given patient always on the same level in order to be able to compare successive measurements.

Conclusions

A well-functioning VA is mandatory for the adequate hemodialysis therapy. As compared to catheter-based approach, AVF creation is associated the lowest rate of complications [32], and a vast majority of the patients tolerate it very well.

However, the ESRD population is polymorbid, and the access flow could be one of the mechanisms involved in the development of heart failure or pulmonary hypertension, which might shorten their lives. Although there is limited hard evidence, clinical series and case reports suggest this causal relationship. The reduction of an inappropriately high access flow may lead to considerable improvements in patients' hemodynamics and symptoms. Only multidisciplinary cooperation can assure the best diagnostics and care.

Acknowledgements

This work was supported by grant NT14161 from the Internal Grant Agency of the Ministry of Health, Czech Republic, and the Research project of Charles University P25/LF1/2

Disclosure Statement

The authors have no conflicts of interest to declare.

References

1 Collins AJ: Cardiovascular mortality in end-stage renal disease. Am J Med Sci 2003;325:163–167.
2 Malik J, Tuka V, Mokrejsova M, Holaj R, Tesar V: Mechanisms of chronic heart failure development in end-stage renal disease patients on chronic hemodialysis. Phys Res 2009;58:613–621.
3 Stack AG, Bloembergen WE: A cross-sectional study of the prevalence and clinical correlates of congestive heart failure among incident US dialysis patients. Am J Kidney Dis 2001;38:992–1000.
4 Agarwal R: Prevalence, determinants and prognosis of pulmonary hypertension among hemodialysis patients. Nephrol Dial Transplant 2012;27:3908–3914.
5 Havlucu Y, Kursat S, Ekmekci C, et al: Pulmonary hypertension in patients with chronic renal failure. Respiration 2007;74:503–510.
6 Bolignano D, Rastelli S, Agarwal R, et al: Pulmonary hypertension in CKD. Am J Kidney Dis 2013;61:612–622.
7 Amerling R: Con: on cardiovascular outcomes and the arteriovenous fistula: lesser of evils. Nephrol Dial Transplant 2012;27:3756–3757.
8 Melenovsky V, Skaroupkova P, Benes J, Torresova V, Kopkan L, Cervenka L: The course of heart failure development and mortality in rats with volume overload due to aorto-caval fistula. Kidney Blood Pres Res 2012;35:167–173.
9 Ori Y, Korzets A, Katz M, Perek Y, Zahavi I, Gafter U: Haemodialysis arteriovenous access – a prospective haemodynamic evaluation. Nephrol Dial Transplant 1996;11:94–97.
10 Iwashima Y, Horio T, Takami Y, et al: Effects of the creation of arteriovenous fistula for hemodialysis on cardiac function and natriuretic peptide levels in CRF. Am J Kidney Dis 2002;40:974–982.
11 Malik J, Tuka V, Krupickova Z, Chytilova E, Holaj R, Slavikova M: Creation of dialysis vascular access with normal flow increases brain natriuretic peptide levels. Int Urol Nephrol 2009;41:997–1002.

12 Velez-Martinez M, Weinberg BD, Mishkin JD: Flash pulmonary oedema after relief of haemodialysis graft stenosis. Heart Lung Circ 2013;22:672–676.
13 Movilli E, Viola BF, Brunori G, et al: Long-term effects of arteriovenous fistula closure on echocardiographic functional and structural findings in hemodialysis patients: a prospective study. Am J Kidney Dis 2010;55: 682–689.
14 Johnson G Jr, Blythe WB: Hemodynamic effects of arteriovenous shunts used for hemodialysis. Ann Surg 1970;171:715–723.
15 Chemla ES, Morsy M, Anderson L, Whitemore A: Inflow reduction by distalization of anastomosis treats efficiently high-inflow high-cardiac output vascular access for hemodialysis. Semin Dial 2007;20:68–72.
16 Anderson CB, Codd JR, Graff RA, Groce MA, Harter HR, Newton WT: Cardiac failure and upper extremity arteriovenous dialysis fistulas. Case reports and a review of the literature. Arch Int Med 1976;136:292–297.
17 Vaes RH, Tordoir JH, Scheltinga MR: Systemic effects of a high-flow arteriovenous fistula for hemodialysis. J Vasc Access 2014; 15:163–168.
18 Stanek V, Widimsky J, Hurych J, Petrikova J: Pressure, flow and volume changes during exercise within pulmonary vascular bed in patients after pneumonectomy. Clin Sci 1969; 37:11–22.
19 Beigi AA, Sadeghi AM, Khosravi AR, Karami M, Masoudpour H: Effects of the arteriovenous fistula on pulmonary artery pressure and cardiac output in patients with chronic renal failure. J Vasc Access 2009;10:160–166.
20 Clarkson MR, Giblin L, Brown A, Little D, Donohoe J: Reversal of pulmonary hypertension after ligation of a brachiocephalic arteriovenous fistula. Am J Kidney Dis 2002; 40:E8.
21 Unal A, Tasdemir K, Oymak S, et al: The long-term effects of arteriovenous fistula creation on the development of pulmonary hypertension in hemodialysis patients. Hemodial Int 2010;14:398–402.
22 Elkabbaj D, Hassani K, Bennouk M, et al: Benign intracranial hypertension in a hemodialysis patient: consider the fistula. J Fr Ophtalmol 2012;35:822.e1–e5.
23 Feijoo-Cano C: Giant true aneurysm of the radial artery following ligation of an arteriovenous fistula for haemodialysis. Nefrologia 2012;32:404–406.
24 van Hoek F, Scheltinga MR, Krasznai AG, Cornelissen EA: Retarded hand growth due to a hemodialysis fistula in a young girl. Pediatr Nephrol 2009;24:2055–2058.
25 Nickel P, Gul S, Puhl G, Poellinger A, Schindler R: Acute cardiorenal syndrome by high flow arteriovenous fistula after kidney transplantation. J Vasc Access 2013;14:394–396.
26 Dhingra RK, Young EW, Hulbert-Shearon TE, Leavey SF, Port FK: Type of vascular access and mortality in U.S. hemodialysis patients. Kidney Int 2001;60:1443–1451.
27 Wijnen E, Keuter XH, Planken NR, et al: The relation between vascular access flow and different types of vascular access with systemic hemodynamics in hemodialysis patients. Artif Organs 2005;29:960–964.
28 MacRae JM, Pandeya S, Humen DP, Krivitski N, Lindsay RM: Arteriovenous fistula-associated high-output cardiac failure: a review of mechanisms. Am J Kidney Dis 2004;43:e17–e22.
29 Palecek T, Skalicka L, Lachmanova J, Tesar V, Linhart A: Effect of preload reduction by hemodialysis on conventional and novel echocardiographic parameters of left ventricular structure and function. Echocardiography 2008;25:162–168.
30 Lopot F, Nejedly B, Sulkova S, Blaha J: Comparison of different techniques of hemodialysis vascular access flow evaluation. J Vasc Access 2004;5:25–32.
31 Valek M, Lopot F, Dusilova-Sulkova S, Polakovic V: Physiologic variability of vascular access blood flow for hemodialysis. Blood Purif 2008;26:468–472.
32 Basile C, Lomonte C: Pro: the arteriovenous fistula is a blessing of God. Nephrol Dial Transplant 2012;27:3752–3756.

Jan Malik, MD
3rd Department of Internal Medicine, First Medical Faculty
Charles University and General University Hospital
U nemocnice 1
CZ–128 08 Prague (Czech Republic)
E-Mail malik.jan@vfn.cz

Widmer MK, Malik J (eds): Patient Safety in Dialysis Access.
Contrib Nephrol. Basel, Karger, 2015, vol 184, pp 87–96
DOI: 10.1159/000365825

Simulation in Vascular Access Surgery

Matthias K. Widmer[a] · Ingemar Davidson[b] · Lukas W. Widmer[a] · Jürg Schmidli[a] · Thomas R. Wyss[a]

[a]Department of Cardiovascular Surgery, Swiss Cardiovascular Center, Bern University Hospital, Bern, Switzerland; [b]Department of Surgery, Tulane University, New Orleans, La., USA

Abstract

In the last years, simulation training has become widespread in different areas of medicine due to social expectations, political accountability and professional regulation. Different types of simulators allow to improve knowledge, skills, communication and team behavior. Simulation sessions have been proven to shorten the learning curve and allow education in a safe environment. Patients on dialysis are an expanding group. They often suffer from several comorbidities and need complex surgical procedures with regard to their dialysis access. Therefore, education in evidence-based algorithms is as important as teaching of practical skills. In this chapter, we are presenting an overview of available dialysis access training modalities. We are convinced that simulation will become more important in the near future and has a substantial impact on strategies to improve aspects of patient safety.

Recommendations to Improve Patient Safety

- Simulation training in vascular access should be established rigorously to learn the concepts and technical skills of dialysis access surgery.
- Simulation training and workplace assessments with good quality feedback help to uniform the procedures practiced in an institution and therefore may reduce the risk for errors.
- More and more sophisticated and commercially available models to train dialysis access surgery are ready for use.
- The numbers of professional workshops for simulation with feedback by experts are growing.

Introduction

In the last decade, pressure from political and social institutions and organizations (i.e. the patient safety initiative) as well as new technologies in the clinical setting had a strong impact on educational programs of health care professionals [1]. After simple part-task trainers, more sophisticated simulators were developed. Electronics and informatics made it possible to construct computer-based systems to train in virtual reality and even with haptic systems. Integrated high-fidelity simulators allow, depending on 'deposited' curves and datasets, to make decisions during the exercise. Standardized patients help to train communication skills and to assess professionalism because these persons can give direct feedback to the performer. In simulated environments, like the operating room or an intensive care unit, team training facilitates interprofessional education [2]. Table 1 gives an overview of dimensions of simulation and the characteristics of different simulators with examples. The chapter will focus on training models to improve patient safety in different aspects of vascular access (VA) creation.

Advantages and Benefits of Simulation

For high-reliability organizations like aviation, the nuclear power industry and fire fighters, simulation is vital to train for unexpected situations. In health care, simulation training is important to shorten the learning curve and therefore to improve patient safety. Additionally, simulation is a safe way to teach and learn use of new and innovative technical devices, where risks are involved.

Working hour restrictions, the shift from open surgery towards endovascular procedures and patients with more complex vessel pathology are factors making simulation an additional attractive teaching tool.

In 2012, we performed a study during a 3-day workshop on basics in vascular surgery run by the Vascular International Foundation and School (www.vascular-international.org). The performance of a femoral thrombendarterectomy using a patch plasty by 43 participants was rated using a Likert scale from 1 (= poor) to 10 (= excellent) by 3 tutors. There was an evaluation at the beginning of the course and at the end. Independently, three other raters evaluated the performance and the patch quality after the workshop. A wrong side placement of the patch was rated zero.

Participants improved in median performance from 6 (4–7.5) to 7 (5–9; $p < 0.001$), and median patch quality improved from 3.3 (1–6.7) to 6.7 (1–9; $p < 0.001$; fig. 1). These results are similar to current research in the same field and

Table 1. Dimensions of simulation and types of currently available simulators [1, 3 – 7]

a Dimensions of simulation

	Dimension	Examples of categories
1	Purpose and aims of the simulation activity	Training, assessment
2	Unit of participation in the simulation	Individual, team, organization
3	Experience level of simulation participants	Medical school, residency, continuing medical education
4	Health care domain in which simulation is applied	Radiology, surgery, primary care
5	Health care discipline of personnel participating in the simulation	Aids, nurses, physicians, managers
6	Type of knowledge, skill, attitude, or behavior addressed in the simulation	Conceptual understanding, technical skills, decision making, behaviors
7	Age of the patient being simulated	Infants, adults, elderly
8	Technology applicable or required for simulations	Role playing, standardized patients, part-task trainer, computer patient, electronic patient
9	Site of simulation participants	Home, office, dedicated laboratory, replica of clinical environment, work unit
10	Extent of direct participation in simulation	Remote viewing with verbal interaction, direct on-site hands-on participation
11	Feedback method accompanying simulation	Automatic critique by simulator, real time critique by instructor, video-based post hoc debriefing

b Types of simulators

	Characteristics	Examples and/or goals
Part-task trainer	Skills performance	Models to perform vascular anastomoses
Computer programs	Multimedia programs, independent learning, no technical skills training	Interactive CD-ROMs to train knowledge using graphics, pictures or even videos
Virtual reality and haptic systems	Various level of difficulties, possibility to simulate complications, objective assessment, haptic models with feedback on touch, high initial costs	Models to train endovascular procedures
Integrated simulators (hi-fidelity simulators)	Model or instructor driven, life-like representation of body parts, generating realistic monitoring data	SimMan
Simulated patients	Realism, direct feedback, train nontechnical skills and professionalism	Training of clinical situations (i.e. breaking bad news)
Simulated environments	To train nontechnical and technical aspects	'Virtual' operating room
Human cadaver models	Accurate anatomy, no complications, limited availability, high costs	Exposure of anatomical complex areas, simulation of complex revascularizations
Living animal models	Realism, mimic complications, different anatomy from human, ethical issues, high costs	Soft tissue and vessel preparation, performance of vascular anastomoses, damage control

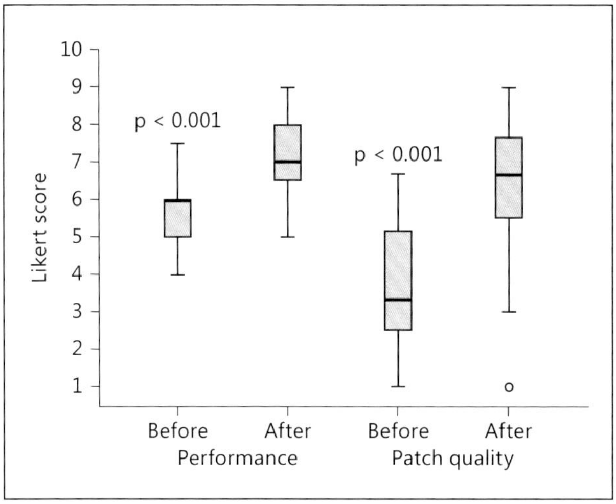

Fig. 1. Simulation significantly improves performance and patch quality.

could also be documented for a thrombendarterectomy using a pulsatile carotid model [8, 9].

Besides the setting and the quality of the models, feedback is a central issue in order to benefit from simulation training. The concept of a practical demonstration of an exercise followed by the performance in a team of two is feasible, as well as to have one experienced tutor supervising 4 participants (fig. 2). Teachers should symbolize operative skills and be trained to give adequate feedback with empathy, first outlining the excellent performance and second correct and add points of potential improvements [10, 11].

As far as we know, in VA surgery only a limited number of models in few institutions are available at the moment. So far, this made it impossible to conceptualize a dedicated course in which all aspects of VA surgery could be covered as a whole, preparing a technical manual and providing theoretical background information. We think that especially in access surgery, where decision-making is so important, 'the mind behind' is key.

Simulation Models and Training Opportunities

In this paragraph, we will present some simulation models which we are familiar with, knowing that there may exist others. In order to push the effort in simulation, the authors would be grateful to gather more information of available facilities and models for VA training.

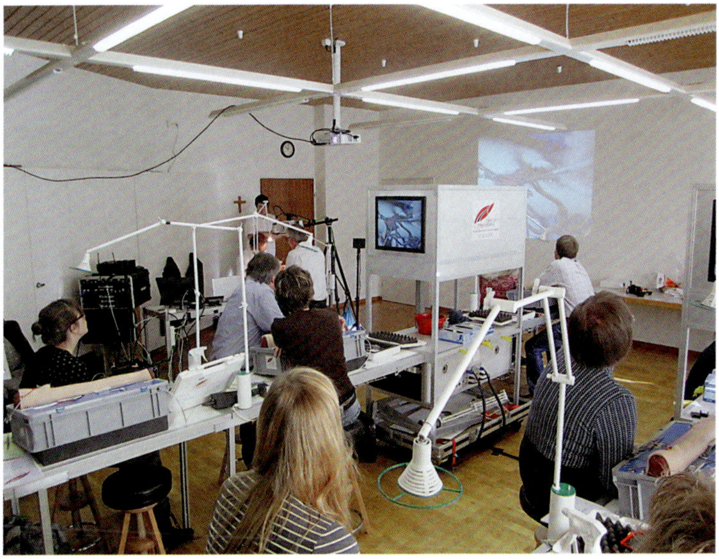

Fig. 2. Live demonstration by video transmission to show technical details in VA creation during a workshop.

Training in Duplex Ultrasound, Catheter Placement and Cannulation

All guidelines stated that duplex ultrasound (US) is an important tool in the decision making process of VA creation. In the last years, many societies developed curricula in which duplex US training takes part. It is reasonable that organizations and institutions offer workshops to teach the basics of duplex US with a focus on VA. This would allow the surgeon to perform correct vascular mapping including assessment of the arteries before VA creation. Such courses can be easily organized at low costs. First, healthy volunteers can be examined and later patients with end-stage renal disease (ESRD), often highly motivated to participate because there is no risk involved.

In anesthesiology, training models for the placement of central venous lines have been available for years. To improve patient safety, the use of micropuncture sets and/or the use of ultrasonography to puncture the internal jugular vein correctly are standard procedures. In VA surgery, the placement of tunneled catheters is part of the daily caseload. Trainees should be familiar with different types of catheters and advantages or disadvantages of an antegrade and retrograde placement of a tunneled central venous catheter. An internet search for simulation and central venous catheter showed that there are different mannequins on the market to train these interventions (www.simulab.com; www.bluephantom.com; www.limbsandthings.com; www.3-dmed.com). Some of the mannequins have pulsatile flow, different fluids to mark venous and arterial blood and an artificial skin that allows US visualization of the vein.

The peritoneal dialysis access catheter placement simulation is ideal to teach aviation safety principles emphasizing the importance of knowing basic facts, such as the tools and instruments needed for the procedure and how the use of checklists improves patient safety. An abdominal simulator is currently under development for the laparoscopic technique of placing the peritoneal dialysis catheter [12].

Dialysis access cannulation conduit simulators use US guidance to place dialysis needles under pressure and are filled with red-colored fluid to show proper needle placement. The hands-on simulation with a biological VA model consists of performing several US-guided punctures of a large vein or a dialysis access. This phase of the practical session is structured on a step-by-step approach towards the skills that the trainee will progressively achieve: these 'Seven Turkey Steps' use an easy-to-make, inexpensive simulator, consisting of a turkey thigh, with a rubber tube inside. The seven steps, divided into three phases, are detailed elsewhere [13]. This biological simulator is being replaced by completely artificial silicon devices that are less cumbersome to transport and assemble [12].

Simulator for Percutaneous Interventions

The computerized percutaneous interventional simulator coupled with end-of-case metrics promotes consistency and shifts the trainee to a higher level of competency. The simulator recreates the feel (haptic), and visually allows the operator to 'treat' an arteriovenous dialysis graft stenosis by placing a guide wire across the venous stenosis, and to select an appropriately sized angioplasty balloon, perform angioplasty, and finally deploy a suitably sized FDA-approved stent graft at the treatment site. Throughout the simulation exercise, an instructor supervises the trainee, while making decisions and technical maneuvers that will either lead to successful completion or failure (with the opportunity to repeat the steps where errors were made). Upon completion, 'metrics' summarizing performance is provided. The goal is for the trainee to select and use the implantable stent safely and effectively [14].

This is similar to carotid stenting where the FDA requires training using simulation in the certification process to perform such procedures. These FDA standards should also apply to ESRD patients' care and safety [15].

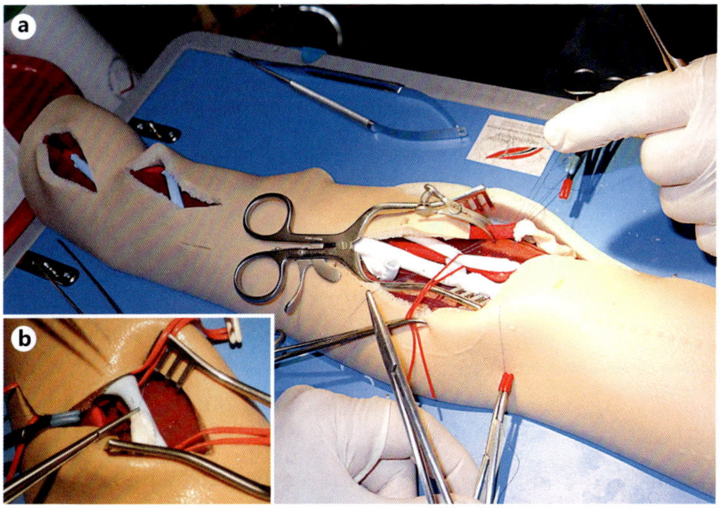

Fig. 3. New pulsatile arm model with more than eight possibilities to create VA. **a** The whole model. **b** Detailed view of how an anastomosis is created.

New Pulsatile Arm Model

During the Charing Cross Symposium in April 2013, Vascular International Foundation and School presented a new pulsatile arm model allowing to perform more than eight different VA modalities like snuff box arteriovenous fistula (AVF), cephalic AVF, basilica transposition or arteriovenous graft placement (fig. 3). Also a DRIL (distal revascularization-interval ligation) procedure and new devices like hybrid prostheses can be placed within this model. All material can be put in an easily transportable box of 50 × 30 × 20 cm. To prepare a training session, the arm model is loaded with inlay vessels, which are then connected to a pump. An artificial skin will cover the whole arm. Using a wedge, the model can be placed in an ideal position. Exercises are performed under pump pressure to check the quality of arteriovenous anastomoses. Important is the knowhow of dedicated workshop leaders and tutors and the mind behind teaching not only the technical details but also concepts of VA creation. Short key lectures to teach VA concepts and decision-making algorithms, a manual with many illustrations, and live demonstrations to introduce each model help trainees to improve their performance. The feedback of the first 1.5-day workshops (11/2013 and 5/2014) with this new model was promising. Vascular International School is willing and interested to run such workshops in collaboration with other organizations dealing with education all over the world [16].

Training on Cadavers

In the past, cadaver training was the only way to perform VA training. Fresh cadavers may pose a hygienic issue, although newer and more expensive technology is available to prepare the human bodies with the 'Thiel' solution, which eliminates bothersome odors. Dissection in the subcutaneous tissue is somewhat different, but the behavior of the blood vessels is quite realistic. It is even possible to prepare a torso and arms to learn how to perform more complex, so called exotic VAs in the neck and breast area. The European Society of Vascular Surgery in collaboration with the Vascular Access Society (www.esvs.org, www.vascularaccesssociety.org) and the European Vascular Course (www.evc.org) offer such workshops.

Communication Skills Simulation consists of prerecorded simulation case videos highlighting communication skills. It emphasizes ways to improve processes, listening skills and patient treatment adherence, thereby improving the quality of patient care [17].

Skills and Knowledge Transfer from Simulation to the Real Operation

Simulation training is only the first step to become a competent VA surgeon. Besides passion for the task and theoretical knowledge, experience and training in the operation theatre is essential. As soon as you are there, you will understand how different reality looks from simulation on a first-generation plastic model. However, in this situation, the trainee should remember the steps he has learned during the workshop. Before taking your knife, check for the landmarks and mark your incision(s). After careful exposure, check that the vessels are well enough prepared to perform an anastomosis without limitations. Be aware not to twist the outflow vessel and to make the anastomosis in the correct anatomical position. As supervising surgeon, give balanced feedback after the procedure. From time to time, a formal workplace assessment with a structured feedback can be helpful [18, 19]. During the performance, trainees have to make their own decisions, building up self-confidence. In the assessment itself, technical aspects can be evaluated and documented, and learning objectives for the next step can be formulated. Finally, institutions can use these assessments to establish a 'unité de doctrine' based on strict policies and procedure manuals, including checklists and briefings to assure patient safety.

Outlook

The trend in peripheral vascular surgery towards endovascular procedures will bring VA surgery in the focus as first-line procedures for young trainees, who have to learn to perform anastomoses in vessels with 2- to 3-mm diameters. In regard of patient safety, hands-on training is mandatory to give an insight into concepts of VA creation and also into technical skills. Such workshops have still not been well established so far. In fact, simulation in dialysis access procedures is still in its infancy. In order to improve this shortcoming, key players of different organizations and vascular societies must collaborate intensely to support and improve simulation training in this field, preventing harm to the vulnerable ESRD patient.

Disclosure Statement

M.K. Widmer is a convenor and tutor at the Vascular International Foundation and School. I. Davidson and L.W. Widmer have no conflicts of interest. J. Schmidli is an Executive Member of the Vascular International Foundation and School. T.R. Wyss has no conflicts of interest.

References

1 Bradley P: The history of simulation in medical education and possible future directions. Med Educ 2006;40:254–262.
2 Davidson IJ, Lok C, Dolmatch B, Gallieni M, Nolen B, Pittiruti M, Ross J, Slakey D: Virtual reality: emerging role of simulation training in vascular access. Semin Nephrol 2012;32: 572–581.
3 Bismuth J, Donovan MA, O'Malley MK, El Sayed HF, Naoum JJ, Peden EK, Davies MG, Lumsden AB: Incorporating simulation in vascular surgery education. J Vasc Surg 2010; 52:1072–1080.
4 Davies J, Khatib M, Bello F: Open surgical simulation – a review. J Surg Educ 2013;70: 618–627.
5 Gaba DM: The future vision of simulation in healthcare. Simul Healthc 2007;2:126–135.
6 Mitchell EL, Sevdalis N, Arora S, Azarbal AF, Liem TK, Landry GJ, Moneta GL: A fresh cadaver laboratory to conceptualize troublesome anatomic relationships in vascular surgery. J Vasc Surg 2012;55:1187–1194.
7 Palter VN, Grantcharov TP: Simulation in surgical education. CMAJ 2010;182:1191–1196.
8 Duschek N, Assadian A, Lamont PM, Klemm K, Schmidli J, Mendel H, Eckstein HH: Simulator training on pulsatile vascular models significantly improves surgical skills and the quality of carotid patch plasty. J Vasc Surg 2013;57:1148–1154.
9 Wilhelm M, Klemm K, Assadian A, Schmidli J, Schumacher H, Merrelaar J, Eckstein HH: Improve your skills!: evaluation of a 2.5-day basic course in vascular surgery for surgical trainees (in German). Chirurg 2013;84:125–129.
10 Ramani S, Krackov SK: Twelve tips for giving feedback effectively in the clinical environment. Med Teach 2012;34:787–791.
11 van der Leeuw RM, Slootweg IA: Twelve tips for making the best use of feedback. Med Teach 2013;35:348–351.

12 Davidson I, Hwang C, Tesfay S, Dolmatch B, Alfrey E, Bargman J, Gallieni M, Jennings W, Kraines K, Lok C, Nolen B, Saad T, O'Rear S, Ross J, Stiffend-Williams A, Vesely T, Wade M: Simulation of Dialysis Access (SoDA) – Hands-On Dialysis Access Simulation. J Vasc Access 2013;14(suppl 6):S50–S51.
13 Davidson IJ, Yoo MC, Biasucci DG, Browne P, Dees C, Dolmatch B, Gallieni M, La Greca A, Korndorffer JR, Nolen B, O'Rear S, Peden E, Pittiruti M, Reed G, Scott D, Slakey D: Simulation training for vascular access interventions. J Vasc Access 2010;11:181–190.
14 Dolmatch B: The interventional simulator. J Vasc Access 2012;13(suppl 5):S7.
15 Levine AI, Schwartz AD, Bryson EO, Demaria S Jr: Role of simulation in U.S. physician licensure and certification. Mt Sinai J Med 2012;79:140–153.
16 Eckstein HH, Schmidli J, Schumacher H, Gurke L, Klemm K, Duschek N, Meile T, Assadian A: Rationale, scope, and 20-year experience of vascular surgical training with lifelike pulsatile flow models. J Vasc Surg 2013;57:1422–1428.
17 Bylund CL, Brown RF, di Ciccone BL, Levin TT, Gueguen JA, Hill C, Kissane DW: Training faculty to facilitate communication skills training: development and evaluation of a workshop. Patient Educ Couns 2008;70:430–436.
18 Norcini JJ, Blank LL, Arnold GK, Kimball HR: The mini-CEX (clinical evaluation exercise): a preliminary investigation. Ann Intern Med 1995;123:795–799.
19 Wragg A, Wade W, Fuller G, Cowan G, Mills P: Assessing the performance of specialist registrars. Clin Med 2003;3:131–134.

Matthias K. Widmer, MD, MME (unibe)
Department of Cardiovascular Surgery, Bern University Hospital
Freiburgstrasse 10
CH–3010 Bern (Switzerland)
E-Mail matthias.widmer@insel.ch

Widmer MK, Malik J (eds): Patient Safety in Dialysis Access.
Contrib Nephrol. Basel, Karger, 2015, vol 184, pp 97–106
DOI: 10.1159/000365826

Team Training to Establish a Safety Culture in Dialysis Access Surgery

Ingemar Davidson[a] · Matthias K. Widmer[d] · Billy Nolen[b] · John Ross[c] · Douglas P. Slakey[a]

[a]Tulane University, New Orleans, La., [b]Flight Safety, American Airlines, Fort Worth, Tex., and [c]The Regional Medical Center, Orangeburg, S.C., USA; [d]Department of Cardiovascular Surgery, University of Bern, Bern, Switzerland

Abstract

Operating room (OR) team safety training and learning in the field of dialysis access is well suited for the use of simulators, simulated case learning and root cause analysis of adverse outcomes. The objectives of OR team training are to improve communication and leadership skills, to use checklists and to prevent errors. Other objectives are to promote a change in the attitudes towards vascular access from learning through mistakes in a non-punitive environment, to positively impact the employee performance and to increase staff retention by making the workplace safer, more efficient and user friendly.

Recommendations to Improve Patient Safety

- A dialysis access global safety mission is: To do the right thing for your patient at the right time, in the right amount, for the right reason within the framework of your conscience, skills, and knowledge modeled by the culture and society laws in which you live.
- A continuous improvement operating room (OR) safety program must change its culture of error management using punitive measures, blaming the individual. Just culture implies a workplace environment where balancing safety and accountability recognizes the human contribution to failure in complex systems.

- Health care safety has much to learn from commercial aviation, with a current unprecedented safety record facilitated by simulation.
- The use of effective customized checklists and briefing at various stages are key components to OR safety.
- Debriefing after surgery is a uniquely effective safety improvement tool, where the lead surgeon conducts a discussion of problems as well as reinforces excellent team performance.

Introduction

Incidents that may harm patients are related to the health organization but also to contributory factors, care delivery problems and missing defenses and barriers (fig. 1). We learned in the past years a lot from civil aviation how a safety culture can be established. In medical education, beside a teaching culture we need a feedback culture to change the behavior and make people report 'unexpected outcomes' in their field, and to end up with a safety culture.

In dialysis access surgery, diagnostic and therapeutic procedures have become increasingly challenging owing to continuously developing innovative techniques and the aging population with concurrently increasingly comorbidity. Behavioral cultural change and error reduction are keystones for a safety program. The outcomes of safety programs will ensure that the participants have a greater awareness and understanding of how human factors (HFs) and performance limitations can lead to unsafe practice. Training of the team identifies clues that reveal an incipient error chain and select and apply appropriate intervention strategies. For maximum effectiveness, complete organizational involvement is required. A key challenge for leaders is to communicate the need to the rest of the organization and to establish a strong commitment from top management down.

Lessons from the Flight Deck

The HF training, also known as crew resource management, is mandatory for all commercial airlines by the International Civil Aviation Organization, the regulatory body of the United Nations. As with high-liability industrial settings, many medical institutions now are also adopting safety practices and training concepts proven successful in aviation, particularly in the operating room (OR), emergency rooms and ICU settings [2–5]. HF training helps workers avoid operational errors that have led to accidents, and identifies existing

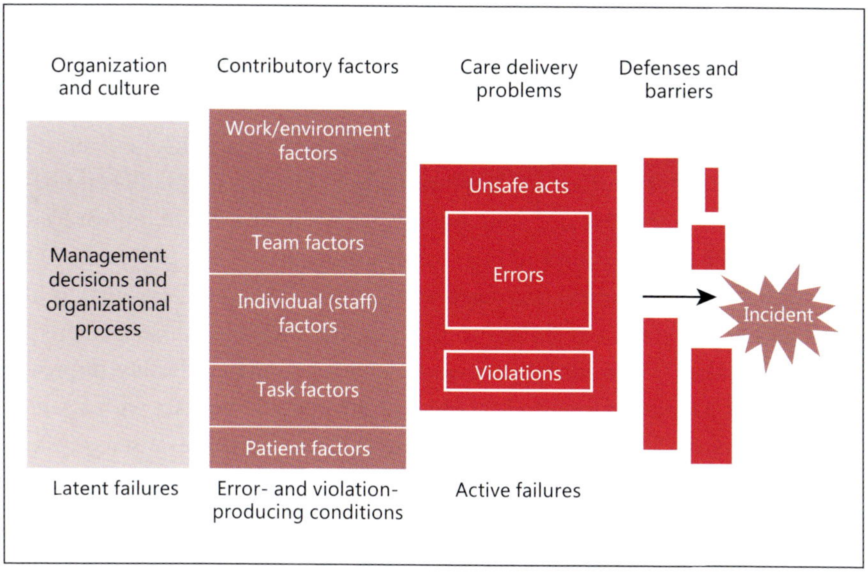

Fig. 1. Organizational accident model modified from Reason [1].

and potential safety threats. Furthermore, it facilitates development, communication, and implementation of plans and actions to avoid and mitigate errors. Secondary benefits are improved morale and enhanced efficiency of operations. OR safety is an interdependent process carried out by teams of individuals with advanced skills training in different roles and decision making responsibilities.

The Dialysis Access Team Training Concept

Three basic components constitute dialysis access OR safety team training. First, team members must have knowledge from formal medical school and continuous postgraduate training. Second, workplace safety comes from skills, training on the job, experience from practice, and more recently by incorporating simulation as part of skills training [6]. There is no substitute for knowledge and skills to achieve safety. In fact, many medical institutions use more training and more knowledge as a means of dealing with 'mistakes' and 'near misses' in a blame and shame culture that still commonly prevails in health care, mainly targeting the individual [2, 3]. The third component deals with the HF role contributing to safety. It entails many things related to human nature, behavior and drive [7–9]. James Reason has written extensively in this field [1, 2]. Cultural shifts in medicine are necessary if the HF approach is to be effective as medical professional training and education have traditionally focused on developing technical proficiency rather than facilitating human interaction. Sidney Dekker bridges the success of the aviation safety records into the medical field in his book entitled *Just Culture* [3]. Over the last 40–50 years, there has been a shift in the emphasis of root causes of accidents and consequently what can be done to improve safety. While in the past aviation and high liability industries in the 1960s and 1970s concentrated on mechanical (hardware) failure (often for good reasons), in the 1980s and 1990s emphasis shifted to blaming the individual for accidents by making mistakes. More recently, accident investigations and safety improvement experts have been focusing on HF and how people interact with systems and cultural issues [2]. The health care industry is also starting to discuss system problem. However, it continues to lag behind aviation and has much to learn from previous experience.

Safety training improves overall patient care, yet OR teams do not routinely engage in simulation training [10]. Dialysis access simulators range from simple suturing learning devices, inexpensive pressurized tunneled graft conduits systems for central vein catheter insertion and cannulation of the access, to computer-designed simulators to teach interventional procedures and simulated case learning. Simulation introduces new techniques in dialysis access through a variety of hands-on experiences. Each training module utilizes simulation technology, delivering examples of how simulation training can advance the field of dialysis access management [11].

The Error Chain and Root Cause Analysis

OR crisis events are often the results of unforeseen internal or external problems, and can frequently be attributed to human cognitive error or complex system safety cultures. There is seldom a single cause leading to an accident. The 'error chain' is a concept to describe human error accidents as the result of a sequence of events that, uninterrupted may culminate in serious injury and death. The links of these error chains are identifiable by means of up to ten 'clues' (table 1). Recognizing and breaking one link in the error chain will likely prevent the potential adverse event.

Root cause analysis (RCA) of adverse surgical outcomes is used in high-liability industries, but still not widely applied to analyze and resolve and improve adverse medical outcomes. Conventional RCA works linearly and backwards to identify root causes with limitations by the traditionally deterministic thinking, creating bias. In contrast, simulation RCA places the investigation in the context

Table 1. Examples of OR surgical 'error chains' as applied to dialysis access surgery

1	Ambiguity: two or more independent information sources disagree on when the patient was last dialyzed.
2	Fixation or preoccupation: the anesthesia crew is trying to address a faulted ECG cable, while missing a severe hypoxic episode.
3	Empty feeling: unsure of the condition. 'A diabetic patient doesn't look right'. Patient is pale and incoherent.
4	Violating lower and upper limits: intentionally ignoring upper and lower norms, i.e. blood pressure measurements, blood glucose levels, or a significant blood loss.
5	Undocumented procedures: 'Cutting corners', i.e. using tools and instruments for which they are not intended or fitted.
6	No one is in charge of the patient: Loss of clear command. 'I thought you were doing this'. (For example DVT prophylaxis was not implemented.)
7	Nobody is looking at the patient: 'Socializing' in the OR and not paying attention to the patient, missing a sudden change in vital signs.
8	Failure to meet targets: no palpable thrill after dialysis access completion.
9	Unresolved discrepancies: preoperative electrocardiogram shows new T-wave abnormality, but no potassium level available.
10	Not adhere to standard procedures: preoperative 'time out' or team briefing is bypassed.

in real time with simulation team members. Therefore, simulation RCA may facilitate the implementation of preventive measures to decrease risk and improve patient safety. Communication errors and medical decision paradigms are most appropriate for simulation presentations [12].

Communication is the mainstay of safety. Effective communication must be clear, crisp, concise and timely. There must be feedback or a response. Without feedback, there is no communication and safety is jeopardized. A briefing is a scripted conversation facilitated by a team leader to establish a shared understanding of the operation ahead. The 500 most commonly used English words have 14,000 dictionary meanings. They mean different things to different people. Poor communication among clinicians is a leading source of adverse events in health care. A safety program will have a set of verbalism or phraseology that is unequivocal for minimizing misunderstanding. Instructions, written policy and procedures and checklists must reflect this clarity. This becomes crucially important as much communication between OR team members occurs under stress [13].

The Dialysis Access OR Team

Team building capitalizes on trust and cooperation [14]. Synergy recognizes that it is not possible to separate individual performance from that of others. This is best described by the term interdependent mindset where each team member feels part of a larger purpose. In contrast, the independent person is not a team player, thinking: 'I don't need you – I know it all and can do everything myself'. HF teaches how to manage conflict, evaluate performance and provide feedback and support to meet commitment to the team and the organization. Team performance is best evaluated with a model of excellence against which to measure performance. Team building will occur more easily when all team members train jointly on tasks of mutual importance. This allows each member to provide their technical knowledge and skills in helping to solve the problem, complete the project, and develop new programs.

Each team member should understand all aspects of the task at hand even if they will not be performing those steps directly. This is not to take away from the team member who normally performs this task, but it is a safety check to ensure that the correct steps are being followed in every procedure, every time. In the OR, the surgeon, the anesthesiologist, the circulator nurse, and scrub technician all must understand the steps in a particular procedure. The surgeon, for example, should be able to start the electrocautery devices and know instrumentation including the details of suture material and where to find it.

Practical Implications

Briefings are fundamental to OR patient safety. A briefing is a scripted conversation facilitated by a team leader to establish a shared understanding of the operation ahead. There are three dialysis access OR-related basic briefings. First, a briefing meeting takes place with all team members in the OR prior to a procedure often also called 'time out' (patient-centered briefing). Second, de-briefing must take place after the procedure to share with the team what went well and what can be improved upon (patient-centered briefing). The purpose is to communicate a shared understanding and to voice concerns regarding all relevant procedure-related and/or patient care issues (table 2). The goal is to maximize learning from a recent experience. Third, an administrative briefing is a staff meeting to communicate all relevant issues and new policies in the management of patient care in the OR (system-centered briefing).

Table 2. Effective leadership in the OR: an example of a 'time out' or a briefing checklist conversation between the OR team led by the surgeon and the anesthesiologist before the start of the dialysis access procedure

1	Introduce your OR team by name and explain the role of each one, for example: I am Dr. Steve Miller, I will be the operating surgeon and Dr. Mary Powel, will assist me. She is a 3-year trainee. Our anesthesiologist is Dr. Stein. Our OR nurses are Mary and Judy both well known to all of us.
2	State the correct procedure: We are going to place a left forearm loop graft. Mary and I went through the instruments following the checklist and everything is correct. The correct PTFE graft is in the room.
3	Confirm the correct extremity side is marked. Dr. Miller: Again, we are operating on the left arm.
4	Consent forms are signed? Consent is correctly signed both for placement of a left forearm graft and anesthesia. Dr. Miller: Yes, that is correct.
5	Beta-blocking agent to be given? Dr. Miller: No, we will not give beta-blocking agent because the patient has some bradycardia.
6	Allergies. Dr. Miller: There are no allergies.
7	Antibiotics given? Dr. Miller: I just gave 2 g of cephalosporin.
8	Is the patient positioned correctly? Dr. Miller: Yes, I checked the position myself before scrubbing.
9	Expect to give blood products? Dr. Miller: The hematocrit is 38%. We do not expect any bleeding, and no blood or plasma should be given.
10	Expected blood loss? Dr. Miller: Blood loss should be 20 ml or less.
11	DVT prophylaxis? Nurse Judy: Yes, TED hoses have been placed.
12	Is the patient being actively warmed? Dr. Miller: Yes, by warm air to upper body.
13	Fire risk. Dr. Miller: There is no fire hazard. Besides we are using bipolar electrocautery today, as always.

Safety Issues in the OR

Successfully implemented safety programs must have a well-designed follow-up plan. Research shows a significant skills decay, suggesting the need for interval refreshment simulation training [15, 16]. The successful leader will ensure the employees are equipped with teamwork and communication skills. Second, project leaders will ensure those teamwork behaviors are hardwired into daily operations by creating and using processes, protocols briefings and checklists. These tools will evolve into the way business is done in the organization. Third, a successful leader will prove that the project has been successful by creating and following a

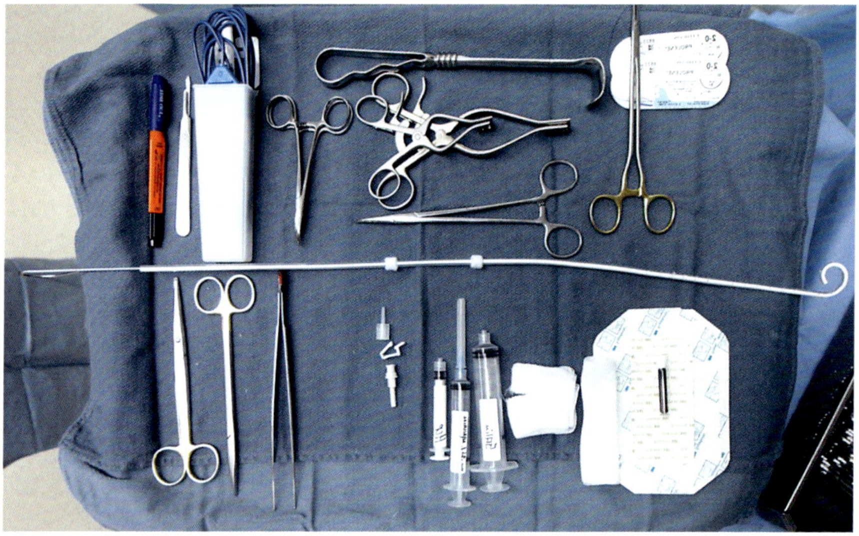

Fig. 2. This image depicts an example of a visual checklist instrument tray (in this case an open peritoneal dialysis placement procedure) for a two-cuff peritoneal dialysis catheter. This is an example of our approach to a consistent, efficient, and safe working environment, where instruments are kept in the same place at all times and in the order of anticipated use. Reproduced with permission from Davidson et al. [17].

measurement plan. However, how we 'bridge the gap' successfully from classroom to the real world environment depends on two vital elements and should be considered as software and hardware, one is useless without the other. The initial safety training provides motivation and skills practice. Follow up (annual) training provides reinforcement [15]. These programs should be mandatory.

A safety culture is key. No matter how advanced the technological system, if humans are involved, errors are inevitable. The key to patient safety and accident prevention is managing the inevitable error by doing two things: First, by training to use specific teamwork and communications behaviors, and second to implement safety tools (policy and procedures, protocols, checklists, briefings) to complement behaviors to detect and trap (small) errors before they become a 'chain' creating a serious or even fatal accident (table 1).

Each dialysis access surgery itself follows steps which is in fact a memorized checklist [17]. This approach enables practitioners to use a standardized approach to checking equipment before use to ensure that the delivery system is correctly adjusted and functional (fig. 2). The checklist procedures are carried out by 2 people (fig. 3). One calls out the individual item on the checklist, and the other is responsible for performing the check and read back. Each has a joint responsibility for the proper execution of this task.

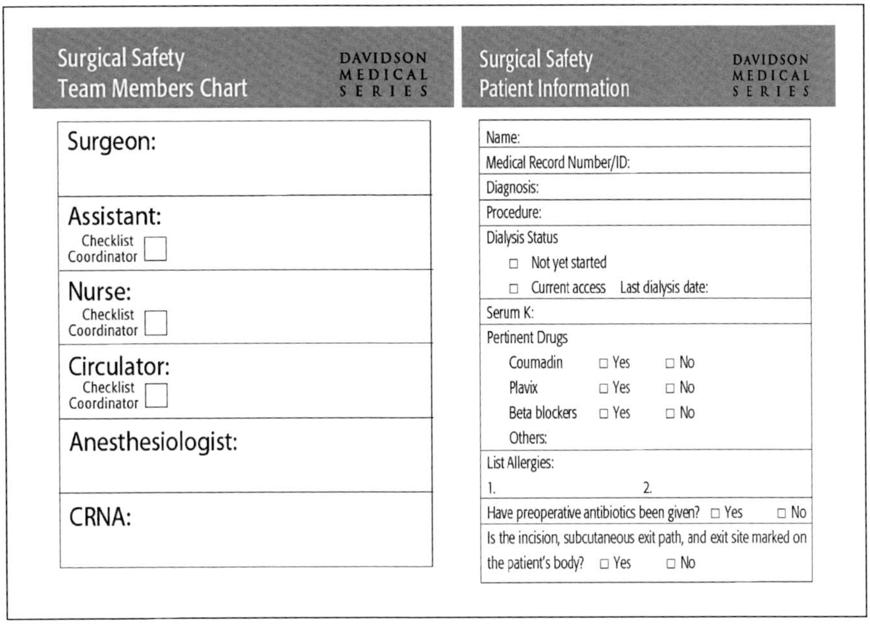

Surgical Safety Team Members Chart — DAVIDSON MEDICAL SERIES

Surgeon:
Assistant: Checklist Coordinator ☐
Nurse: Checklist Coordinator ☐
Circulator: Checklist Coordinator ☐
Anesthesiologist:
CRNA:

Surgical Safety Patient Information — DAVIDSON MEDICAL SERIES

Name:
Medical Record Number/ID:
Diagnosis:
Procedure:
Dialysis Status ☐ Not yet started ☐ Current access Last dialysis date:
Serum K:
Pertinent Drugs Coumadin ☐ Yes ☐ No Plavix ☐ Yes ☐ No Beta blockers ☐ Yes ☐ No Others:
List Allergies: 1. 2.
Have preoperative antibiotics been given? ☐ Yes ☐ No
Is the incision, subcutaneous exit path, and exit site marked on the patient's body? ☐ Yes ☐ No

Fig. 3. Example of surgical safety. Team members chart with patient information charts are best mounted on the wall for easy access. Reproduced with permission from Davidson et al. [17]. CRNA = Certified registered nurses in anesthesiology.

In general, checklists systematically organize your work to obtain a condition of efficiency, to identify team members' roles and accountability. As a consequence of checklists, error rates will decrease and patient safety will be maximally ensured. In the broadest sense, checklists are used to describe the entire surgical procedure [18] or more specifically, critical segments of the OR procedures. In an international multicenter study of 3,733 controls and 3,855 patients subjected to a simple checklist in 8 hospitals, mortality dropped from 1.5 to 0.8% ($p = 0.003$) and in-hospital complication rate fell from 11 to 7% ($p = 0.001$) [19].

Debriefing after a surgical procedure offers an effective safety improvement tool, where the lead surgeon conducts a discussion of case-specific issues and ways to improve. This includes confirming the procedure performed, correct counts, equipment issues, urinary catheter, immediate plans for recovery, continued antibiotics, beta-blockers to mention a few. Each procedure should have an approved debriefing checklist ideally visible to everybody on the wall. He or she also should take the opportunity to reinforce excellent individual and team performance improvements. In contrast to the morbidity and mortality conference format, the debriefing discussion is immediate and palpable and therefore a more effective OR team safety learning tool.

Disclosure Statement

The authors have no conflicts of interest to declare.

References

1 Reason J: Managing the Risks of Organizational Accidents. Aldershot, Ashgate, 1997.
2 Reason J: The Human Contribution. Unsafe Acts, Accidents and Heroic Recoveries. Farnham, Ashgate, 2008.
3 Dekker S: Just Culture, Balancing Safety and Accountability. Aldershot, Ashgate, 2007.
4 WHO: Better knowledge from safer care. Human factors in patient safety. Review of topics and tools. Report for Methods and Measures Working Group of WHO Patient Safety. Geneva, WHO, 2009.
5 Leape LL: Error in medicine. JAMA 1994; 272:1851–1857.
6 Davidson I, Hwang C, Tesfay S, et al: Simulation of Dialysis Access (SoDA) – Hands on dialysis access simulation. J Vasc Access 2013;6:S50–S51.
7 Pink DH: Drive: The Surprising Truth about What Motivates Us. New York, Riverhead Books, 2009.
8 Goleman D, Boyatzis B: Social intelligence and the biology of leadership. Harvard Business Rev, September 2008.
9 Goleman D: Social Intelligence: The New Science of Human Relationships. London, Bantam Books, 2006.
10 Reznick RK, MacRae H: Teaching surgical skills. Changes in the wind. N Engl J Med 2006;355:2664–2669.
11 Davidson I, Lok C, Dolmatch B, et al: Virtual reality: emerging role of simulation training in vascular access. Semin Nephrol 2012;32: 572–581.
12 Slakey DP, Simms ER, Rennie KW, et al: Using simulation to improve root cause analysis of adverse surgical outcomes. Int J Qual Health Care 2014;26:144–150.
13 Patterson K, Grenny J, McMillan R, Swizler A: Crucial Conversations. Tools for Talking when Stakes are High. New York, McGraw Hill, 2002.
14 Covey S: The Seven Habits of Highly Effective People. New York, Free Press, 1989.
15 Ahya SN, Barsuk JH, Cohen JR, et al: Clinical performance and skill retention after simulation-based education for nephrology fellows. Semin Dial 2012;25:470–473.
16 Catchpole K: Toward the modelling of safety violations in healthcare systems. http://qualitysafety.bmj.com/.
17 Davidson I, Paramesh A, Peden E, et al: Open surgical placement of a two cuff, coiled catheter; in Davidson I, Gallieni M, Saxena R (eds): Peritoneal Dialysis. Surgical Technique and Medical Management. Dallas, Divadi LLC, 2012, pp 13–57.
18 Davidson I, Hwang C, Paramesh A, et al: Laparoscopic placement of a two cuff, coiled catheter; in Davidson I, Gallieni M, Saxena R (eds): Peritoneal Dialysis. Surgical Technique and Medical Management. Dallas, Divadi LLC, 2012, pp 69–90.
19 Haynes AB, Weiser TG, Berry WR, et al: A surgical safety checklist to reduce morbidity and mortality in a global population. N Engl J Med 2009;369:491–499.

Ingemar Davidson, MD, PhD
Tulane University Medical School
1430 Tulane Avenue, SL22
New Orleans, LA 70112 (USA)
E-Mail drd@ingemardavidson.com

Widmer MK, Malik J (eds): Patient Safety in Dialysis Access.
Contrib Nephrol. Basel, Karger, 2015, vol 184, pp 107–122
DOI: 10.1159/000367905

How to Perform Safe Anesthesia in Patients with End-Stage Renal Disease

Christian Seidl · Balthasar Eberle

University Department for Anesthesiology and Pain Therapy, Inselspital, Bern University Hospital, Bern, Switzerland

Abstract

Vascular surgical patients and especially those with end-stage renal disease are exposed to a high risk of preventable adverse events. Typically, a combination of organizational and technical deficiencies, human error or ineptitude and patient comorbidity leads to inadvertently poor outcome. Patient safety in perioperative environments requires permanent effort in organizational improvement, staff training, and maintenance of high standards in patient care and technical equipment. Even in multimorbid patients, anesthesia for vascular access surgery can be performed at low to moderate risk if safety problems are minimized.

Recommendations to Improve Patient Safety

- Preoperative preparation for anesthesia should identify individual risks and areas for optimization. An interdisciplinary perioperative plan should be developed and communicated to the entire team.
- Institutionalized surgical safety checks and OR safety precautions help to reduce and manage unexpected adverse events.
- Locoregional anesthesia offers, as an advantage, transient regional sympathectomy and blood flow enhancement without cardiopulmonary depression. General anesthesia avoids interaction with anticoagulant regimes and allows, if required, extension of surgery. Local anesthesia may require supportive sedation and monitoring.

- The use of 2-D ultrasound imaging and guidance is state of the art for vessel cannulation and nerve blocks.
- Proficiency and teamwork of the providers appear more important than anesthesia technique itself, but typical risks and complications need to be anticipated.

Preoperative Evaluation and Planning

Patients requiring vascular access surgery are frequently multimorbid, and surgery is often nonelective. Efficient preoperative planning requires communication of accurate data, dates and details of schedules and procedures. This includes planned location and type of vascular access, patient preparation and positioning, use of grafts or distal perfusion, etc.

Practice guidelines and standard operating procedures of each service should be available. Documentation of individual perioperative surgical requirements should precede clinical evaluation by anesthesiology.

Responsibilities for management of chronic and preoperative medication need to be clearly defined and communicated between all involved caregivers. Timely prescription (e.g. treatment of preoperative anemia), reliable continuation (e.g. beta-blockers, aspirin, statins) [2], timely discontinuation (e.g. metformin, platelet inhibitors, new oral anticoagulants), and effective bridging (insulin, unfractionated heparin) of preoperative medications increase patient safety by reducing risks of myocardial ischemia, bleeding and transfusion, and help to avoid case cancellations.

Preanesthetic evaluation assesses the patient's physical status (American Society of Anesthesiologists ASA PS; table 1) [3] according to relevant active comorbidity, medical, surgical and anesthetic history. Results of diagnostic testing are reviewed, and a focused physical exam is obtained [4]. Factors with relevant impact on perioperative management are identified.

The overall aim is to predict a patient's tolerance to the perioperative stress of his/her specific surgical procedure. Whereas peripheral reconstructive vascular surgery carries a particularly high risk of perioperative cardiac morbidity and mortality, peripheral vascular access surgery is classified as low or moderate risk surgery.

Impaired kidney function is a robust indicator of increased perioperative risk. Patients with end-stage renal disease (ESRD) requiring vascular access surgery are thus usually ASA class 3 or 4, related to their overall health status. ASA classification does not take surgical risk into consideration; this needs to be categorized separately using appropriate scoring systems [5].

Table 1. Anesthesiologic risk classification for the determination of perioperative risk and quick estimation of physical fitness using MET values [6]

ASA physical status classification	
ASA 1	Normal healthy patient
ASA 2	Patient with mild systemic disease
ASA 3	Patient with severe systemic disease
ASA 4	Severe systemic disease that is a constant threat to life
ASA 5	Moribund patient who is not expected to survive without the operation
ASA 6	Declared brain-dead patient (organ donor)
Essential MET values	
1–3 MET	Walking around in the flat, taking care of oneself (eating, getting dressed, cleaning)
4–6 MET	Climbing more than one flight of stairs without stopping, walking >100 m on plain ground, easy homework
≥10 MET	Sports activities (tennis, swimming, football, skiing)

Preoperative assessment of coronary status and cardiovascular function is based on clinical evaluation, noninvasive and invasive diagnostic testing. Physical performance is evaluated according to simple exercise tasks (e.g. walking up stairs), and is quantified by grading their metabolic equivalent (MET, table 1). At a performance of 4 MET or more, the patient is usually fit for vascular access surgery in locoregional anesthesia (LRA) without further cardiac evaluation [6].

If MET cannot be evaluated, the presence of clinical risk factors (renal dysfunction, ischemic heart disease, congestive heart failure, stroke or TIA, diabetes mellitus requiring insulin) is relevant. If up to 2 risk factors are present, noninvasive testing may be considered, but only if it will change management. If 3 or more risk factors are present, cardiology consultation and further cardiac testing are considered.

In patients with a cardiac implantable electrical device (CIED), such as an internal cardiac pacemaker or defibrillator (ICD), some basic information needs to be gathered preoperatively (e.g. indication, current mode of action, underlying cardiac rhythm, type and model of device, accessibility by cardiologist, response to magnetic influence, last function control).

Clinical assessment of pulmonary status is based on history, auscultation and noninvasive pulse oximetry/arterial blood gas analysis on room air. Chest radiography and spirometry are indicated only in patients with known or suspected significant pulmonary disease. Chronic pleural effusion may require preoperative drainage to support respiratory compensation of renal acidosis, the more so if sedation is planned. Current medication regimens should be optimized.

In preexisting severe or acutely exacerbated lung disease, expert pulmonology consultation should be obtained. Radiological imaging, body plethysmography and CO diffusion capacity are indicated only if results would substantially influence perioperative management.

Patients with moderate to severe pulmonary disease requiring vascular access surgery will benefit most from a LRA technique. General anesthesia (GA) with intermittent positive pressure ventilation (IPPV) and use of muscle relaxants impairs respiration more than LRA with maintained spontaneous breathing. IPPV may cause dynamic overinflation or barotrauma to lungs, promote atelectasis and impair mucociliary clearance [7]. This may be associated with increased pulmonary morbidity, prolonged hospital stay, resource utilization and cost.

Questions of specific anesthetic interest in a patient's history should address allergies [e.g. to local anesthetics (LA), antibiotics, disinfectants, radiocontrast, protamine]. Previous experiences with general and LRA, the risk of postoperative nausea and vomiting, chronic steroid medication and relevant substance abuse should be explored. Substitution therapy may be necessary.

Proactive patient blood management implies pre-, intra- and postoperative issues. Timely preoperative conventional or noninvasive hemoglobin testing should be routine in order to allow anemia workup and treatment. Anemia associated with ESRD should be treated appropriately in advance of elective surgery. If indicated, hematopoietic stimulation with recombinant erythropoietin and concomitant iron substitution should be instituted to avoid or minimize perioperative allogeneic transfusion as well as related immunomodulation, infection and cost. This is particularly important in patients awaiting renal transplantation. Nevertheless, type and screen should be available in any patient undergoing vascular access surgery.

Screening for coagulation disorders or impairment, as well as for active anticoagulant and/or antiplatelet medication relies first on history and physical exam. Preoperatively, pertinent conditions and medications must be meticulously reviewed. Focused laboratory testing should follow only if indicated (INR, aPTT, fibrinogen level, platelet count; platelet function testing; thromboelastometry).

Adequate orders for discontinuation, bridging or timing of anticoagulants must be written to avoid interference with the planned surgery and LRA, but also in order to avoid thromboembolic complications [8]. In patients with recently stented coronaries, mechanical valves or chronic atrial fibrillation, a cardiology consult should be obtained.

The most common substances that are suitable in patients with renal insufficiency are listed in table 2, together with pertinent lab tests and recommended

Table 2. Widely used anticoagulants and their safe perioperative management [8]

Mode of action	Antagonist	Lab test	Substance	Stop prior to			Bridging	Pause after operation
				operation	single-shot regional block	GA		
COX 1 inhibition	no specific	platelet function test	**ASS**	continue – stop may be harmful	continue – stop may be harmful	no	no	no
ADP receptor blocker	no specific	platelet function test	**clopidogrel** **prasugrel** **ticagrelor**	7 days 7–10 days 5 days	7 days 7–10 days 5 days	no	no	no
Xa antagonist	no specific	F Xa activity	**apixaban** **rivaroxaban**	2 days 1–2 days	2 days 1–2 days	no	heparin	no
Vitamin K antagonist	vitamin K	INR	**coumadin**	stop assure INR <1.4	stop assure INR <1.4	no	heparin	continue or bridging
AT III activator	protamin	aPTT/Xa activity	**heparin**	4–6 h	4–6 h	no	no	at least 1 h
Prostaglandin inhibition	no specific	platelet aggregation test	**iloprost** **prostacyclin**	2 h 0.5 h	2 h 0.5 h	no	no	no

ASS = Acetylsalicylic acid.

discontinuation intervals. The field of anticoagulant and antiplatelet medication is evolving rapidly. Practitioners may benefit from guideline-based smartphone applications (e.g. CoaguSafe® for iPhone®) to support clinical judgment when balancing risks of bleeding and thrombosis.

Preoperative serum electrolyte status should be known in patients with ESRD. Hemodialysis is indicated prior to surgery, if relevant hyperkalemia (6.0 mEq/l or more) is present, to protect the patient from life-threatening arrhythmia. Severely abnormal serum sodium or chloride needs further workup and slow correction. In emergencies, electrolyte correction is initiated without delaying life-saving surgery.

In insulin-dependent diabetics, presurgical fasting and possible delays in the OR schedule may complicate blood glucose management, and will require close blood glucose and insulin control. Perioperative glucose control is recommended in the range of 100–180 mg/dl or 5.6–10.0 mmol/l to decrease complications (e.g. wound infections) without running risks of hypoglycemia and stroke.

Patient and nursing team information about smoking, food and drink restrictions as well as preoperative medication is mandatory. Smoking should be stopped at least 24 h prior to the operation to enhance tracheal clearance. Fasting is recommended for a minimum of 6 h prior to anesthesia for food and 2 h for clear liquids [9].

Pharmacological premedication is usually prescribed for patients with planned overnight hospital stay. Low-dose benzodiazepines provide anxiolysis, light sedation and anterograde amnesia. Especially at advanced age, benzodiazepines may elicit paradoxical reactions or predispose to postoperative delirium. Alternatives for oral premedication are clonidin or haloperidol. Ambulatory patients usually do not receive preoperative sedatives.

Preoperative Safety Precautions

Good interdisciplinary communication between surgeon and anesthesiologist minimizes delays and cancellations in the schedule and helps to prevent or anticipate critical situations. Charts and records should be made accessible to all perioperative caregivers. Ideally, they should review scheduled patients together in advance.

Anesthesia must be clearly informed of surgical positioning, access or cannulation sites in order to plan their monitoring and instrumentation. If necessary, postoperative hemodialysis, intermediate or intensive care should be organized at this time.

At this point, the decision about the planned anesthesia technique (e.g. GA, regional block, local anesthesia with or without sedation) and monitoring must be made by the anesthesiologist in accordance with surgical requirements and with the patient's informed consent.

Throughout the preoperative and preincision periods, a Surgical Safety Checklist should be completed according to the standardized, structured three-tiered 'Team Time Out' process recommended by the World Health Organization [10]. All steps are documented in the patient's record.

Part 1: Prior to transfer to the OR, the patient is personally identified and the surgeon marks the site of surgery. A hospital-wide implemented patient identification bracelet with patient name, date of birth and identification number ensures correct patient verification.

Part 2: Prior to anesthesia induction, the patient is identified again by name and birth date, which are compared with ID bracelet and records. The scheduled surgical procedure is confirmed by the patient, and the surgical site marking by the OR staff. A brief review of patient's written informed consent, allergies, fasting interval, airway anatomy, ordered antibiotic prophylaxis, availability of blood products and readiness of anesthesia equipment is completed. Specifically in these patients, preoperative information is verified on correct medication intake, on fluid restriction orders, the interval since last hemodialysis and residual urinary output.

Part 3: Immediately prior to incision, the entire OR team performs a team time-out. Team members briefly introduce themselves and their role. The surgeon explains the procedure; the anesthetist mentions any special concerns. The team rehearses conceivable critical situations and their prospective management. Antibiotic administration and the availability of special surgical and anesthesia equipment are confirmed.

Special attention in such patients focuses on the presence and function of preexisting arteriovenous fistulae, hemodialysis central venous catheters, or access for peritoneal dialysis. Arms with vascular accesses are kept free from blood pressure cuffs, pulse oximeters, tourniquets and peripheral venous cannulae.

Gastric emptying is delayed in chronic renal failure [11] or diabetes, which presumptively increases the risk of regurgitation and pulmonary aspiration of gastric contents on induction of GA or during deep sedation. pH of gastric secretions can be raised by oral administration of sodium tricitrate (30 ml, 0.3 mol/l) within 1 h of induction. Also, peritoneal dialysate liquid should be drained from the peritoneal cavity prior to OR transfer and induction of anesthesia. If GA is planned, precautions for rapid airway control on induction should be taken.

If perioperative antibiotic prophylaxis is indicated, responsibility for drug choice, timing and administration must be clear to all. Typical antibiotics for perioperative prophylaxis in vascular surgery target bacterial colonization at the surgical site, such as cephalosporin (e.g. cefazoline, cefuroxime). To achieve adequate tissue concentration, a time interval between i.v. administration and skin incision of 30–60 min is mandatory. The dose of a single shot antibiotic prophylaxis is not adapted to renal clearance, but repetition doses may require adaptation.

Life-threatening allergic responses to medication are rare, with antibiotics, relaxants, latex and colloid infusions as the main culprits. Preoperative team awareness of known allergies can avoid most major incidents. Minor reactions such as skin rash, pruritus or wheals may remain the only manifestation (class I), requiring symptomatic treatment only. As first or co-manifestation, life-threatening symptoms like oropharyngeal swelling, bronchospasm, hypotension, or shock may ensue (class II–IV). Such symptoms are a clear indication for adrenalin (100 μg i.v. bolus), with repetition as needed until the situation improves. In patients without anticoagulation, 0.3–0.5 mg of adrenalin can be given intramuscularly to provide a continued effect [12]. Exposure to all suspected agents is stopped immediately, 100% oxygen is given, and additional help (resuscitation team) is called for.

LA intoxication from inadvertent intravascular injection or rapid systemic absorption of a large LA dose manifests itself by acute changes in CNS function (dysesthesia, drowsiness, tremor, generalized convulsions). This may be followed by myocardial depression and bradyasystole or ventricular fibrillation. Such incidents require immediate institution of Basic and Advanced Life Support, and an attempt to attenuate toxic LA action by a trial of Lipid Rescue Therapy (Intralipid® 20% 1.5 ml/kg i.v., repeatable to a maximum of 8 ml/kg) [13]. Ropivacaine appears less cardiotoxic than bupivacaine and may thus be preferable in patients with cardiovascular comorbidity. Prilocaine can cause significant methemoglobinemia, making it a poor choice in an anemia-prone population.

An increasing number of patients present for vascular access surgery carrying a CIED (e.g. internal pacemaker, defibrillator ICD, or cardiac resynchronization therapy) [14]. In these patients, the surgeon needs to brief the team ahead of time about the use of electrocautery. If monopolar cautery is needed, the pathway of the cautery current should be directed far away from the CIED, and the device should be reprogrammed or deactivated temporarily. Depending on the device and indication, the pacemaker function may be adjusted to a reasonable rate and mode of action [15].

Line placement for monitoring and medication in peripheral or central venous or arterial locations is often challenging. Numerous previous surgeries, preexisting fistulae, failed cannulation attempts, hematoma, venous collapse after hemodialysis, thrombotic vessel occlusion or the presence of CIEDs in central veins reduce options and prolong preparation time.

Frequently, central line or venous dialysis catheter placement under residual anticoagulation cannot be avoided. Ultrasound guidance of vessel puncture and cannulation facilitates line placement and reduces complication rate (futile punctures, hematoma, accidental arterial puncture and injection, nerve damage). Use of ultrasound imaging to guide central venous catheter insertion has been recommended as a measure to improve patient safety by national health care guideline organizations (www.ahrq.gov 2001; www.nice.org.uk 2002). Central venous catheterization (CVC) requires full barrier precautions (mask, cap, scrubbing, sterile gown and gloves, sterile equipment handling) to reduce risk of CVC-related bloodstream infection.

Ultrasound guidance for nerve blocks has revolutionized LRA, and has become state of the art (www.nice.org.uk 2009). Precise identification of nerve structures minimizes risk of inadvertent vessel injury, intravascular injection and complicating hematoma. It improves block success, allows reducing LA dose and dose-related toxic effects [16, 17]. Table 3 gives an overview of maximum recommended dose of LA.

As a consequence, use of ultrasound guidance for anesthesia preparations is strongly recommended as an important safety feature in vascular access surgery.

Table 3. Maximum dose of LA for regional nerve blocks in adults

	Type	Main metabolism	Onset of anesthesia (depending on injection site), min	Duration of action, h	Maximum dosage
Lidocaine	amide	liver	15–30	max. 5	max. 4.5 mg/kg body weight per single injection; cumulative dose 300 mg/day
Bupivacaine	amide	liver > kidney	15–30	4–6	cumulative dose max. 400 mg/day
Mepivacaine	amide	liver	15–30	1.5–2	max. 5 mg/kg body weight per single injection; cumulative dose max. 1,000 mg/day
Ropivacaine	amide	liver/kidney	10–25	6–10	max. 250 mg/single injection; cumulative dose 800 mg/day

These data are based on Swissmedic information. Recommendations may vary between different countries due to local drug regulations. Rescue strategy: lipid rescue therapy can be used intravenously to absorb circulating LA.

Adequate training of ultrasound anatomy and needle navigation skills and dedicated equipment should be provided for and maintained by institutions and services involved.

Intraoperative Safety Precautions

In vascular access surgery, there is usually a choice between local, locoregional or GA. Although anesthesiological considerations apply, the type of anesthesia must be suitable for the planned surgery, should be accepted by the surgeon and also authorized by the patient with his/her written informed consent. Standard operating procedures should be established based on practice guidelines and scientific evidence.

During any type of anesthesia care, an ECG monitor, pulse oximetry, non-/invasive blood pressure measurement and a reliable peripheral i.v. access are standard. If airway tools are employed, capnography is standard of care to prove correct placement of the artificial airway and the presence of respiration, gas exchange and circulation [18].

GA is suitable for all procedures in vascular access surgery patients. Renal insufficiency affects clinically relevant pharmacokinetics of some hypnotics, analgesics and relaxants.

Intravenous sedatives and nonopioid hypnotics (midazolam, propofol, etomidate, ketamine, dexmedetomidine) undergo mainly hepatic biotransformation to inactive metabolites. Their prolonged excretion owing to renal insufficiency is clinically not relevant. Nevertheless, in patients with renal failure a

25–50% dose reduction appears advisable due to alterations in blood volume, protein binding and pharmacodynamics.

Clinical pharmacology of synthetic opioid analgesics (fentanyl, sufentanil, remifentanil) is not substantially altered by renal failure. In contrast, morphine is a poor choice in patients with severe renal impairment, particularly when given repetitively. Morphine effects may be prolonged due to very slow elimination of active metabolites. Postoperative analgesic regimens should also avoid nonsteroidal anti-inflammatory drugs.

Among volatile anesthetics, isoflurane and desflurane are safe for use in patients with renal impairment and cardiovascular disease. These agents undergo minimal (hepatic) metabolism.

Nondepolarizing muscle relaxants are highly dependent on renal elimination if not inactivated otherwise. Degradation pathways of the relaxants atracurium or cisatracurium bypass renal function, making them preferable in renal insufficiency. Rocuronium has an increased elimination half-life in renal failure, but its action is swiftly and reliably terminated by i.v. administration of sugammadex.

Safe induction of GA for vascular access surgery should take specific risk constellations among these patients into account:

- In chronic renal failure, risks of pulmonary aspiration may be increased due to gastroparesis or abdominal distension from residual peritoneal dialysate.
- There is a significant risk of marked arterial hypotension, particularly on GA induction. Considerate selection and dose reduction of induction anesthetics, and titrated use of vasopressor drugs (ephedrine, noradrenaline or phenylephrine) will mitigate hypotensive episodes and prevent fluid overloading. Volemic effects of crystalloid solutions are limited to a short period of time, and fluid overloading may be associated with worse outcome [19]. Artificial colloid solutions appear obsolete due to their renal elimination. Alpha-adrenoceptor agonists should be used conservatively, with the goal to normalize low systemic vascular resistance only. Unnecessary vasoconstriction may adversely affect outcome of peripheral vascular surgery.

LRA is ever gaining popularity for vascular access surgery due to its sympatholytic and venodilatory effect, overall cardiovascular stability and safety, and a potentially positive impact on surgical outcome [20]. The incidence of vasospasm and early thrombosis may be reduced [21]. The site of the regional block needs to be selected such as to adequately anesthetize the projected vascular access site (table 4). For vascular access surgery on the upper extremity, supraclavicular, infraclavicular or axillary nerve blocks are typically performed.

Despite the advantages of LRA, a survey of National Surgical Quality Improvement data (NSQIP; 2007–2010) still found a distribution of anesthesia

Table 4. Covered areas of possible LRA procedures

Type of regional block	Area of adequate surgical anesthesia				
	shoulder	upper arm	elbow	forearm	hand
Interscalene nerve block	+	+ (proximal)	–	–	–
Supraclavicular nerve block	–	+	+	+	+
Infraclavicular nerve block	–	+	+	+	+
Axillary nerve block	–	+ (distal)	+	+	+

techniques for new arteriovenous fistula creation of 85% GA, 3% local anesthesia with monitored anesthetic care, and only 12% LRA [22].

Compared to GA, an overall better safety profile of LRA has not been proven so far. Anesthesia planning in patients with ESRD and typical cardiovascular comorbidity must pay close attention to the coagulation system. When coagulation is compromised, regional nerve blocks are associated with a higher neurological complication rate than GA [13]. Ultrasound guidance to navigate nerve and vessel structures is highly recommended, with the aims to reduce accidental vessel injury and amount of LA required [18]. Still, this will not completely eliminate block-induced nerve lesions or hematoma formation.

Local anesthesia (LA) is a reasonable alternative if patients are compliant and cooperative, or when all other anesthesia options are either not applicable or increase risk more than LA. The sympathicolytic effect of LRA and its motor block cannot be reproduced using an LA technique. On the other hand, residual anticoagulant effects are less of an issue with LA than with LRA. For patients who are uncooperative or may become so during surgery (e.g. owing to substance dependency, paradoxical reactions, anxiety, delirium), LA is the least preferable option.

Basic monitoring standards apply as mentioned above. Depending on the patient's overall health status, it is advisable to combine surgical LA with monitored anesthesia care (MAC). Intraoperatively, MAC allows the anesthetist to diagnose and treat upcoming clinical problems adequately while the surgeon can concentrate on his work. When LA is managed without a professional dedicated to nonsurgical intraoperative patient care, risks from incomplete or discontinuous monitoring and inadequate sedation are inherent. In this field, most adverse outcomes arise from respiratory or cardiocirculatory depression. Therefore emergency equipment, medication and expertise to support or restore vital functions should be available in the procedure room, with advanced life support expert assistance available within 1–5 min [23].

Intraoperative Environment

During any operation, the ambient noise level should be minimized such to ensure safe communication between OR team members. This reduces distraction from their tasks as well as adverse effects (e.g. infections) [24]. Changes in patient condition or critical intraprocedural requirements (e.g. call for heparin) must be clearly communicated within the team in the closed-loop mode. Anybody who has important information should be allowed to speak up at any time to inform the other team members.

The workplace should be organized ergonomically to facilitate the workflow of the OR team (fig. 1). Equipment should be arranged such as to allow adequate logistics for supplies, give access to the patient without breaking sterility, avoid tripwire incidents and cable disconnections, and to allow everybody a view to monitors. Urgent interventions should be possible without delay. Emergency equipment must be available and accessible at all times.

Perioperative normothermia avoids excessive sympathetic activation, shivering, coagulopathy and patient discomfort. Core temperature should be monitored continuously under GA. All patients should be kept normothermic with warming OR table mattresses or forced air warming systems. Patients with LRA or LA are clinically observed and asked whether they feel comfortable.

Allogenic blood product transfusion should be unnecessary in vascular access surgery with adequate preoperative preparation and surgical technique. Transfusion indications should be restrictive and take patients' preoperative chronic stable baseline into consideration. A valid transfusion trigger should combine hemoglobin concentration with the presence of clinical indicators of critical anemia or risks for critical end-organ ischemia (e.g. coronary or cerebrovascular disease [25–28]).

Postoperative Care

In the postoperative period, any patient emerging from GA or LRA should be observed in a postanesthesia care unit (PACU). Staff must be familiar with typical anesthesia- and surgery-related complications and postoperative surgical treatment. Postanesthetic and surgical orders (e.g. pain management, hemodynamic targets, antibiotics, anticoagulation, fluid regime, drains and dressings, positioning, chronic medication) must be documented in writing and actively communicated to PACU staff. Patency and function of a newly established vascular access as well as distal perfusion and sensorimotor function should be controlled regularly by clinical means and Doppler technique. After a regional nerve

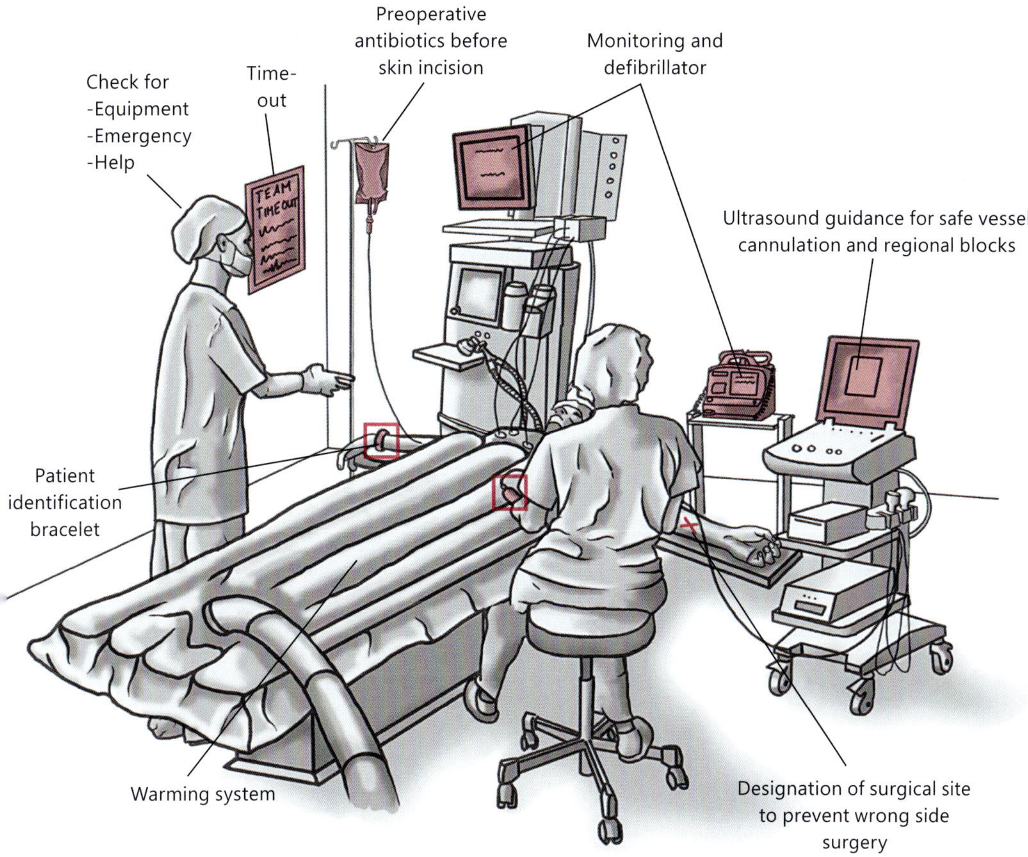

Fig. 1. OR setup and equipment for safe anesthesia performance in vascular access surgery.

block, at least the motor block should be regredient prior to discharge from PACU. Following GA, patients are released from the recovery area when awake and oriented, with vital functions stable, and with pain and postoperative nausea and vomiting under control.

Critical incident-reporting systems play an important role in identifying errors that are related to structural problems. Institutions can improve patient safety in vascular access surgery, as in any perioperative field, by improving OR and equipment ergonomics, by collective open-minded learning from each critical incident [29], by supporting training of technical and nontechnical skills (fig. 2) and critical incident management, and by promoting close interdisciplinary communication and good teamwork behavior [30].

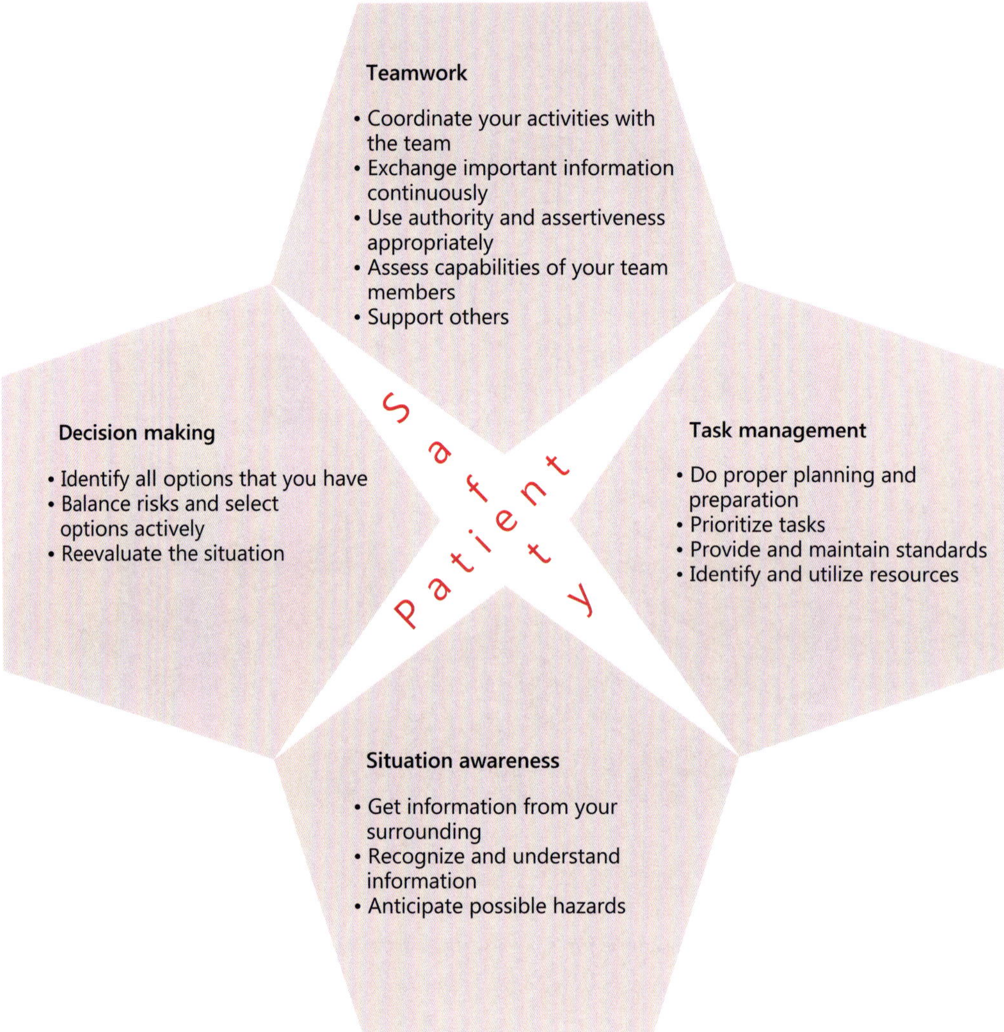

Fig. 2. Nontechnical skills that impact patient safety during the perioperative process [1].

Disclosure Statement

The authors have no conflicts of interest to declare.

References

1 Rall M, Gaba DM: Human performance and patient safety; in Miller R (ed): Miller's Anesthesia, ed 7. Philadelphia, Churchhill Livingstone, 2009, pp 93–150.
2 Kristensen SD, Knuuti J, Saraste A, Anker S, Botker HE, De Hert S, et al: 2014 ESC/ESA Guidelines on non-cardiac surgery: cardiovascular assessment and management: The Joint Task Force on non-cardiac surgery: cardiovascular assessment and management of the European Society of Cardiology (ESC) and the European Society of Anaesthesiology (ESA). Eur Heart J 2014;35:2383–2431.
3 American Society of Anesthesiologists: ASA Physical Status Classification System. https://www.asahq.org.
4 De Hert S, Imberger G, Carlisle J, Diemunsch P, Fritsch G, Moppett I, et al: Preoperative evaluation of the adult patient undergoing non-cardiac surgery: guidelines from the European Society of Anaesthesiology. Eur J Anaesthesiol 2011;28:684–722.
5 Glance LG, Lustik SJ, Hannan EL, Osler TM, Mukamel DB, Qian F, et al: The Surgical Mortality Probability Model: derivation and validation of a simple risk prediction rule for noncardiac surgery. Ann Surg 2012;255:696–702.
6 Poldermans D, Bax JJ, Boersma E, De Hert S, Eeckhout E, Fowkes G, et al: Guidelines for pre-operative cardiac risk assessment and perioperative cardiac management in non-cardiac surgery. Eur Heart J 2009;30:2769–2812.
7 Lumb A, Biercamp C: Chronic obstructive pulmonary disease and anaesthesia. Contin Educ Anaesth Crit Care Pain 2014;14:1–5.
8 Gogarten W, Vandermeulen E, Van Aken H, Kozek S, Llau JV, Samama CM: Regional anaesthesia and antithrombotic agents: recommendations of the European Society of Anaesthesiology. Eur J Anaesthesiol 2010;27: 999–1015.
9 Smith I, Kranke P, Murat I, Smith A, O'Sullivan G, Soreide E, et al: Perioperative fasting in adults and children: guidelines from the European Society of Anaesthesiology. Eur J Anaesthesiol 2011;28:556–569.
10 WHO's patient-safety checklist for surgery. Lancet 2008;372:1.
11 Hubalewska A, Stompor T, Placzkiewicz E, Staszczak A, Huszno B, Sulowicz W, et al: Evaluation of gastric emptying in patients with chronic renal failure on continuous ambulatory peritoneal dialysis using 99mTc-solid meal. Nucl Med Rev Cent East Eur 2004;7: 27–30.
12 Soar J, Perkins GD, Abbas G, Alfonzo A, Barelli A, Bierens JJ, et al: European Resuscitation Council Guidelines for Resuscitation 2010 Section 8. Cardiac arrest in special circumstances: electrolyte abnormalities, poisoning, drowning, accidental hypothermia, hyperthermia, asthma, anaphylaxis, cardiac surgery, trauma, pregnancy, electrocution. Resuscitation 2010;81:1400–1433.
13 Weinberg GL: Lipid emulsion infusion: resuscitation for local anesthetic and other drug overdose. Anesthesiology 2012;117:180–187.
14 Santoro D, Benedetto F, Mondello P, Pipito N, Barilla D, Spinelli F, et al: Vascular access for hemodialysis: current perspectives. Int J Nephrol Renovasc Dis 2014;7:281–294.
15 Crossley GH, Poole JE, Rozner MA, Asirvatham SJ, Cheng A, Chung MK, et al: The Heart Rhythm Society (HRS)/American Society of Anesthesiologists (ASA) Expert Consensus Statement on the perioperative management of patients with implantable defibrillators, pacemakers and arrhythmia monitors: facilities and patient management this document was developed as a joint project with the American Society of Anesthesiologists (ASA), and in collaboration with the American Heart Association (AHA), and the Society of Thoracic Surgeons (STS). Heart Rhythm 2011;8:1114–1154.
16 Eichenberger U, Stockli S, Marhofer P, Huber G, Willimann P, Kettner SC, et al: Minimal local anesthetic volume for peripheral nerve block: a new ultrasound-guided, nerve dimension-based method. Reg Anesth Pain Med 2009;34:242–246.
17 Marhofer P, Eichenberger U, Stockli S, Huber G, Kapral S, Curatolo M, et al: Ultrasonographic guided axillary plexus blocks with low volumes of local anaesthetics: a crossover volunteer study. Anaesthesia 2010;65:266–271.
18 Buhre W, Rossaint R: Perioperative management and monitoring in anaesthesia. Lancet 2003;362:1839–1846.

19 Doherty M, Buggy DJ: Intraoperative fluids: how much is too much? Br J Anaesth 2012; 109:69–79.
20 Malinzak EB, Gan TJ: Regional anesthesia for vascular access surgery. Anesth Analg 2009; 109:976–980.
21 Shemesh D, Raikhinstein Y, Orkin D, Goldin I, Olsha O: Anesthesia for vascular access surgery. J Vasc Access 2014;15(suppl 7):S38–S44.
22 Siracuse JJ, Gill HL, Parrack I, Huang ZS, Schneider DB, Connolly PH, et al: Variability in anesthetic considerations for arteriovenous fistula creation. J Vasc Access 2014, Epub ahead of print.
23 American Society of Anesthesiologists Task Force on Sedation and Analgesia by Non-Anesthesiologists: Practice guidelines for sedation and analgesia by non-anesthesiologists. Anesthesiology 2002;96:1004–1017.
24 Kurmann A, Peter M, Tschan F, Muhlemann K, Candinas D, Beldi G: Adverse effect of noise in the operating theatre on surgical-site infection. Br J Surg 2011;98:1021–1025.
25 Carson JL, Grossman BJ, Kleinman S, Tinmouth AT, Marques MB, Fung MK, et al: Red blood cell transfusion: a clinical practice guideline from the AABB*. Ann Intern Med 2012;157:49–58.
26 Carson JL, Duff A, Poses RM, Berlin JA, Spence RK, Trout R, et al: Effect of anaemia and cardiovascular disease on surgical mortality and morbidity. Lancet 1996;348:1055–1060.
27 Spahn DR, Moch H, Hofmann A, Isbister JP: Patient blood management: the pragmatic solution for the problems with blood transfusions. Anesthesiology 2008;109:951–953.
28 Kozek-Langenecker SA, Afshari A, Albaladejo P, Santullano CA, De Robertis E, Filipescu DC, et al: Management of severe perioperative bleeding: guidelines from the European Society of Anaesthesiology. Eur J Anaesthesiol 2013;30:270–382.
29 Mahajan RP: Critical incident reporting and learning. Br J Anaesthesia 2010;105:69–75.
30 Wahr JA, Prager RL, Abernathy JH 3rd, Martinez EA, Salas E, Seifert PC, et al: Patient safety in the cardiac operating room: human factors and teamwork: a scientific statement from the American Heart Association. Circulation 2013;128:1139–1169.

Balthasar Eberle, MD
University Department for Anesthesiology and Pain Therapy
Inselspital, Bern University Hospital
Freiburgstrasse, CH–3010 Bern (Switzerland)
E-Mail balthasar.eberle@insel.ch

Widmer MK, Malik J (eds): Patient Safety in Dialysis Access.
Contrib Nephrol. Basel, Karger, 2015, vol 184, pp 123–135
DOI: 10.1159/000365827

Careful and Safe Vascular Access Creation

Thomas R. Wyss • Matthias K. Widmer

Department of Cardiovascular Surgery, Swiss Cardiovascular Center, Bern University Hospital, Bern, Switzerland

Abstract

Morbidity and mortality are significant in hemodialysis patients, and every vascular access (VA) is prone to complications – some more, some less. The risk of complications rises from arteriovenous fistulae to arteriovenous grafts and peaks in nontunneled central lines. Strategies to achieve complete evaluation of the patient and precise planning mark the start of successful VA creation. Furthermore, preoperative considerations include safety checklists, team time-out procedures, and antibiotic prophylaxis. Intraoperative technical features and postoperative aspects of documentation and surveillance schemes complete careful and safe VA creation.

Recommendations to Improve Patient Safety

- Clinical evaluation and duplex sonography examination are important in preoperative decision making.
- Safety checklists and team time-out are standard protocol.
- Fistula first concept should be constantly encouraged.
- Synthetic and biological grafts are important adjuncts to arteriovenous fistulae.
- Artery-side-to-vein-end anastomosis is the preferred type.
- Perform careful and meticulous surgical preparation to avoid tissue and vessel trauma.
- Patient education is essential for outcome.

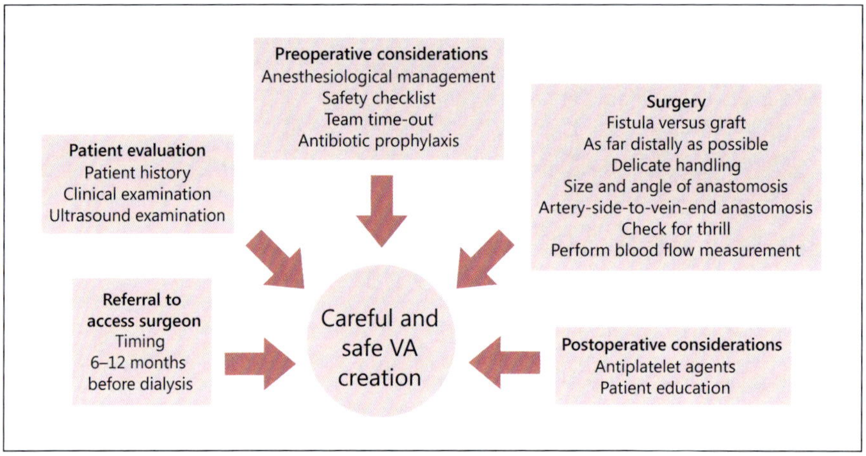

Fig. 1. Tasks for careful and safe VA creation.

Introduction

Considerable morbidity exists when dealing with vascular access (VA) creation. Native arteriovenous fistulae (AVF) are the desired VA for patients on dialysis due to their comparably low morbidity and fairly good long-term patency. However, they are also at risk for nonmaturation, stenosis, thrombosis, infection, aneurysm formation, and steal syndrome [1]. Fistula success is dependent on the center of access creation. Hence, the vascular surgeon's skills and decisions are key [2]. Furthermore, success is also determined by preoperative, technical, and postoperative factors that will be discussed in this chapter (fig. 1).

Preoperative Decision Making

First of all, one has to respect that future hemodialysis calls for sufficient timing of VA creation. AVF require a period of ideally 4–6 weeks [3], sometimes even months, of maturation to become suitable for cannulation. Early decision making is needed to guarantee enough time to have a functioning access ready at the start of hemodialysis. Therefore, patients with advanced chronic kidney disease (glomerular filtration rate <20–25 ml/min, late stage 4) should be referred to an access surgeon [4]. Six to 12 months prior to the expected first hemodialysis, fistula creation should be initiated on the nondominant extremity.

A certain blood flow is necessary to make hemodialysis possible and to avoid recirculation of dialyzed blood: fistulae should have a blood flow of >600 ml/

min, and the majority of proper fistulae report a blood flow of 800–1,200 ml/min [5, 6]. Serving only as a rough guide, criteria for fistula maturation have been summarized as the 'rule of 6s': >6 mm diameter, <6 mm deep from the skin surface, >600 ml/min blood flow, and if after 6 weeks the fistula does not meet these criteria, evaluation for nonmaturation should be commenced. However, many AVF (up to 50%) never mature properly or early thrombosis occurs [3, 5]. In order to avoid nonmaturing AVF and to have enough time for the growth process, certain measures have to be taken. For this purpose, we are referring to the chapter by Malovrh [this vol., pp. 13–23]. Malovrh elaborates on the mandatory preoperative physical and noninvasive duplex ultrasound examination of patients and their vessels. All of these variables affect the surgeon's decision.

When comparing the outcome of fistulae created after using physical examination alone versus physical examination and ultrasound vein mapping, it has been shown that the rate of successfully constructed AVF increased significantly with preoperative ultrasound imaging. Furthermore, the surgical site for fistula creation and type of procedure were considerably modified by ultrasound results and negative surgical explorations were eliminated. Fistula patency rates at 6 months were higher when ultrasound mapping was used [7].

Arteriosclerosis for example can possibly limit fistula maturation due to restricted capacity of the vessel to accommodate the higher flow that is needed for a cannulable hemodialysis access [6].

Consequently, preoperative vessel mapping adds valuable information concerning the choice of fistula type [8]. All this supplementary information eliminates risks of surgical failure and increases the proportion of AVF over arteriovenous grafts (AVG), contributing to the widely accepted 'fistula first' concept. It is generally believed that AVF are preferred over AVG due to better long-term patency. VA is placed as far distally in the upper extremity as possible, beginning with posterior radial branch-cephalic direct wrist access (snuffbox), then radial-cephalic forearm (Cimino-Brescia) fistulae and so on. This leaves more proximal sites for future access [4].

However, if there is limited maturation time available, AVF have failed, suitable vessels are lacking and central venous catheters have to be avoided, AVG represent a good option. Key features of the ideal graft include early access, rapid hemostasis, good long-term patency, and resistance to infection. Generally, grafts can be divided into synthetic or biological vascular substitutes. Expanded polytetrafluorethylene (ePTFE) is the most widely used synthetic graft. Its recommended minimum waiting time until first cannulation is 2 weeks. This period is required for adequate attachment to the subcutaneous tissue surrounding the graft and contributing to hemostasis after puncture. Ideally, immediate graft puncture is possible to evade temporary dialysis catheter placement. Myointimal hyperplasia leading to stenosis and finally thrombosis and therefore access failure is more prominent in AVG than AVF. Development of modified graft materials is important to counteract these issues. A few examples: Heparin bonding aims at reducing the graft's intrinsic thrombogenicity through impregnation of the luminal surface. Multilayer graft wall structures, alterations in graft pore size and mesh configuration as well as changes in material composition try to reduce excess formation of neointima and enable cannulation within 24 h after AVG creation (so-called early stick grafts). Geometrical modifications (e.g. cuffed grafts, swirl/spiral grafts, venous cuffs/collars) have been developed to decrease AVG neointima formation and stenosis, however with variable success compared to standard ePTFE [9]. All of the available artificial implants put the patient at a higher risk of fistula failure, compared to AVF, mainly due to thrombosis and infection, venous hypertension and steal syndrome. These aspects have to be kept in mind when making decisions for different VA models.

Drug-eluting perivascular wraps, intended to reduce myointimal hyperplasia, are under investigation. Paclitaxel- or Sirolimus-eluting and endothelial cell-loaded wraps have shown some benefit in reducing PTFE graft stenosis [10].

Biological and bio hybrid materials (e.g. cryopreserved veins, bovine grafts, ovine matrix collagen grafts) mainly come to use in infected situations due to their lesser susceptibility to reinfection. Rerouting concepts (i.e. using a new subcutaneous tunnel) and biological grafts are advisable when infections of VA are present [11]. Myointimal hyperplasia also seems to be rare in these grafts. Still, data are inconsistent when it comes to patency rates and infections, and surgical handling of synthetic and biological grafts can be difficult as well [12].

Central venous catheter placement can be performed in emergency cases that most likely will need immediate and serial dialysis. Risk of bleeding and pneumothorax as well as higher infection rates, shorter service life and often prolonged hemodialysis treatment times have to be taken into account.

Anesthesia, Safety Checklist and Antibiotic Prophylaxis

Anesthesiological impact is generally small in VA surgery, although often dealing with multimorbid patients. Local anesthesia is sufficient for the majority of procedures if the patient is compliant and an outpatient setting is usually adequate. When dealing with more extensive procedures, regional nerve blocks such as brachial plexus anesthesia offer patient and surgeon comfort as well. Furthermore, a desired advantage of regional block anesthesia is the marked increase in venous diameter of the superficial veins, which may improve the rate of native fistula placement [13]. General anesthesia is rarely needed.

In order to promote a safety culture, the World Health Organization has introduced a so-called surgical safety checklist aiming at reducing the number of surgical deaths across the world. Events of inadequate anesthetic safety practices, avoidable surgical infection and poor communication among team members in the operating theatre put the patient at risk. A list of safety checks has been designed to address this issue. It consists of three parts: (a) sign in (before induction of anesthesia), (b) time-out (before skin incision), and (c) sign out (before the patient leaves the operating room). Each part is made up of multiple questions that need to be checked before the next part can be initiated. For example, the 'sign in' reconfirms patient identity and mentions possible allergies. The 'time-out' introduces all team members and possible critical events during the procedure. Finally, the 'sign out' lists instrument counts, labelling of pathological specimens, and planned postoperative patient management. Adhering to a pattern like this should reduce the number of avoidable risks endangering the lives and well-being of surgical patients [14].

The possibility to develop a surgical site infection depends on bacterial colonization of the operative field. Perioperative antibiotics are central to prevent postoperative surgical wound infection [15]. To reach the best effect, timing of administration of the single-shot antibiotic prophylaxis is crucial: 30–60 min before skin incision is adequate. Errors due to too early or too late medication put the patient at risk for an infection.

General Technical Aspects

A multitude of factors has been identified to affect patency of AVF. Results from a recent review show that nonmodifiable patient factors such as age, diabetes, peripheral vascular disease, predialysis hypotension and vessel characteristics (<2 mm diameter, reduced distensibility) negatively influence patency. When it comes to modifiable factors, smoking, early referral, ultrasound imaging, anastomosis type, vascular staples/clips, flow assessments, antiplatelet therapy, and timing of first cannulation have an effect on patency. Systemic heparin use, cannulation technique and fistula surveillance do not alter the rate of fistula patency according to latest data [16]. Traditionally, systemic heparin use has been of widespread use to counteract clotting in clamped vessels. However, data show that it only increases bleeding complications without adding to the success of primary fistula creation or fistula patency [16].

Marking the vein with duplex ultrasound before the operation and palpation of the artery can help to place the incision in an ideal area. After having decided at which location the anastomosis will be performed, skin incision under antibiotic prophylaxis follows. A short longitudinal incision is preferred to gain good target vessel access and to avoid damage to neighboring structures such as nerves and lymphatic vessels. Attention should be paid that the incision and the suture line are not lying on the top of the vessel but a little bit aside. S-shaped incisions in the cubital fossa or in areas of grafts are ideal because the incision can be prolonged, and the potential exposure of the underlying AVG is, in the middle part of the incision, very short so that the risk for an infection is low.

Creation of AVF

In surgical preparation of the desired vessels, care must be given to avoid wall damage, which could lead to leakage or stenosis of the vessel. Different ways of blocking blood flow exist (e.g. vascular clamp, local vascular tourniquet, proximal pneumatic tourniquet, balloons, cardiac shunts, and endovascular occlusion gel). The safety of pneumatic tourniquet occlusion over clamps to gain vascular control has been documented and its advantage shown when it comes to shorter operative time and technically easier operation as well, especially in redo cases. It has no impact on complications (e.g. nerve injury, bleeding, hematoma, vascular steal, infection, or swelling) and primary patency rates [17]. It must be remembered that the anesthesiological management also influences the possibilities of available blood flow control.

Flushing the distal end of the venous segment with saline allows the surgeons to assess the properties (e.g. diameter, side branches, stenoses) of the vein [4]. Especially in cases of vein transposition, the dissected vein is dilated with heparinized saline and can be marked with a skin scribe to avoid rotation. The vein has to be released from its surrounding tissue for a certain distance to approach the artery. One has to bear in mind that this mobilization causes tissue damage and can lead to devascularization of the vessel. The vein tends to lengthen a bit during fistula maturation. Kinking (due to excess length) has to be avoided because this could lead to severe postanastomotic stenosis. On the other hand, pulling and stretching of the artery and/or vein causes mechanical trauma to the vessel wall. Torsion of the vein or inadequate tension has to be omitted before performing the anastomosis [18].

Available types of preparation include artery-side-to-vein-end, end-to-end, and side-to-side anastomoses. The preferred mode is artery-side-to-vein-end anastomosis leading to less complications (no distal arterial ligation as in end-

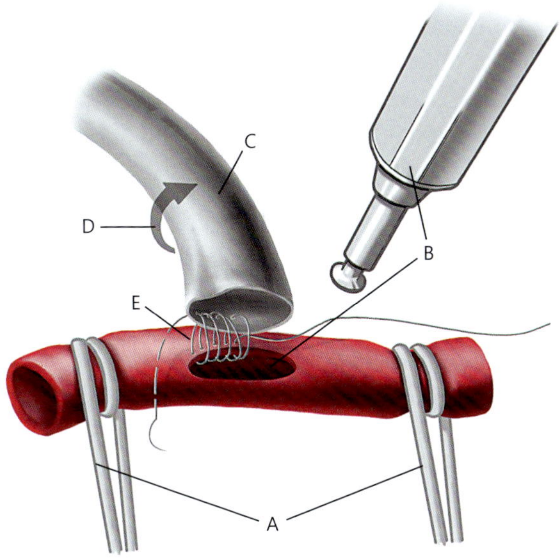

Fig. 2. Safe creation of an arteriovenous anastomosis. A = Control of inflow and outflow using clamps, vessel loops or tourniquets; B = incision of the artery and creating round ends using a punch; C = instillation of heparinized saline solution to check the outflow of the vein and enlarge the vein so it can be marked; D = mild outward rotation of the vein; E = running suture inside artery out in parachute technique.

to-end technique and no hyperemia of the hand as in side-to-side technique) and equal patency rates [19].

The distal end of the vein is ligated and the vein approximated to the artery. This in turn results in varying angles between the artery and the vein at the site of the anastomosis. Hence, the lengths of the arteriotomy and venotomy have to be precisely tailored according to this angle. If the angle is more acute, the length of the arteriotomy/venotomy is longer than if the vein approaches the artery at a right angle [20]. In a rectangular anastomosis, Konner [20] recommends to mildly rotate the vein outward to avoid juxta-anastomotic kinking and stenosis. We prefer the use of a punch to achieve an accurate opening in the arterial wall at the future anastomotic site. It offers good visibility and reduces trauma to the vessel (fig. 2).

Anastomotic technique: surgical telescopes and 6-0 or 7-0 thread for sutures are generally recommended [6]. Vascular nonpenetrating U-shaped clips in an interrupted manner can alternatively be used: maturation and patency rates in forearm fistulae are good [21]. We normally perform a running suture starting at the back wall, then passing the proximal corner, then passing the distal corner with the other end of the thread to complete the anastomosis in the middle of the front wall. In our experience, this offers good visualization during the whole procedure.

Once completed, the arteriovenous connection leads to a drop in peripheral resistance increasing arterial flow. With larger anastomosis size, proximal artery flow increases further. However, larger anastomoses can eventually lead to distal artery flow reversal. Therefore, it is important to respect both size and angle of anastomoses. Van Canneyt showed a distinct hemodynamic impact of anastomosis size and angle in an AVF flow model. For larger anastomoses, arterial inflow and venous outflow increase and arterial outflow decreases. In anastomosis >58°, the arterial inflow was insufficient, leading to distal arterial flow reversal. This in turn could lead to ischemic complications. For larger anastomoses, the pressure drop over the anastomosis decreases at a fixed angle. For more acute anastomosis, the pressure drop was less dependent on anastomosis cross-sectional area [22].

Recently, Bharat et al. [23] showed that their so-called 'piggy back' straight-line onlay technique led to a significant reduction in juxta-anastomotic stenosis, which is the leading cause for fistula failure. In this technique, an anastomosis between the posterior (underside) aspect of the vein and the anterior (upper) aspect of the artery is created and the arterial blood is supposed to flow into a straight cylindrical lumen.

Intraoperative Quality Control

Both, a continuous palpable thrill and a continuous audible (stethoscope) low-pitched bruit should be present upon completion of the fistula. AVF maturation can be predicted by intraoperative blood flow measurement. Low flow calls for immediate revision. Minimal flow values needed for radiocephalic fistulae are 120 ml/min and for brachiocephalic fistulae 310 ml/min. When reaching these values during fistula creation, one can expect maturation [24]. In revision procedures, intraoperative angiography is an essential adjunct. It provides insight into local or distal stenoses that might affect in- or outflow properties. Such issues can be resolved by direct interventional or surgical treatment.

Creation of AVG

If there are no veins available, grafts are an alternative. They can be placed either as straight (= bridge) grafts or as loops. In creating AVG, technical aspects to avoid tissue trauma and infection include gentle and atraumatic soft tissue handling (i.e. no touch technique), avoidance of skin contact of graft materials and

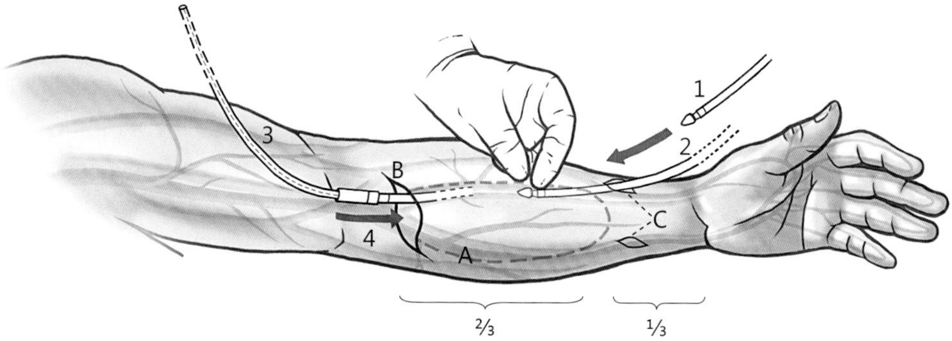

Fig. 3. Instructions for safe AVG placement. A = Mark the planned landing zone for the AVG. The graft length should be about 2/3 of the forearm. B, C = S-shaped incision in the cubital fossa and two incisions far away from the final graft bed. Use of a tunneler: (1) Oversize the olive by 1 mm (e.g. 7 mm for 6-mm graft). (2) Check the tissue depth of your tunneler using your hand. (3) Fix the graft to the tunneler avoiding skin contact. (4) Pull the tunneler and graft through and check to avoid rotation and kinking.

avoidance of scars in the puncture area. A popular tool to limit tissue damage in loop configurations is a tunneler, available in different diameters and lengths. It aids in minimizing skin incisions, and it creates an adequately sized tunnel, avoiding extensive subcutaneous tissue damage as opposed to the use of traditional tunneling forceps (fig. 3). Subsequently, the graft can be pulled through along the tunneler facilitating rotational control.

In graft-vein anastomosis of AVG, Konner recommends a very acute, almost parallel position of the graft along the vein and a length of the anastomosis of up to 20–30 mm. This will result in undisturbed blood flow through the anastomosis without a great change in direction, omitting turbulence which could lead to neointimal hyperplasia [20].

Hand Ischemia and Its Prevention

Steal syndrome can occur after VA creation and put the patient at risk for impaired distal perfusion or even ischemia of the forearm and hand. Accepted risk factors for its development are diabetes, hypertension, smoking, female gender, and coronary artery disease [25]. Two situations have to be distinguished in steal syndrome since they call for different management. If there is a considerably higher than desired blood flow in the arteriovenous segment, flow reduction has to be achieved by narrowing the anastomosis, banding of the postanastomotic venous segment (e.g. narrowing suture, plication, interposition, banding/cuff) or the revision using distal inflow technique which results in a more distal feeding of the venous segment and therefore preserves an antegrade arterial flow pattern. On the other hand, if there is adequate or low blood flow in the arteriovenous segment and blood flow cannot be reduced, angioplasty of arterial in- or outflow vessel stenoses, proximalization of arterial inflow into the arteriovenous segment or proximalization of the post-anastomotic outflow artery by distal revascularization and interval ligation are effective methods. The 'extension technique' by Ehsan is a modified technique for brachiocephalic fistulae to prevent hand ischemia (fig. 4) Anastomosis is performed between the median cubital vein and the radial or ulnar artery just below the brachial bifurcation. This preserves part of the blood supply to the hand avoiding steal syndrome. An additional advantage of this technique is maturation of both, cephalic and basilic, veins [26]. In the case of AVG, the use of a tapered graft is an option to prevent hand ischemia.

Postoperative Management

Cannulation within the first 2 weeks after the operation should be avoided to allow for tissue ingrowth [16]. Consequently, if sufficient fistula maturation has been achieved at that time, access cannulation can start.

Medication that improves patency includes antiplatelet agents, fish oil and calcium channel blockers [27]. A Cochrane review investigated the effect of adjuvant medical treatment to improve patency rates of AVF and AVG. The results of the meta-analysis showed a positive effect of antiplatelet treatment on VA patency in the short term. An included trial comparing low-dose warfarin with placebo was stopped early due to increased bleeding complications in the treatment group [28].

The patient and treating nephrologist have to be well informed about the VA they are dealing with, allowing them to anticipate potential problems in advance and to guarantee best access survival. This can include a schematic drawing of the VA that has been created. Visual understanding of the detailed anatomic conditions supports correct cannulation. Moreover, with every revision procedure, the degree of complexity increases, and therefore it is important to keep track of the structural setting as part of the patient's fistula history (fig. 5). So called 'vascular access passports' represent a helpful documentation tool to achieve this goal (http://heartlandkidney.org/article_resources/passport.pdf). Educational material (http://www.fistulafirst.org/Patients/PatientEducationalMaterials.aspx) for patients is key in raising patient compliance levels and outcome after AV access surgery, implementing correct patient behavior: keeping the wound clean and the fistula protected, touching the access daily to feel the thrill. Additionally, hand squeezing exercises increase the diameter of the outflow vein and seem to help in AVF maturation [29].

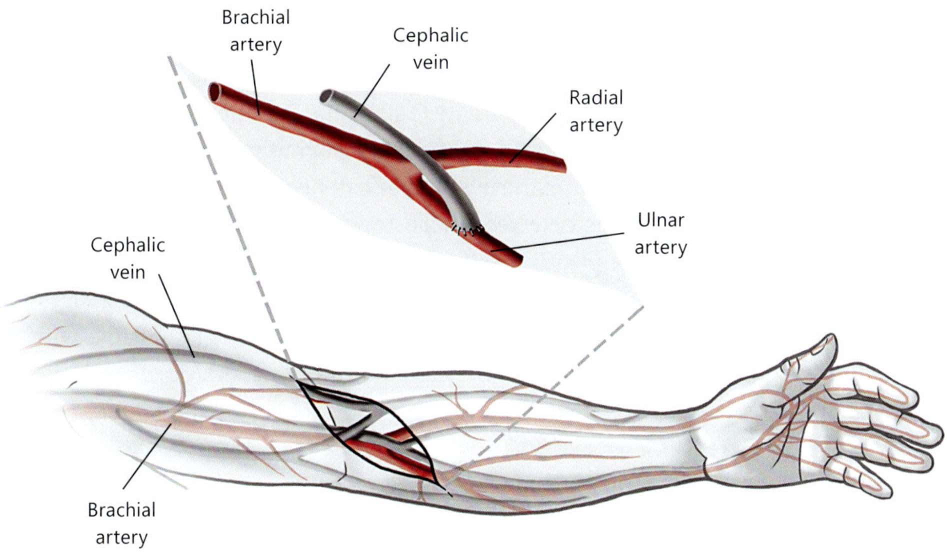

Fig. 4. Cubital AVF in extension technique to avoid hand ischemia in patients with critically diseased arteries.

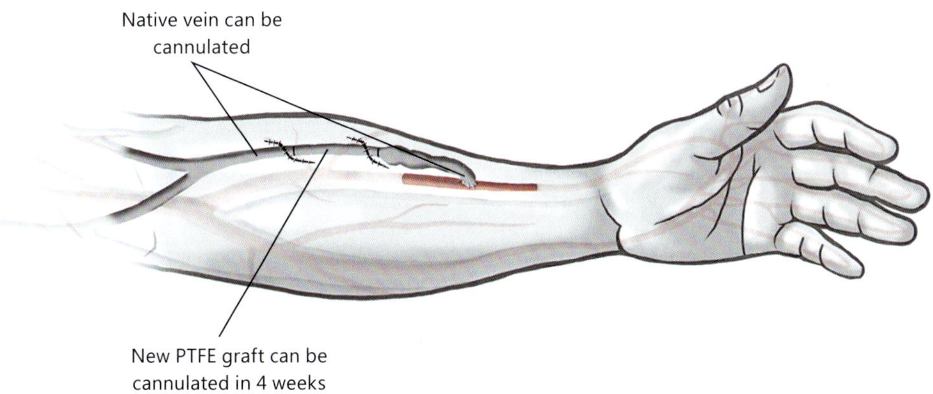

Fig. 5. Visual documentation of VA creation or revision procedures help the dialysis staff to understand where and when they are allowed to puncture.

Evidence regarding the actual benefit of access surveillance is limited. Postoperative surveillance by duplex scanning (detecting inflow or outflow problems) after 6–8 weeks has a high sensitivity (100%) and specificity (85%) for final access outcome [8]. If necessary, endovascular (angiography and angioplasty) or surgical interventions for nonmaturing fistulae can be planned. Preemptive repair of subclinical stenoses detected on postoperative access surveillance by blood flow measurements positively affects access survival [30]. However, only low-quality evidence exists suggesting a potentially beneficial effect of access surveillance followed by interventions to restore patency [31]. Surveillance with blood flow measurements may prevent fistula thrombosis, but does not influence the risk of access loss [32].

Disclosure Statement

T.R. Wyss declares no conflicts of interest. M.K. Widmer is a convenor and tutor at the Vascular International Foundation and School and consultant of Bio Nova International and MAQUET GETINGE GROUP.

References

1 Yu Q, Yu H, Chen S, Wang L, Yuan W: Distribution and complications of native arteriovenous fistulas in maintenance hemodialysis patients: a single-center study. J Nephrol 2011;24:597–603.

2 Huijbregts HJ, Bots ML, Moll FL, Blankestijn PJ: Hospital specific aspects predominantly determine primary failure of hemodialysis arteriovenous fistulas. J Vasc Surg 2007;45: 962–967.

3 Asif A, Roy-Chaudhury P, Beathard GA: Early arteriovenous fistula failure: a logical proposal for when and how to intervene. Clin J Am Soc Nephrol 2006;1:332–339.

4 Sidawy AN, Spergel LM, Besarab A, Allon M, Jennings WC, Padberg FT Jr, Murad MH, Montori VM, O'Hare AM, Calligaro KD, Macsata RA, Lumsden AB, Ascher E: The Society for Vascular Surgery: clinical practice guidelines for the surgical placement and maintenance of arteriovenous hemodialysis access. J Vasc Surg 2008;48(suppl 5):2S–25S.

5 Huijbregts HJ, Blankestijn PJ: Dialysis access-guidelines for current practice. Eur J Vasc Endovasc Surg 2006;31:284–287.

6 Shenoy S: Innovative surgical approaches to maximize arteriovenous fistula creation. Semin Vasc Surg 2007;20:141–147.

7 Ilhan G, Esi E, Bozok S, Yurekli I, Ozpak B, Ozelci A, Destan B, Gurbuz A: The clinical utility of vascular mapping with Doppler ultrasound prior to arteriovenous fistula construction for hemodialysis access. J Vasc Access 2013;14:83–88.

8 Ives CL, Akoh JA, George J, Vaughan-Huxley E, Lawson H: Pre-operative vessel mapping and early post-operative surveillance duplex scanning of arteriovenous fistulae. J Vasc Access 2009;10:37–42.

9 Day JC, Glickman M: Prosthetic graft design to prevent access stenosis formation; in Tordoir J (ed): Best Practice in Vascular Access. Turin, Edizioni Minerva Medica, 2010, pp 73–79.

10 Roy-Chaudhury P, El-Khatib M, Campos-Naciff B, Wadehra D, Ramani K, Leesar M, Mistry M, Wang Y, Chan JS, Lee T, Munda R: Back to the future: how biology and technology could change the role of PTFE grafts in vascular access management. Semin Dial 2012;25:495–504.

11 Stellmes AW, Schmidli J, Widmer MK: Biological grafts in infected patients; in: Tordoir J (ed): Best Practice in Vascular Access. Turin, Edizioni Minerva Medica, 2010, pp 169–177.
12 Mailey BK, Wilson SE: New synthetic grafts and early access; in: Wilson SE, (ed): Vascular Access: Principles and Practice. Philadelphia, Lippincott Williams & Wilkins, 2010, pp 114–119.
13 Reynolds TS, Kim KM, Dukkipati R, Nguyen TH, Julka I, Kakazu C, Tokhner V, Chauvapun JP: Pre-operative regional block anesthesia enhances operative strategy for arteriovenous fistula creation. J Vasc Access 2011;12: 336–340.
14 WHO: Surgical Safety Checklist and Implementation Manual 2013. http://www.who.int/patientsafety/safesurgery/ss_checklist/en/ (accessed October 22, 2013).
15 Bandyk DF: Vascular surgical site infection: risk factors and preventive measures. Semin Vasc Surg 2008;21:119–123.
16 Smith GE, Gohil R, Chetter IC: Factors affecting the patency of arteriovenous fistulas for dialysis access. J Vasc Surg 2012;55:849–855.
17 Dickson CS, Gregory RT, Parent FN, Wheeler JR, Snyder SO, Gayle RG, DeMasi RJ: A new technique for hemodialysis access surgery: use of the pneumatic tourniquet. Ann Vasc Surg 1996;10:373–377.
18 Konner K, Lomonte C, Basile C: Placing a primary arteriovenous fistula that works – more or less known aspects, new ideas. Nephrol Dial Transplant 2013;28:781–784.
19 Wedgwood KR, Wiggins PA, Guillou PJ: A prospective study of end-to-side vs. side-to-side arteriovenous fistulas for haemodialysis. Br J Surg 1984;71:640–642.
20 Konner K: The anastomosis of the arteriovenous fistula – common errors and their avoidance. Nephrol Dial Transplant 2002;17:376–379.
21 Lin PH, Bush RL, Nelson JC, Lam R, Paladugu R, Chen C, Quinn G, Lumsden AB: A prospective evaluation of interrupted nitinol surgical clips in arteriovenous fistula for hemodialysis. Am J Surg 2003;186:625–630.

Thomas R. Wyss, MD
Department of Cardiovascular Surgery
Swiss Cardiovascular Center
Bern University Hospital
Freiburgstrasse 10, CH–3010 Bern (Switzerland)
E-Mail thomas.wyss@insel.ch

22 Van Canneyt K, Pourchez T, Eloot S, Guillame C, Bonnet A, Segers P, Verdonck P: Hemodynamic impact of anastomosis size and angle in side-to-end arteriovenous fistulae: a computer analysis. J Vasc Access 2010;11:52–58.
23 Bharat A, Jaenicke M, Shenoy S: A novel technique of vascular anastomosis to prevent juxta-anastomotic stenosis following arteriovenous fistula creation. J Vasc Surg 2012;55: 274–280.
24 Berman SS, Mendoza B, Westerband A, Quick RC: Predicting arteriovenous fistula maturation with intraoperative blood flow measurements. J Vasc Access 2008;9:241–247.
25 Gupta N, Yuo TH, Konig Gt, Dillavou E, Leers SA, Chaer RA, Cho JS, Makaroun MS: Treatment strategies of arterial steal after arteriovenous access. J Vasc Surg 2011;54:162–167.
26 Ehsan O, Bhattacharya D, Darwish A, Al-khaffaf H: 'Extension technique': a modified technique for brachio-cephalic fistula to prevent dialysis access-associated steal syndrome. Eur J Vasc Endovasc Surg 2005;29:324–327.
27 Gibbons CP: Primary vascular access. Eur J Vasc Endovasc Surg 2006;31:523–529.
28 Osborn G, Escofet X, Da Silva A: Medical adjuvant treatment to increase patency of arteriovenous fistulae and grafts. Cochrane Database Syst Rev 2008;CD002786.
29 Oder TF, Teodorescu V, Uribarri J: Effect of exercise on the diameter of arteriovenous fistulae in hemodialysis patients. ASAIO J 2003; 49:554–555.
30 Tessitore N, Lipari G, Poli A, Bedogna V, Baggio E, Loschiavo C, Mansueto G, Lupo A: Can blood flow surveillance and pre-emptive repair of subclinical stenosis prolong the useful life of arteriovenous fistulae? A randomized controlled study. Nephrol Dial Transplant 2004;19:2325–2333.
31 Casey ET, Murad MH, Rizvi AZ, Sidawy AN, McGrath MM, Elamin MB, Flynn DN, McCausland FR, Vo DH, El-Zoghby Z, Duncan AA, Tracz MJ, Erwin PJ, Montori VM: Surveillance of arteriovenous hemodialysis access: a systematic review and meta-analysis. J Vasc Surg 2008;48(suppl 5):48S–54S.
32 Tonelli M, James M, Wiebe N, Jindal K, Hemmelgarn B, Alberta Kidney Disease N: Ultrasound monitoring to detect access stenosis in hemodialysis patients: a systematic review. Am J Kidney Dis 2008;51:630–640.

Widmer MK, Malik J (eds): Patient Safety in Dialysis Access.
Contrib Nephrol. Basel, Karger, 2015, vol 184, pp 136–142
DOI: 10.1159/000367680

Improving Patient Safety in Vascular Access: A Role for Individualization and Patient Preferences

Prabir Roy-Chaudhury • Ashish Verma

Dialysis Vascular Access Research Group, Division of Nephrology, University of Cincinnati and VA Medical Center, Cincinnati, Ohio, USA

Abstract

Patient safety is central to the practice of medicine. Traditional pathways to improve patient safety have included better education of patients and better training of health care professionals. In this chapter, we make the case for a nontraditional approach to patient safety in the setting of dialysis vascular access which focuses on (a) the development of a patient-centric process of care, (b) individualization of care (personalized medicine), and (c) the use of novel and safer therapies.

Recommendations to Improve Patient Safety

- Provide opportunities for the patient to participate in their own care through pathways for self-cannulation and voicing of patient preferences (what is important to the patient).
- Develop pathways for individualization of care (personalized medicine).
- Focus on the process of care with well-defined roles and responsibilities for all team members.
- Advocate for the use of new technologies that reduce complications.

Introduction

Dialysis vascular access is currently the 'lifeline' for hemodialysis patients. Unfortunately, due to the many complications associated with dialysis vascular access, it is also the 'Achilles heel' of hemodialysis. A relatively ignored aspect of dialysis vascular access pertains to patient safety. The first part of this chapter will describe patient safety issues in the traditional context of arteriovenous fistulas (AVFs), arteriovenous grafts (AVGs) and tunneled central venous catheter (tCVC). In the second half of this chapter, however, we will make the case that a nontraditional approach which emphasizes (a) individualization of care, and (b) patient preferences and patient involvement may be our best opportunity to improve patient safety in hemodialysis patients.

Traditional Patient Safety Issues in Dialysis Vascular Access

Arteriovenous Fistulas

AVFs remain the preferred form of dialysis vascular access due to their superior long-term patency and lack of infection. The main disadvantage of AVFs is a very high incidence of maturation failure (defined as the inability to use the AVF for dialysis due to inadequate flow and diameter), likely due to a combination of neointimal hyperplasia and inadequate outward remodeling in the perianastomotic region [1, 2]. This stenotic lesion can at times also result in thrombosis. A long period of AVF maturation, however, often results in prolonged dependence on tCVCs with all their attendant risks of infection, thrombosis and central vein stenosis. The prolonged presence of a tCVC could also push health care professionals towards more aggressive cannulation regimens. While this is not a bad idea, early cannulation could potentially result in large infiltrations, which would necessitate resting the AVF and so prolong even further the duration of tCVC dependence and the risk of infection [3, 4]. An additional issue that has recently come to light in the context of cannulation is an increased risk of infection with the buttonhole technique, although there is likely to be a well-selected and defined patient population that could benefit from this approach, especially with the right infrastructure, training and process of care [5–8].

Arteriovenous Grafts

In marked contrast to AVFs, AVGs do not have a problem with early maturation failure, with the vast majority being cannulated between 3–6 weeks after surgery. Unfortunately, they do have significant problems with stenosis (most commonly at the graft-vein anastomosis) and thrombosis, with a recorded one year unassisted primary patency as low as 23% [9]. In addition, polytetrafluroethylene (PTFE) grafts have an infection rate of approximately 10% over the lifetime of the graft.

Tunneled Central Venous Catheters

Although tCVCs allow for the immediate initiation of patients onto hemodialysis, they can result in very significant complications as a result of catheter-related bloodstream infections, thrombosis, inadequate dialysis and central venous stenosis. Recent data also document a very significant increase in mortality, especially within the first 90 days of hemodialysis in patients initiating dialysis with a tunneled dialysis catheter as compared to those starting dialysis with an AVF or AVG [10]. Despite these statistics, almost 80% of patients starting dialysis in the US do so with a tCVC, with only a quarter of these patients having a maturing AVF. Thus, 60% of all patients starting dialysis in the US do so with no real plan for permanent dialysis vascular access. We believe that this epidemic of incident tCVC use is perhaps the biggest safety risk associated with dialysis vascular access at the current time. How can we best address this problem?

Is There a Solution?

The best solution would of course be for every patient to start hemodialysis with an AVF that was ready to use. This would require significant focus on the process of care in the chronic kidney disease (CKD) stage, including early referral to nephrology and to the access surgeon, aggressive programs for vein preservation and venous mapping, the services of a dedicated vascular access surgeon, identification and early intervention in the setting of AVF nonmaturation and the use of master cannulators for the initial cannulations. More than anything else, we believe that spending resources on vascular access coordinators would result in the greatest potential impact on successful AVF placement and maturation during the CKD phase. In our minds, this would likely have a huge positive impact on patient safety in the context of dialysis vascular access.

Individualization of Care

While trying to ensure that every patient has a functional AVF at the time of starting hemodialysis is a laudable goal, it is important to do this in the context of individualization of vascular access care. Thus, while an AVF would be the vascular access of choice in young to middle-age patients with adequate vessel size and estimated glomerular filtration rates around 25–30 ml/min, this may not hold true for a middle-aged patient with extensive comorbidities and small vessels who is already dialyzing through a tCVC. In this latter instance, placement of a PTFE graft (perhaps even an early cannulation graft) may be a more appropriate plan of action from the patient safety aspect since this would result in earlier removal of the tCVC.

Similarly, recent data suggest that patient survival is similar for octogenarians who initiate dialysis with either a PTFE graft or an AVF, with catheters doing far worse. This is particularly important information in the context of the large numbers of unnecessary procedures that are often performed in elderly patients who have AVFs placed during the CKD stage, in that these patients often die prior to the initiation of hemodialysis [11]. Based on the papers by DeSilva et al. [12, 13], PTFE grafts placed within a month of the initiation of hemodialysis might be the preferred option both at the clinical and the patient safety level in older patients with CKD.

Another approach that could optimize patient safety related to vascular access in the future could be the use of novel therapies to enhance vascular access survival. Thus, the best vascular access care plan for the middle-aged man with multiple comorbidities, small vessels and a tCVC already in place as described above may in the future not just be a PTFE graft, but rather an AVF in combination with a wrap or other device to improve AVF maturation and subsequent rapid tCVC removal.

Patient Involvement and Patient Preferences

Finally, we strongly believe that the best way to reduce patient safety issues related to dialysis vascular access is to actively involve patients in the whole process of vascular access care. This could be at the level of patient involvement or patient preferences.

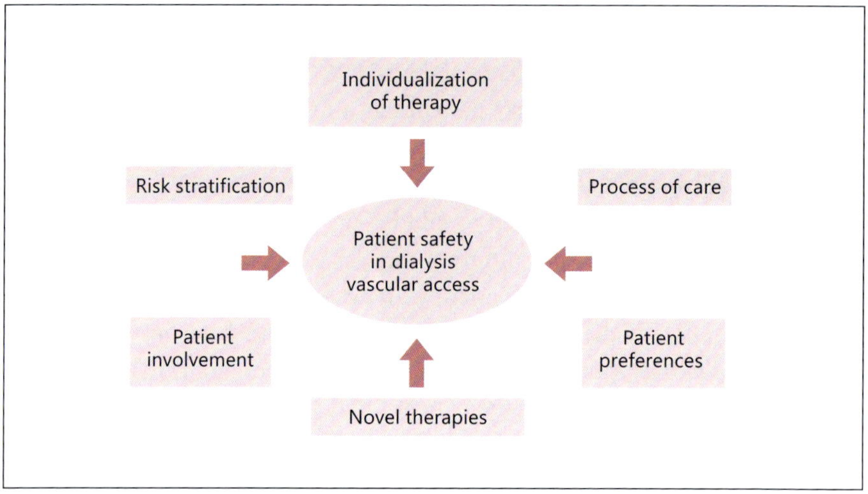

Fig. 1. A nontraditional approach to patient safety in dialysis access.

Patient Involvement

Active patient involvement and education about the pros and cons of the different types of dialysis vascular access including the concept of individualization of vascular access care as described above could go a long way towards the enhancement of patient safety in vascular access. Another important aspect of patient involvement could be the use of self-cannulation. This could potentially not only reduce the incidence of infiltrations, but also give 'ownership' of the vascular access to the patient.

Patient Preferences

Linked to the concept of patient involvement is the adoption of patient preferences. We believe that an individual patient's perception of the risks and benefits of the different forms of dialysis vascular access may be quite different from those of the health care professionals. An older patient with multiple comorbidities and limited survival may feel that the use of a tCVC which avoids needle sticks may be preferable to an AVF which may need multiple procedures to be able to support dialysis. Although the concept of bringing patient preferences into the decision making mix for dialysis vascular access is new, we believe that it could allow us to develop a much more holistic and patient-centric approach to dialysis vascular access safety.

Conclusions

Patient safety in dialysis vascular access cannot be considered to be a stand-alone field in its own individual silo.

We have therefore described a nontraditional, albeit more holistic approach to patient safety for dialysis vascular access (fig. 1), which emphasizes process of care pathways, individualization of therapy through risk stratification and the use of novel technologies, active patient involvement and identification of individual patient preferences.

We strongly believe that adoption of such a *patient-centered* approach to dialysis vascular access could have a very positive impact on patient safety in dialysis vascular access.

Disclosure Statement

Dr. Roy-Chaudhury is supported by NIH-5U01-DK82218, NIH-1R21-DK089280, NIH-1R01DK088777 (MPI), NIH-R21-EB016150, NIH-R21-EB16737-01, NIH-R41-DK100156, NIH-R41-DK101206, NIH/NCCR UL1RR026314 and a VA Merit Review.

References

1 Dember LM, Beck GJ, Allon M, et al: Effect of clopidogrel on early failure of arteriovenous fistulas for hemodialysis: a randomized controlled trial. JAMA 2008;299:2164–2171.

2 Roy-Chaudhury P, Sukhatme VP, Cheung AK: Hemodialysis vascular access dysfunction: a cellular and molecular viewpoint. J Am Soc Nephrol 2006;17:1112–1127.

3 Lee T, Barker J, Allon M: Needle infiltration of arteriovenous fistulae in hemodialysis: risk factors and consequences. Am J Kidney Dis 2006;47:1020–1026.

4 Lee T, Barker J, Allon M: Tunneled catheters in hemodialysis patients: reasons and subsequent outcomes. Am J Kidney Dis 2005;46: 501–508.

5 Ball LK: The buttonhole technique: strategies to reduce infections. Nephrol Nurs J 2010;37: 473–477; quiz 478.

6 Birchenough E, Moore C, Stevens K, Stewart S: Buttonhole cannulation in adult patients on hemodialysis: an increased risk of infection? Nephrol Nurs J 2010;37:491–498, 555; quiz 499.

7 Chow J, Rayment G, San Miguel S, Gilbert M: A randomised controlled trial of buttonhole cannulation for the prevention of fistula access complications. J Ren Care 2011;37:85–93.

8 Labriola L, Crott R, Desmet C, Andre G, Jadoul M: Infectious complications following conversion to buttonhole cannulation of native arteriovenous fistulas: a quality improvement report. Am J Kidney Dis 2011;57:442–448.

9 Dixon BS, Beck GJ, Vazquez MA, et al: Effect of dipyridamole plus aspirin on hemodialysis graft patency. N Engl J Med 2009;360:2191–2201.

10 Perl J, Wald R, McFarlane P, et al: Hemodialysis vascular access modifies the association between dialysis modality and survival. J Am Soc Nephrol 2011;22:1113–1121.
11 O'Hare AM, Bertenthal D, Walter LC, et al: When to refer patients with chronic kidney disease for vascular access surgery: should age be a consideration? Kidney Int 2007;71: 555–561.
12 DeSilva RN, Sandhu GS, Garg J, Goldfarb-Rumyantzev AS: Association between initial type of hemodialysis access used in the elderly and mortality. Hemodial Int 2012;16:233–241.
13 DeSilva RN, Patibandla BK, Vin Y, et al: Fistula first is not always the best strategy for the elderly. J Am Soc Nephrol 2013;24:1297–1304.

Prabir Roy-Chaudhury, MD, PhD
Division of Nephrology, University of Cincinnati
MSB G-251, 231, Albert Sabin Way
Cincinnati, OH 45267-0585 (USA)
E-Mail prabir.roychaudhury@ucmail.uc.edu

Widmer MK, Malik J (eds): Patient Safety in Dialysis Access.
Contrib Nephrol. Basel, Karger, 2015, vol 184, pp 143–152
DOI: 10.1159/000366122

How to Prolong the Patency of Vascular Access

Sidney Glazer[a] · Lindsey Saint[b] · Surendra Shenoy[b]

[a]Division of Vascular Surgery, Department of Surgery, University of California at Irvine, Orange, Calif., and [b]Section of Abdominal Organ Transplantation, Department of Surgery, Barnes Jewish Hospital, Washington University School of Medicine, Saint Louis, Mo., USA

Abstract

Prolonging the patency and limiting the complications of a functioning hemodialysis (HD) access require a multidisciplinary approach. It begins with careful access planning that is executed and continually reinforced by physicians and facility staff encouraging active patient participation. Vascular access (VA) dysfunctions identified by regular monitoring and surveillance need further evaluation. Color duplex ultrasound is evolving as the primary tool to evaluate functional implication of the structural problems in the VA. While ease of scheduling makes endovascular management attractive, definitive surgical management provides better longevity and should be used when indicated. Timing of intervention and selection of technique depend on optimal use of available expertise and the nature of the problem. Avoiding a bridging HD catheter should be a priority while prolonging access patency and improving patient safety.

Recommendations to Improve Patient Safety

- Prolongation of access patency begins with developing and implementing a strategy to provide vascular access (VA) for the entire end-stage renal disease life by a VA specialist and constant reinforcement by a multidisciplinary dialysis care team along with active patient participation.
- The aim of monitoring and surveillance programs is to prolong access patency and function using minimum intervention.

- Training dialysis personnel to perform physical exam before every cannulation and educating patients regarding its importance are critical to prolong patency and increase patient safety.
- While venography is a reliable tool to assess central veins, color duplex ultrasound provides both structural and functional evaluation of peripheral vessels and the VA.
- Timely intervention to prolong access patency provides uninterrupted dialysis by averting access complications.
- Repeated angioplasty is associated with decreasing efficacy; hence, it should be used judiciously.
- Surgical intervention for stenosis correction maintains options for future treatment and should be considered prior to placement of an endovascular stent.

Introduction

Advances in patient care have increased prevalence despite a decline in incidence of the end-stage renal disease (ESRD) population [1]. Hemodialysis (HD) remains the commonest mode of renal replacement therapy in the majority of countries [1]. Longevity on HD is dependent on its adequacy which is dependent on vascular access (VA) function. Arteriovenous fistula (AVF), the preferred access, has a high maturation failure rate leading to loss of multiple sites to achieve one working access. Arteriovenous graft (AVG) has better early success, but a shorter lifespan, resulting in use of multiple sites. The limitations of sites available to create a VA coupled with longevity of patients on HD highlights the importance of prolonging patency of a functioning VA. The goal of prolonging patency is to maintain access that provides adequate dialysis for the life of an ESRD patient using least number of interventions.

This chapter reviews current concepts regarding access creation, monitoring and surveillance as well as their impact on prolonging the VA patency. A focus is placed on stenotic and thrombotic complications. We discuss tools available to evaluate problems detected during monitoring/surveillance and the impact of treatment strategies on long-term patency in the context of patient safety.

VA Planning and Placement

Failure rates of VA are variable but relatively high [2, 3]. Loss of standard VA options necessitates unusual procedures (exotic access) as a desperate measure [4]. From a patient safety perspective, this represents a system failure. Reasons for failure are multifactorial with elements contributed both by the patient (education, comorbidities, compliance and follow-up) and the providers (expertise, evaluation, planning and follow-up). Proper VA planning and timely execution can often remedy the situation.

The goal of access planning is to design a sequence of surgical options for providing VA all through the lifespan of an ESRD patient. The intention is to provide a durable VA in a timely fashion with minimal future interventions and preserve future access options [5]. Involvement of the multidisciplinary team in the patient care, and reinforcement of the plan throughout the ESRD lifetime are important. Patient's acceptance and participation are critical components to execute such a plan.

Stenosis in the circuit is the commonest cause for VA failure. Stenosis is a result of myointimal hyperplasia (MIH) narrowing the lumen of the vessel to the point of occlusion. Pathophysiology demonstrates a fibromuscular thickening of the vessel wall initiated by platelet adhesion and activation, leukocyte recruitment and migration followed by myofibroblast proliferation [6]. Attempts to mitigate this response targeting one or more elements of the causative pathway using systemic agents such as aspirin, dipyridamole, clopidogrel and fish oil or topical treatments such as paclitaxel, perivascular endothelial cell wrap or pancreatic elastase have not resulted in significant clinical benefit [2, 3, 7, 8]. Recent studies using computational fluid dynamics provide compelling evidence that the ongoing injury response to shear stress caused by increased blood flow is the primary driving force for MIH. Increasing blood flow is a primary goal for VA. Fistulae that mature normally provide evidence that many veins are capable of handling increased flow [9]. Evolving data suggest that modulating flow-induced stress by altering anastomotic configuration may provide a significant benefit in prolonging access patency [10]. From the patient safety perspective, evaluation and access creation should be performed by practitioners who specialize in this field and are aware of evolving concepts. This is critical to obtain higher prolonged patency in a given access.

Access Monitoring/Surveillance

A well-functioning VA provides the prescribed blood flow (without recirculation) that ranges from 200 to 500 ml/min during dialysis treatment. Over 90% of VA dysfunction is a result of stenotic problems developing in the access circuit. Manifestation of dysfunction depends on the location of stenosis in the circuit, its diameter relative to volume of blood flow and the outflow pattern [11]. A stenosis located in the juxta-anastomotic artery or vein tends to reduce inflow. A stenosis located in the outflow vein beyond the needling segment tends to in-

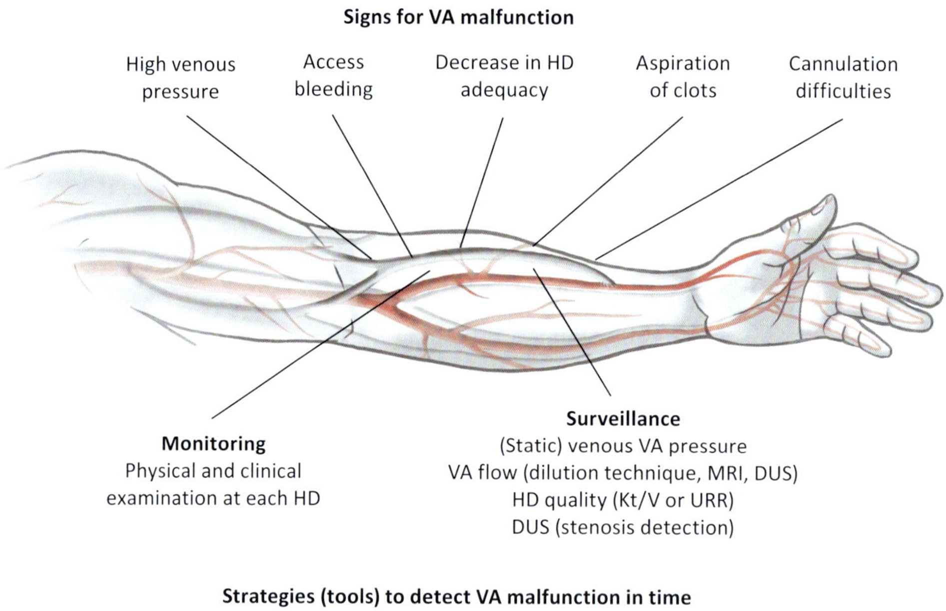

Fig. 1. Signs and tools to recognize VA dysfunction.

crease pressure within the needling area. Due to gradual development, subtle early symptoms often go unnoticed. Patient safety is enhanced by raising awareness of this problem in patients and care providers and identifying this problem when symptoms are mild. A successful monitoring/surveillance program intends to detect and follow evolving access problems and help plan timely interventions to prolong patency and ensure delivery of adequate uninterrupted dialysis (fig. 1).

The term access monitoring refers to physical examination (PE) and clinical assessment of the VA. PE has a sensitivity and specificity of 92 and 86% for outflow stenosis and 85 and 71% for inflow stenosis, respectively, in detecting AVF dysfunction [12]. PE also has up to 80% positive predictive value in detecting AVG dysfunction [13]. Limitation of PE is subjectivity and reliance on dedication for regularity and expertise of treating personnel.

The term access surveillance refers to device-based measurements (such as VA pressures and blood flow) that have been developed to overcome the limitations of PE. Serial measurements of adequacy parameters (Kt/V or urea reduction ratio – URR) of HD have not proved very useful in detecting stenosis. An acute decrease in Kt/V >0.2 units with AVG has shown a positive predictive value of 69% in detecting significant graft stenosis [13]. Clinical signs of dysfunction such as difficulty in cannulation, aspiration of clots or prolonged needle access site bleeding often prompt evaluation. Attempts to correlate these symptoms to stenosis showed a positive predictive value of 76% for prolonged bleeding, 50% for difficulty in cannulation and 30% for aspiration of clots [13]. Surveillance attempts to detect stenosis based on pressure and flow measured in the needle access segment (in the absence of other etiologies e.g. kinked tubing, poor needle position etc.). Prospective studies indicate a positive predictive value of 92% for abnormally high static VP/MAP in detecting outflow stenosis [14]. Access flow can be measured with a US dilution technique (UDT), magnetic resonance imaging, differential conductivity or duplex ultrasound (DUS). Flow monitoring shows a high positive predictive value in detecting significant stenosis [15]. It is favored over static pressure monitoring in VA. UDT is the most common surveillance method used in the United States.

Color DUS (CDUS) provides accurate and reproducible data when used for access surveillance. It provides direct visualization of the stenosis and measurement of velocity changes indicative of hemodynamic stress at the stenosis [15]. CDUS can be performed in the dialysis units, though currently it is performed in hospital laboratories or clinic settings.

Studies using flow surveillance in AVG have shown 87–100% positive predictive value in detecting hemodynamically significant stenosis. However, prophylactic intervention has failed to show a reduction in thrombosis and prolongation of AVG survival. Flow surveillance has shown benefit in reducing thrombosis with a trend towards increased longevity in AVF [16].

For AVG, NFK-KDOQI recommends PE for access monitoring. It lists use of intra-access flow, direct or derived static venous pressures and US as preferred techniques for access surveillance. For AVF, direct flow measurements, physical findings of persistent swelling of the arm, presence of collateral veins, prolonged bleeding on needle withdrawal, altered characteristics of pulse or thrill in the outflow vein and US are preferred techniques of surveillance [17].

In summary, evolving stenotic problems in VA that risk thrombosis and access loss can interfere with dialysis but go unnoticed. A recent prospective blinded AVF study has shown PE exam to rank close to flow (Qa) measurement in detecting >50% inflow stenosis and just behind VP in detecting outflow obstruction [18]. As surveillance with pressure and flow are effective in detecting stenotic problems only after they exceed a critical threshold, there is controversy about their cost effectiveness and utility in prolonging the life of an access. Training and education of patients and care providers to evaluate the access at every dialysis treatment can make significant improvement in early detection of access dysfunction at no additional cost.

Patient safety is enhanced by dialysis facilities adopting protocols for access monitoring and surveillance coupled with timely referral for evaluation based on local practices. Access dysfunction that impairs delivery of adequate dialysis should be further evaluated.

Table 1. Comparison of CDUS with fistulography for dysfunctional access evaluation

CDUS	Angiography
Noninvasive	Invasive
Can be performed in a variety of settings	Requires a specific environment and setup
Provides structural evaluation	Provides structural evaluation
Provides function evaluation	Has a limited ability to evaluate function
Used for intervention	Used for intervention
Reliable for evaluation of peripheral veins	Less reliable for evaluation of peripheral veins
Not reliable for evaluation of central veins	Reliable for evaluation of central veins
Economical	Expensive

Evaluation of Access Dysfunction

VA that is unable to provide adequate Kt/V or URR, or >25% persistent drop in Qa, or persistent elevation in static venous pressure needs to be evaluated. CDUS and fistulography are two modalities to be considered. B mode US provides direct visualization of vessel wall, lumen and surrounding tissue. It provides functional data including luminal diameter and effect on blood flow. DUS is not as reliable in evaluating the central vascular system. Fistulography, on the other hand, is an invasive technique requiring an institution-based expensive setup and provides luminal dimensions limited by the contrast flow in the vessel. A well-conducted fistulogram can provide visualization of the entire VA circuit, starting and ending at the heart. It is still considered the gold standard to evaluate central veins. Table 1 outlines the key differences between US and fistulography. Structural and functional information obtained by CDUS provides an opportunity to avoid angiography and interventions on stenosis that are not hemodynamically significant.

Management of Dysfunction to Prolong Access Patency

Needle Access Site Complications

Prolonged bleeding from the needle puncture in an AVF is often controlled with pressure. Occasionally, a simple skin suture using 3 or 4-0 monofilament nonabsorbable material like nylon or polypropylene on a noncutting needle may be necessary. Prolongation of partial thromboplastin time resulting from heparin administration during dialysis is a common cause of bleeding. Adjustment in

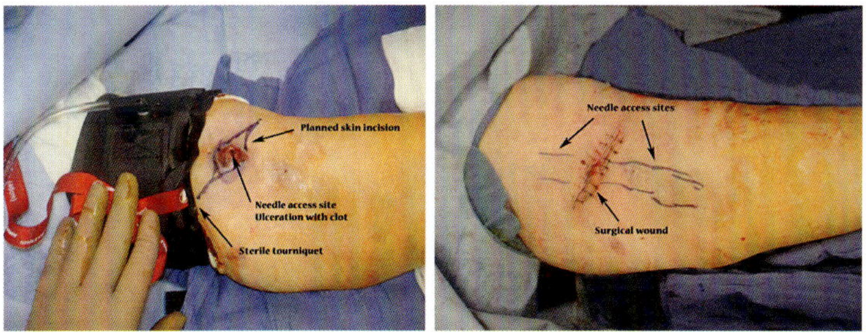

Fig. 2. Local skin excision with vein repair to preserve the same VA.

dosage of anticoagulants or antiplatelet agents may resolve the problem. PE suggesting high pressure (pulsatile access) within the access warrants further evaluation after control of acute bleeding.

A CDUS measurement of brachial artery flow upstream may reveal an outflow stenosis or a high flow (causing high intra-access pressure) risking development of aneurysms. Changing the needle puncture site is an option to prevent further problems in some patients. Avoiding needle access of aneurysms from the top where there is paucity of subcutaneous tissue and approaching them from the sides through healthy skin and subcutaneous tissue often resolves the bleeding problem and provides safe needle access [19]. Treating outflow stenosis or flow reduction should be considered when the problem persists.

Ulceration of the skin caused by infection or a neglected subcutaneous hematoma requires surgical intervention under antibiotic coverage following acute control of bleeding with site compression or suturing. Excision of infected skin, repair of the underlying vein wall defect and provision of a healthy skin cover prolongs access patency and often avoids the use of a bridging catheter. Figure 2 illustrates one such case where the access is in use all through the postoperative healing phase. While endovascular placement of a covered stent has been reported for acute management, it is at a higher risk for infection [20] making it an unsafe clinical practice.

Bleeding problems in AVG, with healthy skin, are managed similar to those in AVF. Using a covered stent is a relatively common practice in the United States for persistent bleeding or thinned out skin with underlying defects in an AVG. While there are reports of successful management of bleeding and threatened rupture, there are also reports of problems (stent fracture, stent infection and exposure through skin) with this approach. None of the covered stents available in the USA are currently approved for this indication by the FDA. Despite this, cover stents have evolved as a viable option for acute management of bleeding from AVG to prolong patency in the absence of infection [20, 21].

Stenosis

Percutaneous transluminal angioplasty (PTA) with or without stent graft placement or surgical revision are tools available to manage stenosis [22, 23]. Surgical approaches include patch angioplasty, excision of the stenotic segment with reconstruction or surgical bypass of the stenosis [24]. Details of surgical management are discussed in the chapter by Lazarides et al. [this vol., pp. 153–163].

Treating stenosis with PTA has an inherent disadvantage of inducing a fibrotic healing response, resulting in decreasing benefit with repeat procedures [25]. Bare metal stents have not shown benefit over PTA alone unless there is >30% residual stenosis or elastic recoil. Covered stents show benefit over PTA alone for stenosis at graft to vein anastomosis but fail to extend graft survival. Their longevity is limited by MIH that develops at the outflow and the inflow of the stent resulting in stenosis/occlusion and loss of proximal vein segment for surgical intervention.

Thrombosis

A thrombectomy should be attempted within 1–3 days to provide uninterrupted dialysis during acute thrombosis which is commonly seen with AVG. All thrombectomy attempts should evaluate the entire access circuit and attempt to treat the cause. Being less invasive and easier to schedule, percutaneous techniques are preferred [26]. Surgical approaches provide safety in removing acute and chronic thrombi within large aneurysms but have the disadvantages of scheduling issues and difficulty in evaluating the entire circuit. Expertise with and availability of hybrid operating rooms that provide the ability to combine the advantages of both options are ideal [27].

While 6 months' primary patency (PP) for surgical thrombectomy is marginally better (50 vs. 40%), its initial success is similar (75–90%) to endovascular technique [28]. It is common practice to consider surgical thrombectomy when the longevity of 2 successive percutaneous interventions is <3 months [29]. For definitive surgical repair, placement of an interposition graft is preferred over patching the stenosis. Recent literature suggests better PP at 1 year with surgery is better than the endovascular approach (70 vs. 50%), especially for forearm fistula. A retrospective cohort study showed better results for the hybrid approach as opposed to endovascular alone [27].

Surgical venoplasty opens the stenosis using autologous vein or artificial patch material such as polytetrafluoroethylene or bovine pericardium. Recurrent MIH results in its eventual failure by restenosis/occlusion but preserves the option for PTA and stenting. As the goal of access management is to maintain the access site for the longest period of time, we prefer surgical repair prior to stent placement for any stenotic lesion that is surgically accessible. This is an important patient safety issue in prolongation of access patency.

Summary

Prolonging the patency of an access circuit is a key element for patient safety. It starts with optimal access planning utilizing DUS and surgical techniques that minimize hemodynamic stress responsible for the development of MIH. Monitoring, surveillance and timely interventions play a key role in prolonging the access patency. It is important that the access plan developed and communicated to the patient gets reinforced by all personnel involved in patient care activities.

Disclosure Statement

The authors have no conflicts of interest to declare.

References

1 US Renal Data System, USRDS 2013 Annual Data report: Atlas of chronic kidney disease and end stage renal disease in the United States. Bethesda, National Institutes of Health, National Institutes of Diabetes and Digestive and Kidney Diseases, 2013, 2.1.1 p 217, 2.12.3 p 338.
2 Dixon BS, Beck GJ, Vazquez MA, et al: Effect of dipyridamole and aspirin on hemodialysis graft patency. N Engl J Med 2009;360:2191–2201.
3 Dember LM, Beck GJ, Allon M, et al: Effect of clopidogrel on early failure of arteriovenous fistulas for hemodialysis: a randomized controlled trial. JAMA 2008;299:2164–2171.
4 Anaya-Ayala JE, Bellows PFH, Ismail N, et al: Surgical management of hemodialysis related central venous occlusive disease: a treatment algorithm. Ann Vasc Surg 2011;25:108–119.
5 Okada S, Shenoy S: Arteriovenous access for hemodialysis: preoperative assessment and planning. J Vasc Access 2014;15(suppl 7):s1–s5.
6 Lee T, Roy-Chaudhury P: Advances and new frontiers in the pathophysiology of neointimal hyperplasia and dialysis access stenosis. Adv Chronic Kidney Dis 2009;16:329–338.
7 Yevzlin AS, Conley EL, Sanchez RJ, Young HN, Becker BN: Vascular access outcomes and medication use: a USRDS study. Semin Dial 2006;19:535–539.
8 Lok CE, Moist L, Hemmelgarn BR, et al: Effect of fish oil supplementation on graft patency and cardiovascular events among patients with new synthetic arteriovenous hemodialysis grafts. A randomized controlled trial. JAMA 2012;307:1809–1816.

9 Remuzzi A, Ene-lordache B: Novel paradigms for dialysis vascular access: upstream hemodynamics and vascular remodelling in dialysis access stenosis. Clin J Am Soc Nephrol 2013;8:2186–2193.
10 Bharat A, Jaenicke M, Shenoy S: A novel technique of vascular anastomosis to prevent juxta-anastomotic stenosis following arteriovenous fistula creation. J Vasc Surg 2012;55:274–280.
11 Hoganson DM, Hinkel CJ, Chen X, Agarwal RK, Shenoy S: Validation of computational fluid dynamics-based analysis to evaluate hemodynamic significance of access stenosis. J Vasc Access 2014;15:409–414.
12 Asif A, Leon C, Orozco-Vargas LC, et al: Accuracy of physical examination in the detection of arteriovenous fistula stenosis. Clin J Am Soc Nephrol 2007;2:1191–1194
13 Robbin ML, Oser RF, Lee JY, et al: Randomized comparison of ultrasound surveillance and clinical monitoring on arteriovenous graft outcomes. Kidney Int 2006;69:7305.
14 Besarab A, Sullivan KL, Ross RP, Moritz MJ: Utility of intra access pressure in detecting and correcting venous outlet stenosis prior to thrombosis. Kidney Int 1995;47:1364–1373.
15 Moist LM, Churchill DN, House AA, et al: Regular monitoring of access flow compared with monitoring of venous pressure fails to improve graft survival. J Am Soc Nephrol 2003;14:2645.
16 Tessitore N, Bedogna V, Verlato G, et al: The rise and fall of access blood flow surveillance in arteriovenous fistulas. Semin Dial 2014;27:108–118.
17 NKF-KDOQI clinical practice guidelines and clinical practice recommendations for vascular access, update 2006. Am J Kidney Dis 2006;48(suppl 1):S177–S247.
18 Tessitore N, Bedogna V, Melili E, et al: In search of optimal bedside screening program for arteriovenous fistula stenosis. Clin J Am Soc Nephrol 2011;6:819–826.
19 Wilson NA, Shenoy S: Managing 'buttonhole' complications. J Vasc Access 2014;15(suppl 7):s91–s95.
20 Kim CY, Guevara CJ, Engstrom BI, et al: Analysis of infection risk following covered stent exclusion of pseudoaneurysms in prosthetic arteriovenous hemodialysis access grafts. J Vasc Interv Radiol 2012;23:69–74.
21 Peden EK: Role of stent grafts for the treatment of failing hemodialysis accesses. Semin Vasc Surg 2011;24:119–127.
22 Falk A: Maintenance and salvage of arteriovenous fistulas. J Vasc Interv Radiol 2006;17:807–813.
23 Cull DL, Washer JD, Carsten CG, et al: Description and outcomes of a simple surgical technique to treat thrombosed autogenous accesses. J Vasc Surg 2012;56:861–865.
24 Georgladia GS, Lazarides MK, Lambidis CD, et al: Use of short PTFE segments (<6 cm) compares favorably with pure autologous repair in failing or thrombosed native arteriovenous fistulas. J Vasc Surg 2005;41:76–81.
25 Chang C, Ko P, Hsu L, et al: Highly increased cell proliferation activity in the restenotic hemodialysis vascular access after percutaneous transluminal angioplasty: implication in prevention of restenosis. Am J Kidney Dis 2004;43:74–84.
26 Bittl JA: Catheter interventions for hemodialysis fistulas and grafts. J Am Coll Cardiol Intv 2010;3:1–11.
27 Hyun JH, Lee JH, Park SI: Hybrid surgery versus percutaneous mechanical thrombectomy for the thrombosed hemodialysis autogenous arteriovenous fistulas. J Korean Surg Soc 2011;81:43–49.
28 Klimach SG, Norris JM: Surgical versus endovascular management of thrombosed autogenous arteriovenous fistulae. Int J Surg 2014;12:237–240.
29 Tordoir JHM, Bode AS, Peppelenbosch N, et al: Surgical or endovascular repair of thrombosed dialysis vascular access: is there any evidence? J Vasc Surg 2009;50:953–956.

Surendra Shenoy, MD, PhD
Section of Abdominal Organ Transplantation, Department of Surgery
Barnes Jewish Hospital, Washington University School of Medicine
Campus Box 8109
660 South Euclid Blvd
Saint Louis, MO 63110 (USA)
E-Mail shenoysu@wustl.edu

Widmer MK, Malik J (eds): Patient Safety in Dialysis Access.
Contrib Nephrol. Basel, Karger, 2015, vol 184, pp 153–163
DOI: 10.1159/000365912

Safety Issues in Surgical and Endovascular Techniques to Rescue Failing or Failed Arteriovenous Fistulas and Arteriovenous Grafts

Miltos Lazarides • George Georgiadis • Christos Argyriou

Department of Vascular Surgery, Democritus University Hospital, Alexandroupolis, Greece

Abstract

A great variety of thrombotic and nonthrombotic events may complicate all types of vascular access (VA) procedures. Thrombotic events are the most frequent complication, caused by stenoses in various locations, representing a common problem for arteriovenous fistulas (AVFs) and arteriovenous grafts (AVGs). Monitoring AVF with physical examination by trained physicians represents an accurate method for diagnosis of malfunction. AVF stenoses >50% in diameter should be treated either by surgical or endovascular means when accompanied with access malfunction. Aneurysms and infections represent the most frequent nonthrombotic VA complications. Access-related aneurysms do not represent per se an indication for intervention; however, anastomotic aneurysms and those with skin erosion should be repaired urgently to avoid rupture. Infections of AVFs are extremely rare, while AVG could be complicated either with postoperative infections attributable to the initial procedure with an early onset and more frequently with late infections caused by punctures, with an annual rate of 5%. Treatment options for AVG infections comprise total or subtotal graft excision or partial excision of the involved segment only, the latter representing a VA salvage procedure but with a significantly higher risk of recurrence.

Recommendations to Improve Patient Safety

- Check after creation of an arteriovenous fistula or arteriovenous graft (AVG) for palpable thrill or a bruit: The presence of a strong pulse in the draining vein without a thrill or bruit indicates a proximal venous stenosis. Patients need an instruction when checking their vascular access (VA) daily for bruit and thrill.

- Failed or failing VA needs revision by surgical or endovascular means depending on the location of the lesion. Check thrombosed accesses after thrombectomy for underlying stenotic lesions that have to be corrected.
- Anastomotic aneurysms and those with skin erosion (mostly false aneurysm of AVG) should be repaired urgently to avoid rupture and life-threatening hemorrhage. Patients should be informed about this complication.
- Aneurysms are often associated with proximal stenosis, and this should be corrected simultaneously.
- The best policy to prevent infection is to limit the implantation of synthetic prostheses only to patients with no autogenous options.

Introduction

The failure of vascular access (VA) represents the major cause of morbidity for those end-stage renal disease patients on hemodialysis, and access maintenance is the most frequent cause of hospitalization for such patients [1]. The subsequent extended length of stay commonly encountered in older patients is also related to further adverse events as hospital-acquired infections and fever, prolonged catheterization predisposing to central venous obstruction and delay in access revision with increased associated costs. The VA maintenance cost increases 5-fold for those patients with a failed autogenous access [2].

A great variety of thrombotic and nonthrombotic events may complicate all types of VA procedures and necessitate a wide spectrum of rescue operations.

Stenoses and Thrombosis in Arteriovenous Fistulas or Grafts

Thrombotic events represent the most frequent complication of all VA with an incidence rate of 0.2/patient/year for arteriovenous fistula (AVF) and 0.8/patient/year for synthetic arteriovenous graft (AVG) [3]. Therefore, redo surgery is the rule rather than exception in VA patients.

Stenosis is a common problem for AVFs and AVGs and represents the main cause of dysfunction and thrombosis, and the choice of the best method for repair depends on the location of the lesion. Access stenosis has been classified based on its location as: juxta-anastomotic (type I), in the cannulable segment (type II) and at the outflow into the deep venous system (type III) [4] (fig. 1). There are two additional categories of stenoses not involving the access itself, those of the central veins caused by longstanding catheters and those of the arterial inflow [5].

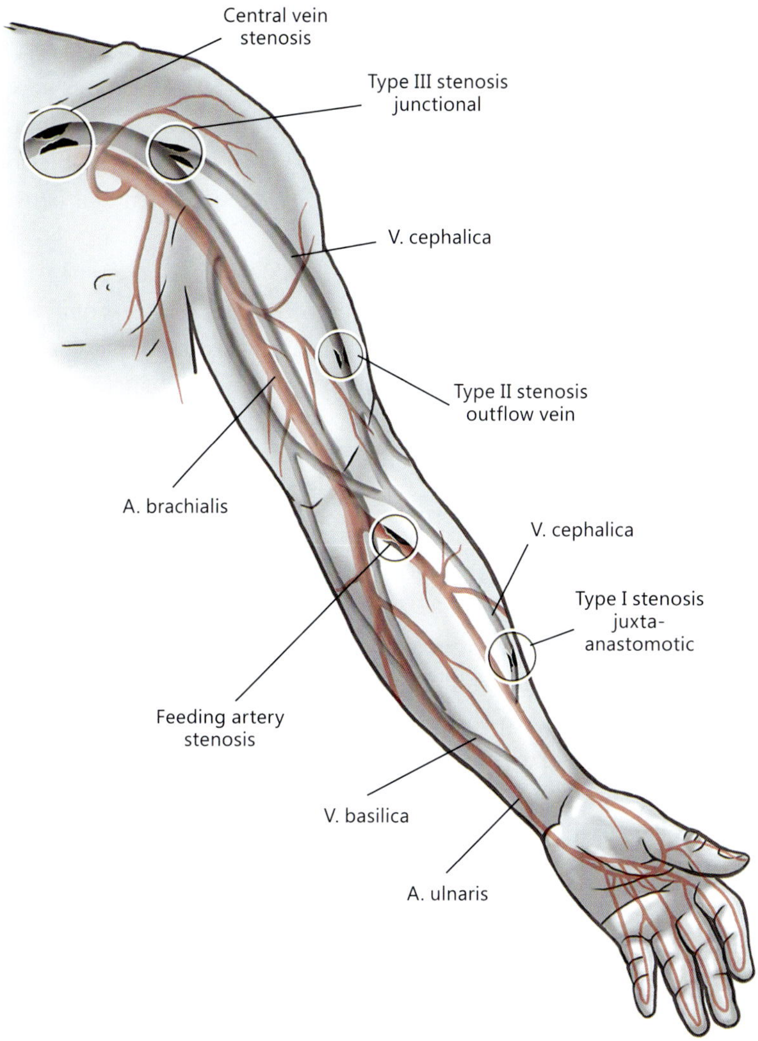

Fig. 1. Schematic representation of the main types of stenotic lesions complicating accesses.

Juxta-anastomotic type I stenosis is the most frequent reason for access dysfunction, especially in the distal radiocephalic AVFs. With endovascular means, in most cases the fibrotic perianastomotic tissue necessitates high-pressure or cutting balloons and prolonged dilatation times, and therefore most authors suggest surgical revision instead, with creation of a new anastomosis a few centimeters proximally; however, in brachiocephalic AVF, a short polytetrafluorethylene segment may be needed to bridge the greater distance between the artery and the vein [5, 6].

Type II is a mid-vein cannulable segment stenosis and should be first treated with PTA (percutaneous transluminal angioplasty) in autogenous accesses in order to preserve the length of the needling site of the vein; however, in case of failure an interposition graft should be inserted [4]. In this type of lesions, the dialysis dose is usually not affected because the stenosis often falls between the arterial and venous needles [5].

Type I and II stenoses are not frequent in AV grafts, where type III stenosis is the predominant type of stenosis causing access failure and should be treated either by endovascular or open surgical means consisting of patch angioplasty or jump graft repair depending of center's experience and availability. Regarding the endovascular methods of treatment, stent grafts have better patency rates in comparison to PTA alone according to a recent randomized study [7]. Cephalic arch stenosis is the equivalent of type III stenosis in AVF; PTA should be the first choice as the use of stents may cause axillary vein obstruction, while surgical cephalic vein transposition is an alternative option with equal patency but fewer reinterventions [8].

Stenoses of central veins principally induced by longstanding catheters can become symptomatic as a result of increased flow when an ipsilateral AV fistula is functioning distally to an obstruction. In case of complete venous outflow obstruction, venous hypertension with intractable upper arm painful edema occasionally involving the breast and head may necessitate urgent intervention to avoid tissue loss of the fingers. Access ligation and abandonment bring immediate relief of the complaints but requires a new access creation, which is not always feasible. Surgical repair of the inflow obstruction is not recommended as first choice because of the significant morbidity and mortality of such 'exotic' major operations, in opposition, PTA is recommended as the treatment of choice, but it is a matter of debate if primary stenting would be a better option [9].

Arterial inflow stenoses represent atherosclerotic lesions proximal to the anastomosis, and their clinical picture is usually characterized by delayed AVF maturation. These lesions usually involving the radial artery are best treated with PTA [10].

All accesses should be evaluated immediately after their creation and then routinely examined during their life span. After creation of an AVF or AVG, there should be a palpable thrill or a bruit; the presence of a strong pulse in the draining vein without a thrill or bruit indicates a proximal venous stenosis. Monitoring AVF with physical examination by trained physicians represents an accurate method for diagnosis of malfunction [11].

AVF stenoses >50% in diameter should be treated either by surgical or endovascular means when accompanied with low flow, difficulties in cannulation, painful edema or prolonged bleeding at puncture sites [12] (fig. 2). None of the

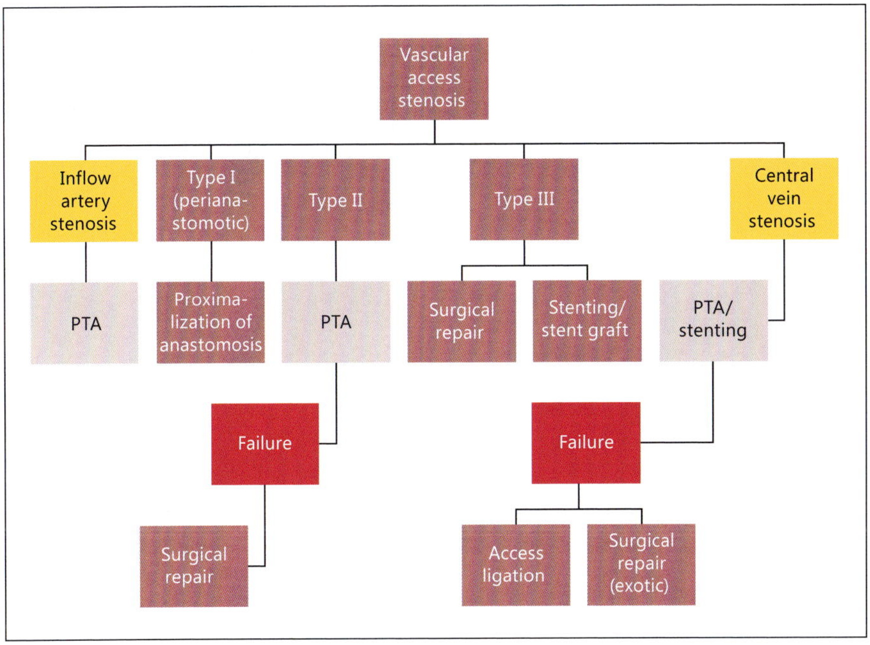

Fig. 2. Algorithm of the preferential treatment methods in failing accesses.

currently available surveillance methods (periodic assessment using technical devices) can reliably distinguish between stenosed VA destined to clot, and those that will remain patent without intervention [13]. As a consequence, a percentage of unnecessary angioplasties are performed based on surveillance findings only.

Thrombosis of AVF necessitates treatment as quickly as possible because delayed intervention allows the thrombus to propagate, and become fixed to the vein wall with a local inflammation, making any thrombectomy attempt difficult and predisposing to arterial wall damage with its risk of re-thrombosis. Thrombosed VA can be treated either by an open or endovascular intervention. Thrombectomy alone is generally insufficient unless the underlying stenotic lesion is corrected.

Aneurysms

Aneurysms may complicate 2–10% of all types of VA [14]. These may be false aneurysms (also called pseudoaneurysms from the Greek word pseudos: false) and true aneurysms caused by degeneration and subsequent dilatation of the

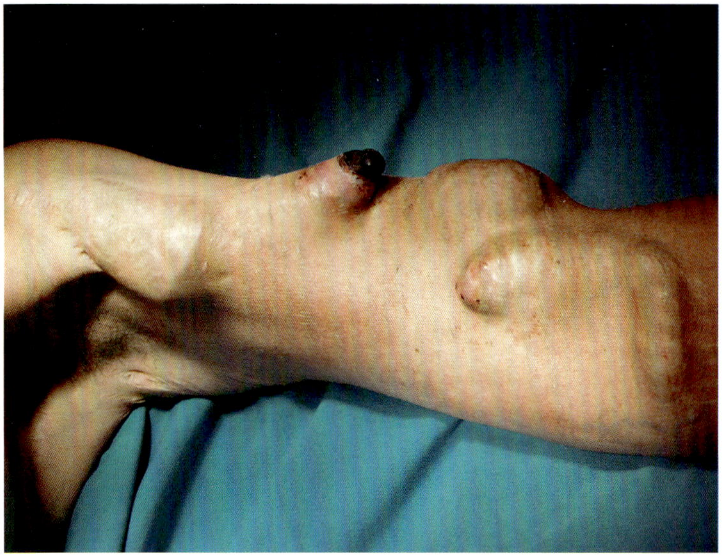

Fig. 3. Skin erosion about to rupture caused by a false aneurysm in a brachiocephalic AVF.

Table 1. Indications for surgical repair of aneurysms in AVG and AVF

	AVGs	AVFs
Size exceeding 2-fold the graft diameter	✓	–
Rapid enlargement	✓	–
Skin thinning or erosion	✓	✓
Rupture	✓	✓
Pain (throbbing)	✓	✓
Large or multiple aneurysms limiting the cannulable area	✓	✓
Signs of infection	✓	–
Wall-adherent thrombus	–	✓
Anastomotic aneurysms	✓	✓
Cosmetic reasons	?	?

whole native vein wall. In contrast to AVF where true aneurysms are the most frequent type, aneurysms in AVG occur mostly as false aneurysms and less frequently as anastomotic aneurysms. The false aneurysms represent a chronic blood extravasation through a circumscribed graft defect surrounded by thrombi encapsulated in a gradually developed fibrous false wall. The updated DOQI guidelines differentiate between true and false aneurysms and suggest surgical treatment of the enlarging false aneurysms and those exceeding twice the diameter of the graft to prevent the risk of acute rupture. The indications for surgical repair of aneurysms summarizing suggestions from guidelines and articles are presented in table 1 [15, 16]. Access-related aneurysms do not represent per se an indication for surgery; however, anastomotic aneurysms and those with skin erosion should be repaired urgently to avoid rupture and life-threatening hemorrhage (fig. 3).

Pseudoaneurysms can be managed either with conventional surgery or with endovascular techniques; however, conventional surgery represents the current standard treatment [17, 18]. Surgical correction includes resection of the involved segment and new graft interposition in situ, or aneurysm ligation/exclusion followed by a bypass graft adjacent to the old one via new route in cases of suspected contamination of the sac [16].

There are many recent series reporting results of stent graft repairs in AVG but with small number of patients and limited follow-up; contraindications of this method include overt graft infection, presence of skin erosion, need to cross the elbow or axilla and lack of adequate landing zones [18, 19]. Aneurysms are often associated with proximal stenosis and both lesions should be treated simultaneously [18].

True aneurysms can be repaired with aneurysmorrhaphy (fig. 4), where the excess sac of the aneurysm is resected, and a new autogenous access is reconstructed by plicating the excess free wall [17].

Infection

Infection of autogenous accesses is extremely rare, while AVG could be complicated with two main types of infections: (1) postoperative infections attributable to the initial access procedure with an early onset (<1 month) and an incidence of 0.8%, representing only 6% of the total AVG infections and (2) late infections caused by punctures, representing >50% of the total, with an annual rate of 5% [20]. Bacteremias are 5 times more frequent in grafts than in AVF (3.1 vs. 0.6 bloodstream infections per 100 patient months) [21]. Staphylococcus species are the most common culprits in over 70% of the cases [22].

The difference between AVF and AVG is that infection in autogenous accesses can be treated successfully with antibiotics (and potential drainage) with the exception of those infections involving the anastomosis because of the risk of suture line bleeding and those complicated with septic emboli necessitating access ligation.

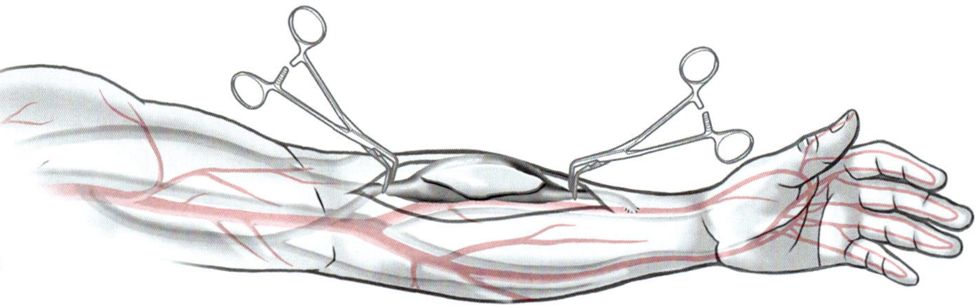

a

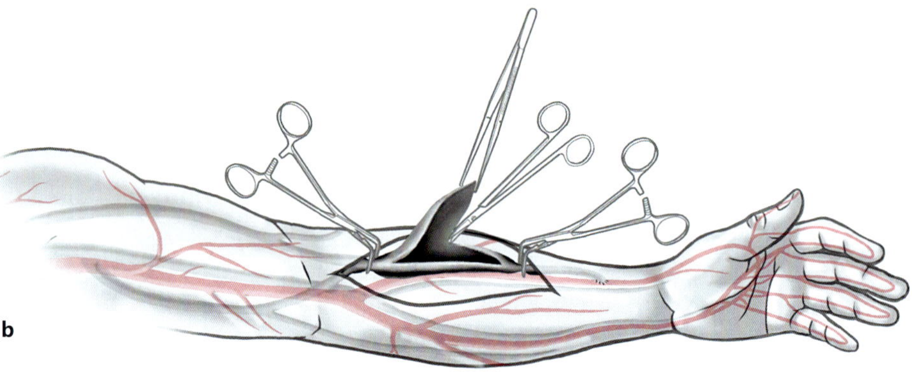

b

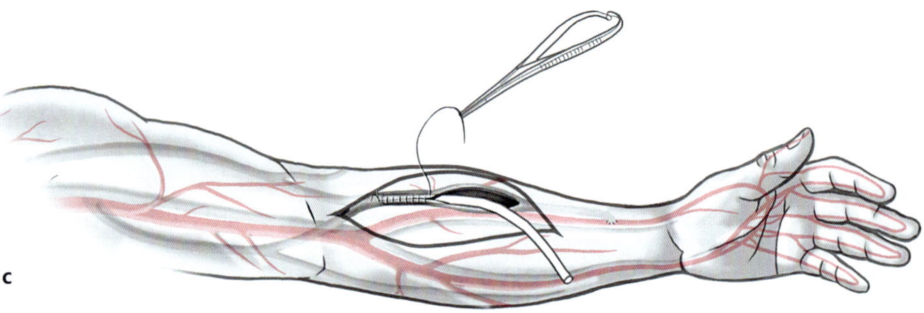

c

Fig. 4. Details how to perform aneurysmorrhaphy to correct true AVF aneurysm: **a** Incision of overlapping skin with preparation of the aneurysm to control in- and outflow. **b** Excision of the aneurysmatic vein wall. **c** Suture line using a tube graft as model to complete a 'new' vein with a diameter of approximately 6 mm.

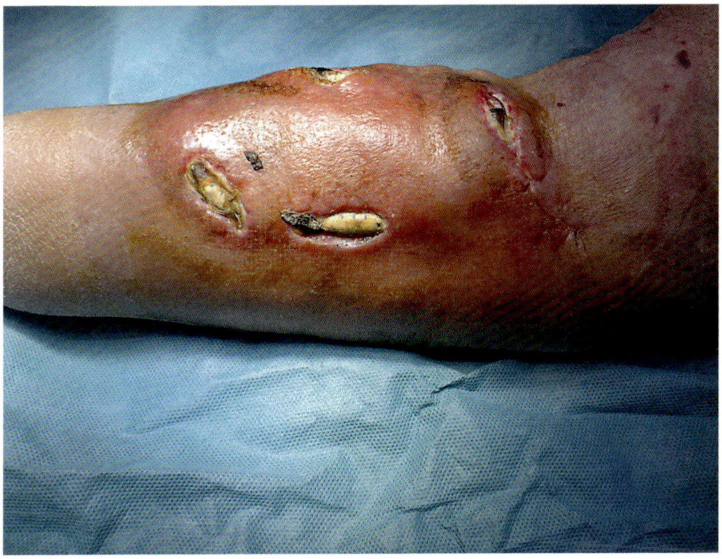

Fig. 5. Infected forearm loop AVG with skin erosion; the inflammatory infiltration involves the entire AVG, and total excision is mandatory.

Treatment options for AVG infections comprise: (1) total graft excision, with optional vein patching of the donor artery anastomotic site; (2) subtotal graft excision with an oversewn cuff of prosthetic material left at the donor artery site; the latter avoids hazardous dissection near an artery fixed in scar tissue, minimizing the risk of accidental adjacent nerve damage or hemorrhage, and (3) partial excision of the involved segment only, with interposition of a new graft through an uncontaminated field via a new route [23].

Total graft excision represents the most effective way to eradicate the infection with a very low recurrence rate of 1.6%. In early infections, in the vast majority of cases the graft is not incorporated in the adjacent tissues, and it is easily removed through multiple short incisions; the latter should be left open to heal by secondary intention. Partial excision of the infected segment rescues the access site but has a 29% risk of recurrence. This method is particularly applicable where the infection is 'late', usually local in nature and cannot easily spread along a well-incorporated graft [23].

Ultrasound is useful to locate fluid collections and determine the extent of the infection; when there is inflammatory infiltration of the entire graft length, total excision should be undertaken (fig. 5). Although theoretically biological grafts should be preferential over polytetrafluorethylene grafts in infected areas, the former did not fulfill expectations regarding patency and frequently are complicated with aneurysmal degeneration [24].

The best policy to prevent infection is to limit the implantation of synthetic prostheses only to patients with no autogenous options, and in these cases meticulous antiseptic measures and use of surgical drapes are crucial. Avoiding premature puncturing of AVG (<3 weeks from creation), perioperative antibiotic prophylaxis and careful needling with a sterile technique after maturation is the recommended policy [24].

Disclosure Statement

The authors have no conflicts of interest to declare.

References

1 Mayers JD, Markell MS, Cohen LS, et al: Vascular access surgery for maintenance hemodialysis. Variables in hospital stay. ASAIO J 1992;38:113–115.

2 Lee H, Manns B, Taub K, et al: Cost analysis of ongoing care of patients with ESRD: the impact of dialysis modality and dialysis access. Am J Kidney Dis 2002;40:611–622.

3 Tordoir JH, van der Sande FM, de Haan MW: Current topics on vascular access for hemodialysis. Minerva Urol Nefrol 2004;56: 23–35.

4 Mickley V: Stenosis and thrombosis in haemodialysis fistulae and grafts: the surgeon's point of view. Nephrol Dial Transplant 2004; 19:309–311.

5 Pirozzi N, Garcia-Medina J, Hanoy M: Stenosis complicating vascular access for hemodialysis: indications for treatment. J Vasc Access 2014;15:76–82.

6 Long B, Brichart N, Lermusiaux P, et al: Management of perianastomotic stenosis of direct wrist autogenous radial-cephalic arteriovenous accesses for dialysis. J Vasc Surg 2011;53:108–114.

7 Haskal ZJ, Trerotola S, Dolmatch B, et al: Stent graft versus balloon angioplasty for failing dialysis-access grafts. N Engl J Med 2010; 362:494–503.

8 Sigala F, Sassen R, Elissaios Kontis E, et al: Surgical treatment of cephalic arch stenosis by central transposition of the cephalic vein. J Vasc Access 2014;15:272–277.

9 Mickley V: Central vein obstruction in vascular access. Eur J Vasc Endovasc Surg 2006;32: 439–444.

10 Turmel-Rodrigues L, Boutin JM, Camiade C, Brillet G, Fodil-Chérif M, Mouton A: Percutaneous dilation of the radial artery in nonmaturing autogenous radial-cephalic fistulas for haemodialysis. Nephrol Dial Transplant 2009;24:3782–3788.

11 Coentrao L, Turmel-Rodrigues L: Monitoring dialysis AVF: it's in our hands. J Vasc Access 2013;14:209–215.

12 Tordoir J, Canaud B, Haage P, et al: EBPG on vascular access. Nephrol Dial Transplant 2007;22 (suppl):88–117.

13 Allon M, Robbin ML: Hemodialysis vascular access monitoring: current concepts. Hemodial Int 2009;13:153–162.

14 Ballard JL, Bunt TJ, Malone JM: Major complications of angioaccess surgery. Am J Surg 1992;164:229–232.

15 National Kidney Foundation KDOQI: Clinical practice guidelines and clinical practice recommendations for 2006 updates: hemodialysis adequacy, peritoneal dialysis adequacy and vascular access. Am J Kidney Dis 2006; 48(suppl):S1–S322.

16 Georgiadis GS, Lazarides MK, Panagoutsos SA, et al: Surgical revision of complicated false and true vascular access related aneurysms. J Vasc Surg 2008;47:1284–1291.

17 Derungs U, Wyss TR, Stellmes A, Schmidli J, Widmer MK: Management von echten und falschen Aneurysmen bei Hämodialyse-shunts. Gefässchirurgie 2012;17:115–121.
18 Shemesh D, Goldin I, Zaghal I, Berelowitz D, Verstandig AG, Olsha O: Stent graft treatment for hemodialysis access aneurysms. J Vasc Surg 2011;54:1088–1094.
19 Zink JN, Netzley R, Erzurum V, Wright D: Complications of endovascular grafts in the treatment of pseudoaneurysms and stenoses in arteriovenous access. J Vasc Surg 2013;57:144–148.
20 Schild AF, Simon S, Prieto J, et al: Single-center review of infections associated with 1574 consecutive vascular access procedures. Vasc Endovasc Surg 2003;37:27–31.
21 Klevens RM, Tokars JI, Andrus M: Electronic reporting of infections associated with hemodialysis. Nephrol News Issues 2005;19:37–43.
22 Ponce P, Cruz J, Ferreira A, et al: A prospective study on incidence of bacterial infections in Portuguese dialysis units. Nephron Clin Pract 2007;107:133–138.
23 Lazarides MK, Georgiadis G, Nikolopoulos E: Surgical intervention for vascular access infection; in Tordoir J (ed): Best Practice in Vascular Access. Turin, Edizioni Minerva Medica, 2010, pp 151–159.
24 Stellmes A, Wyss T, Schmidli J, Widmer M: Biological grafts in infected patients; in Tordoir J (ed): Best Practice in Vascular Access. Turin, Edizioni Minerva Medica, 2010, pp 169–177.

Miltos Lazarides, MD
Marathonos 13, N. Chili
GR–68100 Alexandroupolis (Greece)
E-Mail mlazarid@med.duth.gr

Widmer MK, Malik J (eds): Patient Safety in Dialysis Access.
Contrib Nephrol. Basel, Karger, 2015, vol 184, pp 164–175
DOI: 10.1159/000366050

Vascular Access-Induced Hand Ischemia: Risks and Safe Management

Carmine Sessa[a] • Albéric De Lambert[a] • Augustin Pirvu[a] • Pedro Palacin[c] • Olivier Pichot[b]

Departments of [a]Vascular and Thoracic Surgery and [b]Angiology, University Hospital Grenoble, and [c]Hemodialysis Center AGDUC Grenoble, Grenoble, France

Abstract

Hand ischemia is rare but complex and multifactorial. Distal arteriopathy below the vascular access (VA) is responsible in the vast majority of patients and not a problem of high flow of the VA. Therefore, surgical technique should focus on improving blood flow and pressure instead of reducing blood flow. We present an overview of the standard techniques which are recommended to treat VA-induced hand ischemia. The banding techniques, most of which empirical and not codified, have been abandoned by the majority of the authors because of a high rate of failure and reintervention. Ligation may be necessary in patients with severe ischemia and diffuse arterial lesions and in case of ischemic monomelic neuropathy.

Recommendations to Improve Patient Safety

- Developing severe ischemic symptoms requires prompt recognition and treatment to avoid irreversible neurological damage and extensive tissue loss leading to major amputation.
- Surgical techniques such as distal revascularization and interval ligation aimed to improve blood flow and pressure to the hand without changing flow through the vascular access are key. Other techniques i.e. revision using distal inflow proximalization of arterial inflow/proximalization of the arteriovenous anastomosis are aimed to improve blood flow of the hand by reducing VA flow. Banding is not popular yet.

- Ligation of the distal radial artery below an end-to-side radiocephalic fistula is effective in treating reversal of flow in patients with patent ulnar and digital arteries.
- Ligation may be necessary in patients with severe ischemia and arterial lesions or in case of ischemic monomelic neuropathy.

Clinical Presentation of Hand Ischemia

Hand ischemia is a severe adverse event in vascular access (VA) surgery that has an incidence of 1–10% [1–29]. Symptoms are usually mild with extremity coolness and vague neurosensory changes and, in most cases, resolve within a few weeks and clinical presentation can be classified into 4 stages [1].

Development of severe threatening acute or disabling chronic ischemic symptoms that requires prompt recognition and appropriate treatment occurs in approximately 5% (1–8%) of patients with VA [1–3, 6–8]. Clinical manifestations are most commonly symptoms of chronic critical ischemia such as rest pain, muscle weakness, digital ulcerations and finger or hand gangrene. Patients at risk of developing ischemic symptoms are more likely to be female, diabetics with brachial origin fistula who have forearm and digital arteriopathy [1–3, 16].

Ischemic monomelic neuropathy is a rare cause of severe sensory-motor impairment of the forearm that occurs immediately after fistula creation and where often no clear signs of finger malperfusion can be seen. Such a situation requires immediate ligation of the VA. It is thought to be due to a transient reduction in blood flow that causes ischemia of the vasa nervorum with sudden and permanent sensory and motor impairment involving multiple nerve groups of a distal limb. Ischemic monomelic neuropathy is most commonly associated with diabetes, atherosclerotic vascular disease, and brachiocephalic and prosthetic grafts [3].

The diagnosis of hand ischemia is suspected clinically, and the diagnosis is confirmed by measurement of distal and/or forearm Doppler pressure and flow and by recording digital pulse wave plethysmography, with and without manual compression of the fistula [11, 13]. Increase in distal pressure or improvement of the pulse wave after access compression confirms hemodynamic ischemic symptoms. Digital pulse oximetry has also proved useful in diagnosing VA-induced hand ischemic syndrome. A fistulogram, with and without VA compression, may document the presence of flow reversal and evaluate the arterial status below the VA.

Prompt recognition and appropriate treatment are necessary to avoid irreversible neurological damage and extensive tissue loss leading to finger or major hand and forearm amputation [1, 2, 4].

Treatment Concept of Hand Ischemia

The purpose of treatment is to relieve ischemic symptoms by improving distal perfusion to the hand, while preserving VA. The choice of the more appropriate technique should be based on the underlying hemodynamic mechanism of ischemia and the location of the arteriovenous fistula (AVF) [21–23]. Since the vast majority of patients with hand ischemia do not have VA high flow defined as a flow greater than 1.5 l/min, the choice of the technique should focus on improving distal flow to the hand rather than focusing on reducing the flow of the VA.

The various surgical techniques designed to treat ischemia and to preserve the access include:

(1) Distal radial artery ligation below an end-to-side radiocephalic AVF to treat reversal of flow [10–13].

(2) Techniques aimed to improve blood flow of the hand without changes of the VA flow such as distal revascularization and interval ligation (DRIL) [1–8, 15–23].

(3) Techniques aimed to improve blood flow of the hand by reducing VA flow, i.e. banding, revision using distal inflow (RUDI) [17, 18, 27], proximalization of arterial inflow (PAI) or proximalization of the arteriovenous anastomosis (PAVA) [25, 28, 29].

Treatment of Hand Ischemia at the Wrist

In patients with patent ulnar and digital arteries, occlusion of the distal radial artery below the fistula by ligation or embolization is an easy and simple way of treating the VA-induced hand ischemia (fig. 1) [10–13]. This technique described by Storey et al. [10] effectively eliminates the steal and restores antegrade flow to fingers. Before considering ligation of the artery, evidence of the efficiency of this approach can be documented by relief of symptoms after manual compression of the artery below the AVF [11]. Measurement of distal and/or forearm Doppler pressure and of digital pulse wave plethysmography with and without manual compression of the fistula is also useful. Intraoperative occlusion of the distal radial artery with a ballon catheter with an increase in radial pressure can further demonstrate that occlusion of the radial artery would be beneficial in ischemic symptoms [11, 13]. Miller et al. [13] reported 15 cases; 10 were treated with embolization and 5, in whom embolization was not possible, with ligation. Complete resolution of symptoms was experienced in 100% (10/10) of patients who received distal radial artery embolization and by 3/5 patients who required ligation.

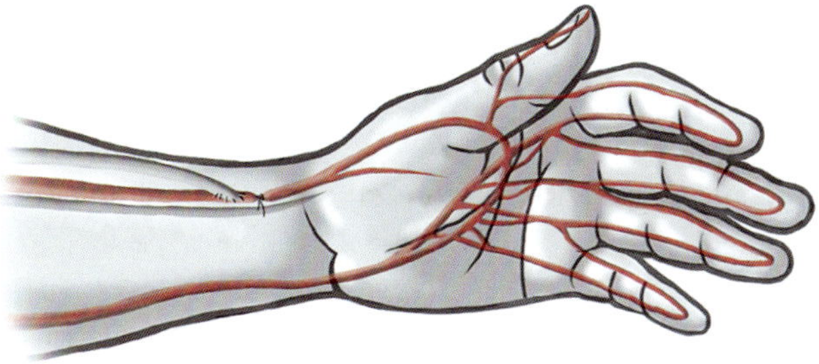

Fig. 1. Treatment strategy of hand ischemia at the wrist – performing a distal radial artery ligation.

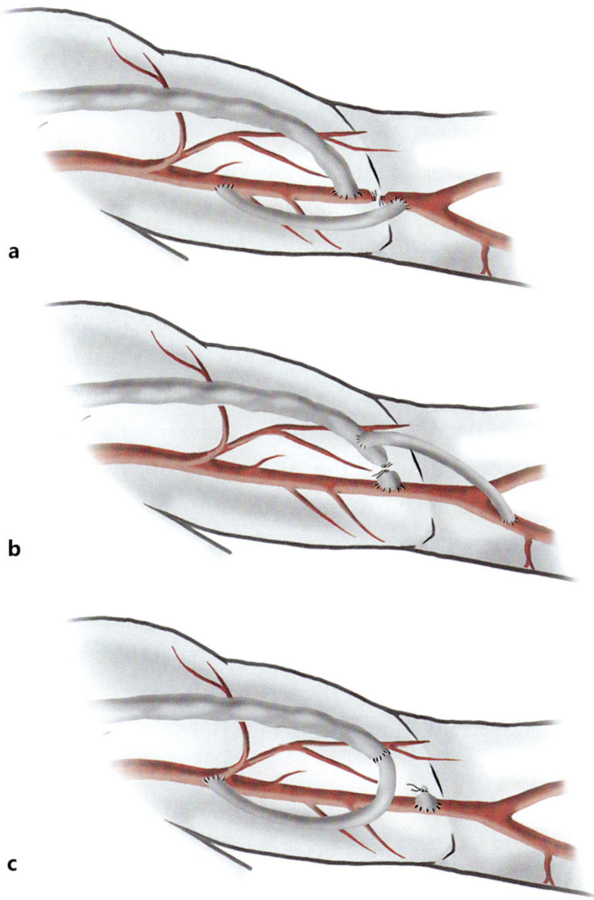

Fig. 2. Schematic representation of the different procedures: DRIL (**a**), RUDI (**b**) and PAVA (**c**).

Another option is a DRIL procedure. The DRIL procedure in the forearm (described in detail for the upper arm below) aimed to improve blood flow to the hand is the best option in patients with severe forearm and digital arteriopathy. If distal ligation and DRIL are not an option or are not successful, fistula ligation is mandatory.

Treatment of Hand Ischemia at the Elbow in Patients with Normal VA Flow

The DRIL Technique and Results

The DRIL technique, which was initially described by Schanzer et al. [2] and subsequently reported by many authors, has clearly shown to improve distal perfusion [7, 21–23], allowing relief of ischemic symptoms and maintenance of fistula function [8, 12, 15–17, 19–26]. The DRIL technique works by establishing anterograde flux in the hand and by eliminating retrograde flow. A bypass constructed of reversed saphenous vein or PTFE is anastomosed to the brachial artery 10 cm above the arteriovenous anastomosis to avoid diastolic retrograde flow from the bypass to the fistula (fig. 2). Gradman and Pozrikidis [30] have shown that performing the DRIL bypass distal to the brachial artery (mid-brachial DRIL) proportionally reduces the forearm blood flow compared to the more proximal DRIL at 10 cm above the fistula. The vein graft is then anastomosed distally in the forearm either to the brachial, ulnar or radial artery. The artery is then ligated just below the AVF to eliminate retrograde flow towards the fistula (fig. 2) and directs flow in the bypass to the distal arterial network. Ligation prevents flow inversion from the collaterals to the AVF and maintains antegrade perfusion to the hand.

After the initial descriptions of the DRIL technique by Schanzer et al. [2], an increasing number of publications in the literature [3–8, 12, 15–17, 19–23] have reported impressive results with a success rate approaching 80–90% in terms of relief of symptoms, healing of lesions, arterial bypass patency and maintenance of VA, as summarized in table 1. About 75% of patients are cured, 15% are improved and 0–5% require fistula ligation. The DRIL technique can be used to treat ischemia involving fistulas of the wrist and elbow as well as the lower extremity [4]. The material of choice for the DRIL bypass is the greater saphenous vein [4], although PTFE grafts, cephalic or basilic veins, lesser saphenous vein and femoral vein have also been used. Cryopreserved arterial material was the graft of choice in one case series.

However, despite good results, some surgeons are still reluctant to ligate a 'normal' brachial artery because of the risk of acute ischemia in the case of bypass thrombosis [25, 26], although this has never been reported in the literature be-

Table 1. Clinical presentation of hand ischemia

Stage	Description	Indication
I	pale/blue and/or cold hand without pain	expectation
II	pain during effort and/or hemodialysis	diagnostics/intervention
III	rest pain	intervention
IV	ulcers/necrosis/gangrene	urgent intervention

cause of the collaterality at the level of the shoulder and elbow. In case of recurrence of ischemic symptoms due to thrombosis or deterioration of a DRIL bypass, repeat venous or prosthetic bypass can be performed. Concerns have also been raised about the long-term durability and effectiveness of the DRIL bypass in a patient population with severe arterial diseases, heavy comorbidities and limited life expectancy.

Two recent reports by Knox et al. [5] and Huber et al. [20] with the largest series of DRIL procedures reported in the literature, not only showed the benefit of the DRIL technique but also demonstrated its long-term durability and effectiveness with a 5-year follow-up.

Aimaq and Katz [3] reported in a recent publication 88 DRIL procedures in 77 patients. Thirty-eight DRIL were performed for ischemic rest pain (46.9%), 21 for digital ulceration (25.9%), 16 for neurological deficits (19.7%), and 6 for digital gangrene (7.4%). Complete symptoms resolution was seen in 31 patients with ischemic rest pain (81.6%), 19 patients with digital ulceration (90.5%), 9 patients with neurological deficits (56.3%), and 5 patients with digital gangrene (83.3%). Interestingly enough, best results were achieved in patients with rest pain and tissue loss compared to patients with neurologic deficits. Among them, 4 underwent fistula ligation and 3 refused further intervention. After ligation, only one patient had complete resolution of symptoms, and 3 had persistent neurological symptoms. However, it is not clear if initial ligation would have been more beneficial than the delay in treatment caused by the attempt of fistula preservation prior to ligation.

Treatment of Hand Ischemia at the Elbow in Patients with Normal or High VA Flow

A variety of techniques, such as the bandings, RUDI and PAVA or PAI, are available to treat hand ischemia in patients with normal or high VA flow. As a matter of fact, most patients in our experience and in the literature do not have high VA flow that is defined as flow greater than 1.5 l/min. However none of these techniques is well codified with varying degrees of success.

The Banding Techniques

Fistula banding or plication is aimed to increase the resistance of the fistula to divert flow below the fistula to the native artery [24–26]. This reduces flow in the fistula and threatens its survival. However, most of these techniques are empirical, not well codified and reproducible and pose many questions: (1) It is not clear where the reduction should be placed, whether on the arteriovenous anastomosis or the vein or both. (2) What is the optimal percentage of surface reduction in order to satisfactorily reduce flow without taking the risk of having a fistula thrombosis? For these reasons, many reports of banding show high rates of fistula thrombosis, and these techniques have been abandoned by most authors [1–8, 16].

Intraoperative pressure or flow monitoring may improve the success of the procedure while preserving fistula flow. In one series, distal artery flow was monitored by digital plethysmography to achieve a digital pressure of greater than 50 mm Hg and a digital to brachial pressure index greater than 0.69. This approach relieved steal symptoms in all 16 patients, but only 10 (63%) had satisfactory graft function for more than 6 months [24]. Zanow et al. [25] reported a series of 78 patients with VA-induced hand ischemia and high fistula flow. Banding was tailored to reduce fistula flow to 400 ml/min in autogenous grafts, and 600 ml/min in prosthetic grafts. Ischemic symptoms were relieved in 86% of patients with 91% of autogenous fistulae remaining patent at 12 months. Primary patency rate for fistula and graft was 91 versus 58% at 12 months and 81 versus 41% at 36 months, respectively. Most interestingly, mean preoperative flow was 1,691 ml/min and dropped postoperatively to 499 ml/min in fistula and to 676 ml/min in grafts. The authors suggested that higher flow rates (>750 ml/min) in the graft were required to prevent thrombosis.

Gupta et al. [16] also reported 62% of thromboses among 22 bandings in a series including other procedures to treat hand ischemia such as DRIL, PAVA and RUDI. Among the 11 reinterventions, 8 (73%) were needed in patients with banding.

More recently, the minimally invasive limited ligation endoluminal-assisted revision (MILLER) technique describes a modified method of banding [26]. In this procedure, the fistula is exposed, and a 4- to 5-mm balloon is introduced into the fistula and inflated. A nonresorbable suture is tied around the inflated balloon and vein to achieve a defined reduction in balloon diameter. In the original report of 16 patients, all had improvement in symptoms, 2 required further revision of their fistulae, and all were patent at a mean of 3 months of follow-up.

The RUDI Technique

This procedure involves ligation of the fistula at its origin followed by reestablishment of the fistula via a saphenous vein bypass from a more distal arterial source to the fistula (fig. 2). By using a smaller distal artery as inflow, RUDI lengthens the fistula, decreases the diameter, and preserves antegrade flow in the brachial artery. In contrast to DRIL, it is the fistula, not the native arterial supply that is placed at risk by ligation and revascularization. However, the overall success rate for radial artery-based access procedures is fairly poor in the elderly and diabetics.

Whether this is effective because of the increase in arterial resistance proximal to the fistula or through other mechanism is yet unknown. Moreover, it is not clear what the ideal length and diameter are of the conduit of the bypass to achieve improvement of distal flow.

Minion et al. [27] reported a small series of 4 patients with 4–14 months of follow-up. Three patients had complete resolution of symptoms, with marked improvement of the average finger pressure. The 4th patient experienced residual paresthesia with no improvement of finger pressure.

Callaghan et al. [17] recently published his experience in 7 patients with autogenous fistula and found that 3 fistulas had failed, 2 within days and one at 8 months. The authors conclude that although RUDI was successful at treating ischemic symptoms, a high rate of AVF failure was seen requiring technical modifications and further experience before becoming a valuable method. Ehsan et al. [18] have suggested a modified technique for brachiocephalic fistula to prevent ischemic symptoms called the 'extension technique'. In this technique, the anastomosis is done between the median cephalic or basilic vein and the ulnar or radial artery 2–3 cm distal to the bifurcation in an end-to-side fashion. This technique was used in 32 upper arms in patients deemed to be at 'high risk' of developing hand ischemia and was found to be safe and effective with good patency rate.

The PAVA or PAI Technique

Two authors have reported their experience with the PAVA or PAI technique that consists of performing proximal anastomosis to a more proximal mid-brachial or axillary artery by using a small-caliber (4 or 5 mm) or a 4–7 tapered expanded PTFE graft as feeder [28, 29]. The more proximal artery has a larger diameter, and theoretically the arterial pressure drop distal to the AVF should be significantly lower. The absence of reversed flow in the forearm arteries makes the PAVA/PAI technique similar to DRIL. However, this technique is not well codified, and the following are not clearly established: (1) What is the optimal site for the proximal anastomosis between the mid-brachial artery and the axillary artery? (2) What is the ideal length and diameter of the bypass? This technique was used by Zanow et al. [28] in 30 patients including tissue loss in 37% of the cases. The symptoms completely resolved in 84% of patients and improved in 16%. The significant hemodynamic improvement was confirmed by an increase in intraoperatively measured mean distal arterial pressure. There was no significant change in VA flow that went from 658 to 634 ml/min after the PAVA procedure. Thermann and Wollert [29] recently published their experience in 23 patients with 18 AVF at the elbow and 5 at the wrist. In 15 cases (65%), ischemic symptoms resolved completely, and in 6 patients (26%) wound healing with improvement of symptoms was achieved. Symptoms were persistent in 2 patients (9%) with severe tissue loss. There was a significant increase in radial artery flow velocity after PAVA with a significant decrease in fistula flow in patients with elbow fistula but not in patients with wrist fistula. Mean pre- and postoperative VA flow was 1.38 and 0.94 l/min, respectively. The authors concluded that PAVA led to good clinical results in patients with small finger necrosis but was unsuccessful in the case of severe tissue loss greater than 1 cm in diameter. In our experience, we use the PAVA technique to treat high VA flow greater than 1.5 l/min regardless of ischemic symptoms.

Which Technique to Choose? DRIL, Bandings, RUDI or PAVA/PAI?

Since most patients do not have high VA flow requiring correction, in our experience and according to the literature, DRIL is the technique of choice in dealing with hand ischemia. In patients with either normal or high flow, the alternative to DRIL is the bandings or the RUDI, PAVA or PAI technique with various clinical success rates. In the literature, there are strong clinical [1, 8, 12, 15–17, 19–29] and hemodynamic data [21–23, 30] to support DRIL as the most effective well-codified, reproducible and durable technique with long-term follow-up. Given the high rate of thrombosis and the number of empirical and not clearly established techniques, the bandings have been abandoned by most authors. Surgeons who are reluctant to do an arterial ligation have a valuable alternative, i.e. the RUDI or PAVA/PAI technique, although these techniques are not well codified with only a few reports published with shorter follow-up and results comparable to DRIL [17, 18, 27–29]. However, on the basis of a sophisticated physiological analysis, Gradman and Pozrikidis [30] described a flow model to analyze and compare the hemodynamic changes associated with the various treatments for access-related hand ischemia and concluded that DRIL was the most effective in restoring adequate hand perfusion, followed by the PAVA technique. Gupta et al. [16] reported a series of 70 patients who underwent 87 procedures for ischemic symptoms. Procedures performed included ligation (n = 27), banding (n = 22), DRIL (n = 21), improvement of proximal inflow (n = 9), RUDI (n = 4), and PAI (n = 3). Early procedures (<30 days from the index fistula) were mostly ligation (50%) or banding (38%), while DRIL was the most frequent choice for late interventions (41%). Banding had a high failure rate (62%) and was the most common reason for reintervention (8 of 11, 73%), and DRIL had a better success rate than banding ($p \leq 0.05$). The authors concluded that among various options to treat ischemic symptoms, banding has a low success rate and high likelihood for reintervention, while DRIL is particularly effective although not uniformly.

VA Ligation

Ligation of the VA might be necessary in the following situations:
(1) Severe arterial lesions, poor general conditions or extended tissue loss in patients in whom revascularization is not feasible.
(2) Ischemic monomelic neuropathy. Immediate ligation of the fistula is required for this acute presentation because revascularization may not prevent permanent nerve damage.
(3) No improvement of symptoms after revascularization.
(4) Patients with kidney transplant.

Conclusions

When severe VA-induced hand ischemia occurs distal to an end-to-side radiocephalic fistula at the wrist in a patient with patent ulnar and digital arteries, ligation of the distal radial artery effectively improves symptoms by eliminating the reversed flow. Data from our experience and the literature suggest that DRIL is the most effective and durable treatment for relieving hand ischemia and preserving the VA compared to other techniques in patients with normal VA flow. It should be proposed as the first-line treatment for hand ischemia following VA at the elbow and at the wrist in patients with forearm and digital arteriopathy. Other techniques such as RUDI, PAVA or PAI are an alternative in patients presenting with ischemia and high VA flow. Banding techniques have been abandoned by most authors given the high rate of thrombosis. Ligation of the VA is an option in patients with severe arterial lesions and extended tissue loss, poor general status or absence of improvement after revascularization, and is mandatory in patients presenting with ischemic monomelic neuropathy.

Disclosure Statement

The authors have no conflicts of interest to declare.

References

1 Tordoir JHM, Dammers R, van der Sande FM: Upper extremity ischemia and hemodialysis vascular access. Eur J Vasc Endovasc Surg 2004;27:1–5.

2 Schanzer H, Skladany M, Haimov M: Treatment of angioaccess-induced ischemia by revascularisation. J Vasc Surg 1992;16:861–866.

3 Aimaq R, Katz SG: Using distal revascularization with interval ligation as primary treatment of hand ischemia after dialysis access creation. J Vasc Surg 2013;57:1073–1078.

4 Berman SS, Gentile AT, Glickman MH, et al: Distal revascularisation-interval ligation for limb salvage and maintenance of dialysis access in ischemic steal syndrome. J Vasc Surg 1997;26:393–404.

5 Knox RC, Berman SS, Hughes JD, et al: Distal revascularization-interval ligation: a durable and effective treatment for ischemic steal syndrome after hemodialysis access. J Vasc Surg 2002;36:250–256.

6 Sessa C, Pecher M, Maurizi-Balzan J, et al: Critical hand ischemia after angioaccess surgery: diagnosis and treatment. Ann Vasc Surg 2000;14:583–593.

7 Sessa C, Riehl G, Porcu P, et al: Treatment of hand ischemia following angio-access surgery using the distal revascularization interval-ligation technique with preservation of vascular access: description of an 18-case series. Ann Vasc Surg 2004;18:685–694.

8 Sessa C, DeLambert A, Cochet E, Pichot O, Palacin P, Magne JL: Ischemia and DRIL procedure; in Tordoir J (eds): EVC Vascular Access. Turin, Editioni Minerva Medica, 2009, pp 161–177.

9 Tynan-Cuisinier GS, Bermann SS: Strategies for predicting and treating access induced ischemic steal syndrome. Eur J Vasc Endovasc Surg 2006;32:309–315.

10 Storey BG, Georges CRP, Stewart JO, et al: Embolic and ischemic complications after anastomosis of the radial artery to cephalic vein. Surgery 1969,66.325–327.

11 Chemla E, Raynaud A, Carreres T, et al: Preoperative assessment of the efficacy of distal radial artery ligation in treatment of steal syndrome complicating access for hemodialysis. Ann Vasc Surg 1999;13:618–662.

12 Sessa C, Guigard S, De Lambert A, Cochet E, Pichot O, Maghlaoua M: Treatment of hand ischemia related to vascular access: DRA (Distal Radial Artery) ligation, DRIL (Distal Revascularization-Interval Ligation), RUDI (Rivascularization Using Distal Insertion) and PAI (Proximalization of the Arterial Inflow) or PAVA (Proximalization of Arterio-Venous Anastomosis); in Becquemin JP (ed): Controversies and Updates in Vascular Surgery. Turin, Editioni Minerva Medica, 2010, pp 179–192.

13 Miller GA, Khariton K, Kerdos SV, et al: Flow interruption of the distal radial artery: treatment for finger ischemia in a matured radiocephalic AVF. J Vasc Access 2008;9:58–63.

14 Kwun KB, Schanzer H, Finkler N, et al: Hemodynamic evaluation of angioaccess procedures for hemodialysis. J Vasc Surg 1979;13:170–177.

15 Diehl L, Johansen K, Watson J: Operative management of distal ischemia complication upper extremities dialysis access. Am J Surg 2003;186:17–19.
16 Gupta N, Yuo TH, Konig G 4th, Dillavou E, Leers SA, Chaer RA, Cho JS, Makaroun MS: Treatment strategies of arterial steal after arteriovenous access. J Vasc Surg 2011;54:162–167.
17 Callaghan CJ, Mallik M, Sivaprakasam R, Iype S, Pettigrew GJ: Treatment of dialysis access-associated steal syndrome with the 'revision using distal inflow' technique. J Vasc Access 2011;12:52–56.
18 Ehsan O, Bhattacharya D, Darwish A, Al-khaffal H: 'Extension Technique': a modified technique for brachio-cephalic fistula to prevent dialysis access-associated steal syndrome. Eur J Vasc Endovasc Surg 2005;29:324–327.
19 Yu SH, Cook PR, Canty TG, et al: Hemodialysis-related steal syndrome: predictive factors and response to treatment with the distal revascularization-interval ligation procedure. Ann Vasc Surg 2008;22:210–214.
20 Huber TS, Brown MP, Seeger JM, et al: Midterm outcome after the distal revascularization and interval ligation (DRIL) procedure. J Vasc Surg 2008;48:926-932.
21 Wixon CL, Mills JL, Berman SS: Distal revascularisation-interval ligation for maintenance of dialysis access and restoration of distal perfusion in ischemic steal syndrome. Semin Vasc Surg 2000;13:77–82.
22 Wixon CL, Hughes JD, Mills JL: Understanding strategies for the treatment of ischemic steal syndrome after hemodialysis access. J Am Coll Surg 2000;191:301–310.
23 Illig KA, Surowiec S, Shortell CK, et al: Hemodynamics of distal revascularization-interval ligation. Ann Vasc Surg 2005;19:199–207.
24 Odland MD, Kelly PH, Ney AL, Andersen RC, Bubrick MP: Management of dialysis-associated steal syndrome complicating upper extremity arteriovenous fistulas: use of intraoperative digital photoplethysmography. Surgery 1991;110:664–669.
25 Zanow J, Petzold K, Petzold M, Krueger U, Scholz H: Flow reduction in high-flow arteriovenous access using intraoperative flow monitoring. J Vasc Surg 2006;44:1273–1278.
26 Goel N, Miller GA, Jotwani MC, Licht J, Schur I, Arnold WP: Minimally Invasive Limited Ligation Endoluminal assisted Revision (MILLER) for treatment of dialysis access-associated steal syndrome. Kidney Int 2006;70:765–770.
27 Minion DK, Moore Z, Endean E: Revision using distal inflow: a novel approach to dialysis-associated steal syndrome. Ann Vasc Surg 2005;19:625–628.
28 Zanow J, Kruger U, Scholz H: Proximalization of the arterial inflow: a new technique to treat access-related ischemia. J Vasc Surg 2006;43:1216–1221.
29 Thermann F, Wollert U: Proximalization of the arterial inflow: new treatment of choice in patients with advanced dialysis shunt-associated steal syndrome? Ann Vasc Surg 2009;23:485–490.
30 Gradman WS, Pozrikidis C: Analysis of options for mitigating hemodialysis access-related ischemic steal phenomena. Ann Vasc Surg 2004;18:59–65.

Carmine Sessa, MD, PhD
Department of Vascular and Thoracic Surgery, University Hospital Grenoble
PO Box 217
FR–38043 Grenoble Cedex 09 (France)
E-Mail c.sessa@ghm-grenoble.fr

Widmer MK, Malik J (eds): Patient Safety in Dialysis Access.
Contrib Nephrol. Basel, Karger, 2015, vol 184, pp 176–188
DOI: 10.1159/000365984

Patient Safety in Peritoneal Dialysis

Douglas P. Slakey · Ingemar Davidson

Department of Surgery, Tulane University Medical School, New Orleans, La., USA

Abstract

Peritoneal dialysis (PD) is effective and safe when patients and caregivers understand the best practices. Health care teams responsible for PD must act in a coordinated and consistent manner to ensure the most effective outcomes. This chapter will review the evidence for PD and discuss the safety implications of the phases of PD from patient selection to education to maintenance.

Recommendations to Improve Patient Safety

- Peritoneal dialysis (PD) has economic advantages compared to hemodialysis.
- Safe PD requires evaluation and education by health care team.
- Patient education to avoid infection during fluid change and catheter maintenance is key.
- PD health care team education should be ongoing, and the team members must advocate for outcome-based care.

Introduction

Patient safety is an increasingly important topic for all patients and for physicians and surgeons worldwide. A clear definition of 'patient safety' remains elusive, and depends upon the perspective of whoever is defining it at the time (i.e. doctor, patient, government – regulatory body). A variety of factors contribute to patient safety and all play a role in patients receiving peritoneal dialysis (PD).

In its most literal interpretation, patient safety is a modern term with roots extending back to Hippocrates who admonished physicians to 'first do no harm'. Certainly, every physician who has recited the Hippocratic Oath has considered the depth of meaning contained in that simple statement.

Today however, the concept of patient safety extends beyond managing risk and not harming a patient. Included in the broad context of patient safety is an understanding that patient treatment must be effective and be economically reasonable. Cost-effective health care is difficult to achieve, but is a goal that is increasingly important worldwide. Physicians and health care teams who monitor outcomes and continuously refine practices, procedures and protocols based on an honest appraisal of results are able to reduce the incidence of complications, improve the outcomes of their patients and, hopefully, reduce costs overall.

PD provides an ideal platform with which to evaluate patient safety and cost-effectiveness. PD can be readily compared to hemodialysis (HD) and even kidney transplantation to determine the safety, patient outcomes and cost [1–4]. For example, PD, when compared to HD, has several potential advantages including better preservation of residual renal function, a flexible dialysis schedule for patients allowing them more normal participation in the activities of daily living, and statistically greater patient survival when compared with HD [1–10]. Overall cost is reported to be lower with PD than HD. As reported by Berger et al. [11], HD is USD 43,510 more for 12 months of care than PD in the United States (USD 173,507 vs. 129,997). Assessing patient safety from these perspectives relies on population studies and public health considerations. The large numbers of patients required to evaluate patient safety in this manner allows investigators to identify statistically valid outcome comparisons that cannot occur on an individual patient level. Application of large population studies to the individual patient and patient care setting are sometimes difficult because of the unique realities of every doctor-patient or patient-health system interaction [12]. This reality underlies a major difficulty in standardizing patient care paradigms across populations of patients. Nonetheless, to improve patient safety and outcomes attention must be paid to larger population evidence, and physicians should use evidence-based decision making as a fundamental way to improve patient safety and outcomes. Best practices for the delivery of patient care require the physician to understand larger population evidence and then determine how to apply that evidence to individual patient care decisions.

At the individual patent level, optimal patient safety requires: (1) a preoperative evaluation to identify any contraindications to PD, (2) a thorough understanding of the methods to place a PD catheter, (3) managing technical and infectious complications, and (4) ensuring thorough and ongoing education for the patient and family with respect to performing PD at home.

Preoperative Evaluation

Each patient with end-stage renal disease (ESRD) should receive an evaluation to assess if they are a good candidate for PD [13, 14]. Before instituting any form of dialysis, a determination of intercurrent medical conditions, expected patient survival, and potential for transplantation should be assessed [15–17]. Relevant issues include visual acuity, ability to follow instructions and to use the equipment and supplies needed, the level of social support and of course patient willingness. The patient and family must have an appropriate location within the home to store equipment and supplies. In addition, cleanliness of the home is important to lessen the risk of infections. Health care staff experienced in home PD should personally evaluate the home setting and document any concerns. Depending upon the local health care payment system, it is important that the physicians and nurses responsible for initiating and maintaining a patient on PD know details of the individual patient's financial considerations as they relate to PD. The patient will need to be assessed for the impact of PD on activities of daily living including work or school, travel, family relations, and activities such as sports.

Providing education to the patient and family is important to ensure success of PD. Patients must be given a basic understanding of how PD works and the risks. The patient needs to be taught the mechanics of PD including strict adherence to sterile technique. Teaching must include both didactic and actual practice in a realistic setting. Didactic teaching is not adequate to ensure that the patient truly understands the details of PD. Careful assessment by an experienced educator should be documented. Follow-up education is helpful in answering questions that arise after beginning PD, and in reinforcing sterile technique.

The primary preoperative surgical consideration is a history of previous abdominal surgery or intra-abdominal infection. If a patient has had multiple abdominal operations or complex surgeries or infections, there may be extensive adhesions which would increase the risk of PD failure. In these cases, an exploratory laparoscopy may identify if there is enough free peritoneal space for PD to be effective.

Obesity is not a contraindication to considering a patient for PD, although some morbidly obese patients may not have enough peritoneal surface area to provide adequate exchange, and this cannot be determined conclusively just by a patient's body mass index. A hernia in the abdomen or groin may be a relative contraindication to PD. If a hernia is large and especially if there are skin changes, cellulitis, or symptomatic incarcerations, then the hernia must be repaired prior to beginning PD. In selected patients, a PD catheter and hernia repair could occur at the same setting.

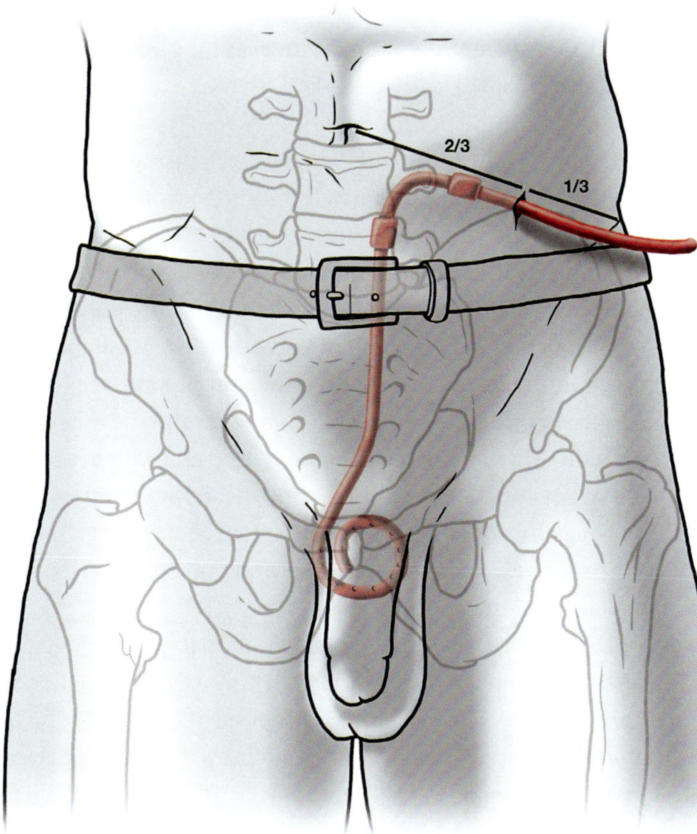

Fig. 1. With your patient wearing a belt in the sitting or lying position, check that the catheter exit area is above or below the belt and that the catheter is placed more in a downwards direction.

It is important to assess the patient preoperatively to ensure the catheter site is easy for the patient to access, away from skin folds and away from the beltline. A patient should be evaluated both sitting and standing, and the patient's skin marked for correct catheter placement (fig. 1).

Catheter Selection

There are four basic designs for the intraperitoneal portion of PD catheters: (1) straight Tenckhoff which is typically 8 or 16 cm containing side holes; (2) coiled Tenckhoff with a coiled 16-cm portion containing side holes; (3) straight Tenckhoff with perpendicular silicone discs, also known as the Oreopoulos-Zellerman or Toronto Western Hospital catheter; (4) T-shaped catheter with grooved limbs that position against the peritoneum.

The subcutaneous portion of the catheter has three basic shapes: (1) straight, (2) with a permanent bend of approximately 150° (Swan-neck catheter), or (3) with a permanent 90° bend (Cruz catheter). The catheter cuffs are designed to allow ingrowth of fibrous tissue reducing the risk of bacteria and fluid migrating along the catheter track. There are three basic designs for the polyester cuff that are attached to the subcutaneous portion of the catheter: (1) a single cuff, in this case usually placed in the rectus muscle or at the anterior surface of the rectus, (2) dual cuffs; the inner one placed in the rectus muscle and the other in the subcutaneous tissue, and (3) a disc/ball combination deep cuff which is placed at the level of the parietal peritoneum/posterior rectus sheaf. Many surgeons who use the disc/ball type of catheter sew the posterior rectus sheaf between the polyester disc and silicone ball. These catheters have a second polyester cuff that is located within the subcutaneous tunnel.

Most adult PD catheters have three possible internal diameters (2.6, 3.1, 3.5 mm). All have an outer diameter of approximately 5 mm. Most catheters currently manufactured are made of silicone rubber. Polyurethane may also be used but much less commonly. The published literature indicates catheters with a coiled intraperitoneal end have a longer, 3-year survival [18, 19]. Similarly, catheters with two cuffs have a lower incident of exit site infection and a longer lifespan than single-cuff catheters. The Swan-neck catheters appear to have lower overall incidents of exit site infection than those with a straight subcutaneous segment, although this is most likely due to a catheter exit that faces caudad as opposed to cephalad.

Operative Techniques

Surgical placement of a PD catheter can be done using an open or a laparoscopic method [20–22]. There are no clear data to suggest that one approach is superior to the other. Patient safety, surgical complications and catheter function rates have not been shown to be different depending upon the method used for placement (table 1). It has been reported that the laparoscopic method is more time consuming and somewhat more expensive (especially if disposable trocars are used), implying that the open technique may be more cost-effective [22]. The functional outcome of the PD catheter is not different when placed either by open or laparoscopic methods.

Patient safety in the operating room requires careful attention to detail, as for any surgical procedure. A timeout (briefing) based on the World Health Organiza-

Table 1. Patient safety considerations of catheter placement techniques

	Advantages	Risks/disadvantages
Blind percutaneous	Local anesthesia 'Office' procedure	Inability to visualize abdominal vasculature or organs Patient may have unrecognized injury Physician cannot manage adhesions or omentum
Seldinger technique with fluoroscopy	Penetration with needle may lessen blind risk of organ or vascular injury	Similar to blind percutaneous
Peritoneoscopy	Allows some visualization of abdominal cavity Does not require formal operating room	Limited visualization Physician cannot manage adhesions or omentum
Open	Identification of adhesions at site of incision Precise placement of cuffs, tunnel Local or general anesthesia	Operating room required Physician cannot manage any remote adhesions without extending incision Physician cannot effectively manage omentum
Laparoscopic	Identification and management of adhesions anywhere in the abdomen are possible Visualization of catheter placement can limit abdominal viscera and vascular injury Omentum can be managed using omental-pexi or resection if needed	General anesthesia needed More expensive equipment if disposable used

tion studies is necessary to promote patient safety [23]. The first portion of the timeout, briefing – the check-in, should ensure correct identification of the patient. In addition, the operating team must be certain that all necessary equipment and supplies are immediately available and functional. Anesthetic choice, antibiotics, and any nonroutine considerations should be acknowledged and discussed by the operating team during the timeout. The planned method of PD catheter placement must be confirmed at this time. If a laparoscopic technique is planned, instrumentation to convert to an open laparotomy must be immediately available if needed.

Irrespective of the method of placing the catheter into the peritoneal cavity, a decision about what to do with the external end must be made prior to the beginning the procedure. If the catheter is to be used within a short time, the exterior end should be attached to a transfer set at the end of the procedure. If the surgeon or physician placing the catheter is not certain about the time to catheter use, the exterior end can be left exteriorized or the Moncrief-Popovich catheter technique can be employed and the end buried. Moncrief and Popovich first described the subcutaneous burial of the external segment of the catheter with subsequent externalization just prior to use [24]. The period of time the catheter remains buried is variable, and can be many months. The theory behind the development of this technique was to prevent colonization of the catheter by skin bacteria prior to the adhesion of catheter cuffs to subcutaneous tissues. Initial reports claimed a reduction in the rate of peritonitis and the rate of the formation of bacteria biofilms in the catheter segment between two cuffs. However, a randomized clinical trial has failed to confirm these claims [25]. The disadvantage to this technique includes a high incidence of seromas, the potential for subcutaneous hematomas, the development of fibrin thrombi in the internal portion of the catheter, and the need for a second procedure [24–26].

The two primary methods are generally used for the placement of PD catheters: surgical and percutaneous.

Percutaneous Technique

For blind percutaneous placement, a large bore trocar is used after provision of local anesthesia. The technique was first developed and described by Tenckhoff. The method is simple and can be performed at bedside. Disadvantages of this method are the inability to effectively tunnel a dual cuff catheter and because it is a blind procedure, therefore subjecting the patient to potentially increased risks of vascular, bowel, or solid organ injury.

The percutaneous method has been simplified with a modified Seldinger technique. Although also a blind procedure, the risk of injury to abdominal structures is reduced because of the use of needle penetration followed by dilation using a blunt plastic dilator. The operator must be certain to aspirate while placing the needle in order to assess for blood or intestinal fluids.

Open PD Catheter Technique

Open surgery for PD catheter placement can be done using local or general anesthetic. Prophylactic antibiotics such as a first-generation cephalosporin should be used. Detailed descriptions of operative techniques are available elsewhere [27].

The open technique is particularly useful for patients who cannot tolerate general anesthetic because local anesthesia and sedation are typically adequate.

Laparoscopic Technique

The laparoscopic PD catheter placement technique is done under general anesthesia because of the discomfort from insufflation of the abdominal cavity [28–30]. Prophylactic antibiotics are administered as for the open technique. As with any laparoscopic procedure, care must be taken during the initial access whether with a Veress needle or a Husain catheter placement. Injury to bowel and major blood vessels are the two most significant complications related to the placement of laparoscopic trocars. If safe access to the peritoneal cavity can be obtained, the laparoscopic approach may be preferred in patients who have had previous abdominal surgeries because of the ability to perform exploratory laparoscopy and possibly lysis of adhesions. In addition, obese patients may benefit from the laparoscopic approach because trocars can traverse a thicker abdominal wall, avoiding a larger incision that may be required if using the open technique in an obese patient. In certain incidences, an experienced laparoscopic surgeon may consider repair of preexisting hernias using a transperitoneal mesh repair at the same setting.

Managing Complications

Optimal patient safety requires that the physicians, surgeons and patient be able to recognize complications or deviations for expected outcomes early and take action to minimize the effect on patient outcomes [31]. Continual assessment for threats to patient safety and prevention of serious adverse outcomes is the goal. Optimization of patient outcomes is more likely if responsible physicians and nurses establish a system of careful follow-up and monitoring. Following operative placement of a PD catheter, the most common complications are infection and malfunctioning of the catheter.

Infections can be limited to the PD catheter exit site, or intraperitoneal potentially causing peritonitis [32]. Early recognition of the sign and symptoms of infection is an essential starting point for the successful treatment of PD-related infection. Education of the patient and other caregivers is necessary, so that if signs and symptoms of an infection become evident, they will rapidly notify the physician and obtain appropriate treatment. Patient safety requires that the patient and caregivers be actively involved in the process of care.

Malfunction of a PD catheter can have many sources. Catheters can have mechanical failure, for example develop holes, cracks and/or leaks. Catheters can develop occlusions due to anatomic reasons such as ingrowth of omentum, malposition, or entrapment in adhesions. In addition, constipation is known to be related to poor catheter function. A careful history and evaluation of a PD catheter will often identify the most likely cause of loss of catheter function and assist the physicians in developing a plan for restoring function.

The health care dialysis team must ensure that the patient has easy access when reporting concerns or changes in health. Protocols for communication including when to call the health care team are important. The patient will almost always be the first person to recognize a change in catheter function or the signs and symptoms of infection. Specific options for managing complications are discussed elsewhere. Establishing and maintaining a system for the active management of patients will help identify and treat complications early and therefore is a key component of the process to optimizing patient outcomes.

Communication and Human Factors

Patient safety is a complex and ever-evolving aspect of providing health care. Optimizing patient outcomes requires active management of the patient by the responsible members of the health care team. This is especially true for patients with chronic diseases such as ESRD and dialysis dependency. The team caring for the patient must develop a system of delivering care that is consistent and patient focused. All too often patient safety is jeopardized because individual members of the health care team (for example the nephrologist and the surgeon) work in isolation from each other, and therefore patient care decisions may not always be well coordinated.

The term 'multidisciplinary care' is often used but not always effective. Frequently, a group of health care professionals interacts with a patient but without ensuring effective communication with all members of the group providing care (fig. 2). This model of care has several problems that lead to ineffectiveness. First, if the care is not patient centered, then each health care professional focuses on their own specialty without always giving consideration to how their decisions affect the interaction of the patient and other providers. For example, if a patient is referred to a vascular access surgeon who never places PD catheters, the patient may not be effectively assessed for PD.

Another potential for failure of the common 'multidisciplinary care' approach is that the financial decision makers, administration, insurance, and

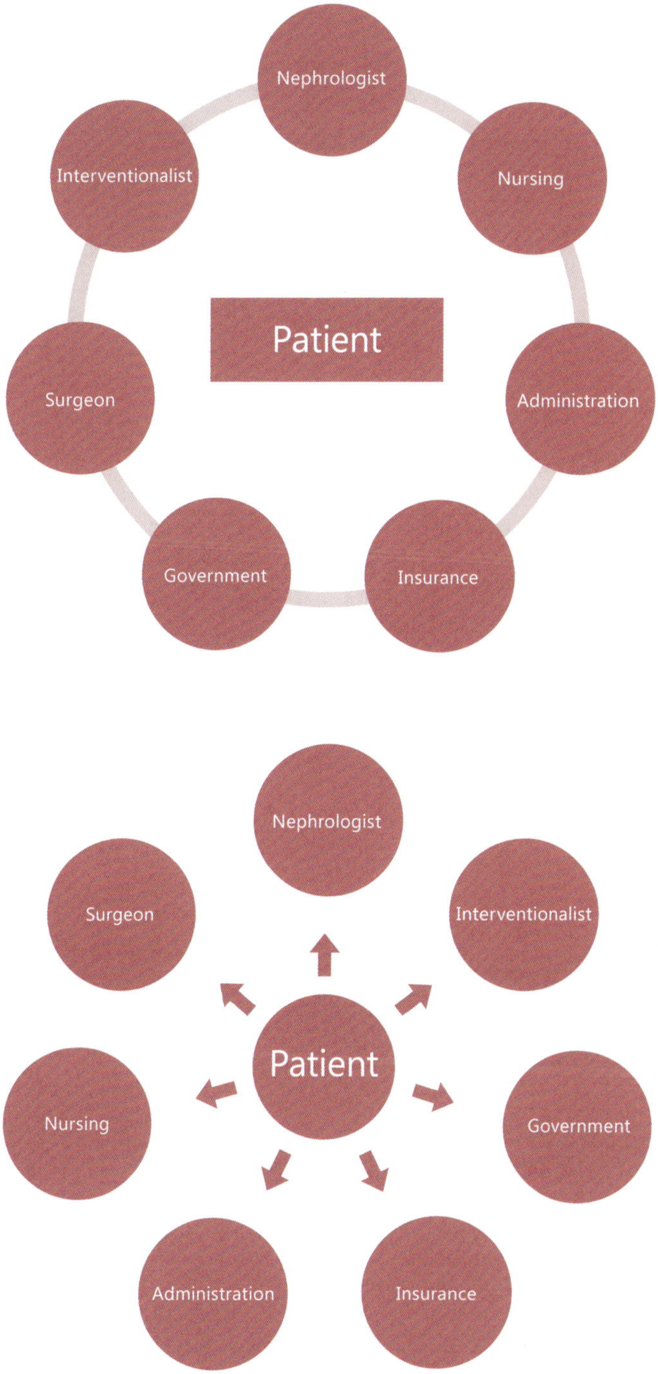

Fig. 2. In the multidiscipline team without being patient centric, the health care team is focused on communication with each other (top). In the patient-centric multidiscipline team, communication is focused on the patient (bottom).

Table 2. Safety-oriented culture shift

Traditional		Modern
Autonomy	⟶	Collaboration
Authority	⟶	Evidence
Assertion	⟶	Measurement
Control	⟶	Transparency
Self-interest	⟶	Public interest

government, are not commonly involved in the patient care process. To maximize patient safety, the efficiency of care delivery, and long-term outcomes, it is important to recognize that for the patient there are many components of the health care system that impact care. If patient safety is truly to be the primary focus of care delivery, then a patient-centric approach that considers all factors that impact the delivery and effectiveness of patient care must be designed and implemented (fig. 2). To do this requires a change in the traditional culture of health care delivery in which each individual provider works primarily in their own specialty in isolation from others who provide care to the patient.

To begin to change the traditional culture, a clear understanding of the complexity of patient interactions with the health care system must be recognized. Patients with end-ESRD are particularly susceptible to a lack of care coordination because they often have so many interactions with various health care specialists. The complexity of the care of ESRD patients makes this group especially at risk of poor outcomes (unacceptable patient safety) due to lack of coordination of care.

Ideally, the system provides a professional to work with the patient to coordinate care and ensure communication between the various components of the system. Of course, this is difficult to achieve, often because it is unclear who is going to pay for the coordination of care. The traditional system of care, even if called 'multidisciplinary' is characterized by each patient-system interaction being quite independent. To improve patient safety, members of the health care system must think and function in a more collaborative culture (table 2). When the culture of care is changed from traditional to modern, patient safety and outcomes become the ultimate measure of success. A health care system that is patient centric and collaborative will be more cost-effective assuming that outcomes are measured and results are shared transparently. In the end, a more cost-effective system of care will result and better serve the public interest by providing optimal care to the greatest number of patients.

Disclosure Statement

The authors have no conflicts of interest to declare.

References

1 Heaf JG, Løkkegaard H, Madsen M: Initial survival advantage of peritoneal dialysis relative to haemodialysis. Nephrol Dial Transplant 2002;17:112–117.

2 Schaubel DE, Morrison HI, Fenton SS: Comparing mortality rates on CAPD/CCPD and hemodialysis. The Canadian experience: act or fiction? Perit Dial Int 1998;18:478–484.

3 Serkes KD, Blagg CR, Nolph KD, Vonesh EF, Shapiro F: Comparison of patient and technique survival in continuous ambulatory peritoneal dialysis (CAPD) and hemodialysis: a multicenter study. Perit Dial Int 1990;10: 15–19.

4 Berkoben M: Patient mortality in chronic dialysis: comparisons between hemodialysis and peritoneal dialysis. Curr Opin Nephrol Hypertens 1999;8:681–683.

5 Saxena R, Caplan NM, Palmer BF: Peritoneal dialysis: a viable renal replacement therapy option. Am J Med Sci 2005;330:36–47.

6 Tokgoz B: Clinical advantages of peritoneal dialysis. Perit Dial Int 2009;29(suppl 2):S59–S61.

7 Lameire N, Van Biesen W: The impact of residual renal function on the adequacy of peritoneal dialysis. Perit Dial Int 1997;17(suppl 2):S102–S110.

8 Jansen MA, Hart AA, Korevaar JC, Dekker FW, Boeschoten EW, Krediet RT; NECOSAD Study Group: Predictors of the rate of decline of residual renal function in incident dialysis patients. Kidney Int 2002;62:1046–1053.

9 Bargman JM, Thorpe KE, Churchill DN; CANUSA Peritoneal Dialysis Study Group. Relative contribution of residual renal function and peritoneal clearance to adequacy of dialysis: a reanalysis of the CANUSA study. J Am Soc Nephrol 2001;12:2158–2162.

10 Bleyer AJ, Burkart JM, Russell GB, Adams PL: Dialysis modality and delayed graft function after cadaveric renal transplantation. J Am Soc Nephrol 1999;10:154–159.

11 Berger A, Edelsberg J, Inglese, et al: Cost comparison of peritoneal dialysis versus hemodialysis in end-stage renal disease. Am J Manag Care 2009;15:509–518.

12 Korevaar JC, Boeschoten EW, Dekker FW, et al: What have we learned about PD from recent major clinical trials? Perit Dial Int 2007; 27:11–15.

13 Jager KJ, Korevaar JC, Dekker FW, et al: The effect of contraindications and patient preference on dialysis modality selection in ESRD patients in the Netherlands. Am J Kidney Dis 2004;43:891–899.

14 Davidson IJA, Gallieni M, Saxena R: Our algorithm for determining the best dialysis access. J Vasc Access 2006;7:143–146.

15 Kinchen KS, Sadler J, Fink N, et al: The timing of specialist evaluation in chronic kidney disease and mortality. Ann Intern Med 2002; 137:479–448.

16 Stack AG: Impact of timing of nephrology referral and pre-ESRD care on mortality risk among new ESRD patients in the United States. Am J Kidney Dis 2003;41:310–318.

17 National Kidney Foundation: K/DOQI clinical practice guidelines for vascular access update 2006. Am J Kidney Dis 2006;48(suppl 1):S176–S322.

18 Blake PG: Peritoneal dialysis in the USA. Perit Dial Int 2006;26:416–418.

19 Tenckhoff H, Curtis FK: Experience with maintenance peritoneal dialysis in the home. Trans Am Soc Artif Intern Organs 1970;16: 90–95.

20 Jwo SC, Chen KS, Lee CC, Chen HY: Prospective randomized study for comparison of open surgery with laparoscopic-assisted placement of Tenckhoff peritoneal dialysis catheter – a single center experience and literature review. J Surg Res 2010;159:489–496.

21 Wright MJ, Bel'eed K, Johnson BF, Eadington DW, Sellars L, Farr MJ: Randomized prospective comparison of laparoscopic and open peritoneal dialysis catheter insertion. Perit Dial Int 1999;19:372–375.

22 Xie H, Zhang W, Cheng J, He Q: Laparoscopic versus open catheter placement in peritoneal dialysis patients: a systematic review and meta-analysis. BMC Nephrol 2012;13:69.
23 Haynes AB, Weiser TG, Berry WR, et al: A surgical safety checklist to reduce morbidity and mortality in a global population. NEJM 2009;360;5:491–499.
24 Moncrief JW, Popovich RP, Dasgupta M, Costerton JW, Simmons E, Moncrief V: Reduction in peritonitis incidence in continuous ambulatory peritoneal dialysis with a new catheter and implantation technique. Perit Dial Int 1993;13:S329–S331.
25 Danielsson A, Blohme L, Tranaeus A, Hylander B: A prospective randomized study of the effect of a subcutaneously 'buried' peritoneal dialysis catheter technique versus standard technique on the incidence of peritonitis and exit-site infection. Perit Dial Int 2002;22: 211–219.
26 Moncrief JW, Popovich RP, Broadrich LJ, He ZZ, Simmons EE, Tate RA: The Moncrief-Popovich Catheter. A new peritoneal access technique for patients on peritoneal dialysis. ASAIO J 1993; 39:62–65.
27 Davidson I, Hwang C, Paramesh A, et al: Laparoscopic placement of a two cuff, coiled catheter; in Davidson I, Gallieni M, Saxena R (eds): Peritoneal Dialysis. Surgical Technique and Medical Management. Dallas, Divadi, 2012, pp 69–90.
28 Nijhuis PH, Smulders JF, Jakimowicz JJ: Laparoscopic introduction of a continuous ambulatory peritoneal dialysis (CAPD) catheter by a two-puncture technique. Surg Endosc 1996;10:676–679.
29 Crabtree JH, Fishman A: Videolaparoscopic implantation of long-term peritoneal dialysis catheters. Surg Endosc 1999;13:186–190.
30 Giannattasio M, De Maio P, La Rosa R, Balestrazzi A: Videolaparoscopy: a new alternative for implantation of peritoneal catheters in ESRD patients with previous abdominal surgeries. Perit Dial Int 1996;16:96–97.
31 Fenton SSA, Schaubel DE, Desmeules M, et al: Hemodialysis versus peritoneal dialysis: A comparison of adjusted mortality rates. Am J Kidney Dis 1997;30:334–342.
32 Goldfarb-Rumyanitzev AS, Hundle JF, Scandling JD, Baird BC, Cheung AK: The role of pre-transplantation renal replacement therapy modality in kidney allograft and recipient survival. Am J Kidney Dis 2005;46:537–549.

Douglas P. Slakey, MD, MPH
Department of Surgery, Tulane University Medical School
1430 Tulane Avenue, SL22
New Orleans, LA 70112 (USA)
E-Mail dslakey@tulane.edu

Widmer MK, Malik J (eds): Patient Safety in Dialysis Access.
Contrib Nephrol. Basel, Karger, 2015, vol 184, pp 189–204
DOI: 10.1159/000365985

Safety Aspects in Patients on Hemodialysis with Catheters

Vladimír Polakovič[a] · František Lopot[a, b]

[a]Department of Internal Medicine – Strahov, General University Hospital Prague, and [b]Institute of Biophysics and Medical Informatics, First Faculty of Medicine, Charles University Prague, Prague, Czech Republic

Abstract

Central venous catheter (CVC)-related problems, risks and safety hazards are partly caused by different characteristics of the CVC-based access and their performance features. This chapter covers those issues in a chronological order, from factors related to the choice of the CVC, insertion site and insertion procedure itself, over those associated with CVC use and their monitoring up to safety hazards of interventional procedures. Not discussed are CVC infections as they are covered in a separate chapter in this book.

Recommendations to Improve Patient Safety

- Medical and nursing staff dealing with central venous catheters (CVC) should be aware of specific risk factors and safety hazards associated with this access type (damage of the vessels and/or surrounding tissue at CVC insertion, fibrin sheath formation, leak of the anticoagulation lock solution into the vascular system, etc.).
- Safety of CVC use is to be regarded as a complex issue starting with proper entry examination of the patient (to discover preexisting risk factors), over selection of the insertion site and CVC type (to avoid anatomically knotty areas), prophylactic care, monitoring of both CVC status and patient condition up to CVC removal. Experienced staff, appropriate instrumentation, and standardized protocols are key safety factors.

- CVC monitoring based on the catheters' pressure/flow characteristics is a proactive measure for the timely detection of CVC malfunction and/or assessment of its severity.
- Research and development in CVC design is focused on prevention of CVC fibrin sheath formation, thrombosis and infection. With lack of sufficiently large studies, true benefits of the innovations should, however, be carefully assessed.
- Forensic implications of CVC insertion and their use should be kept in mind.

Introduction

Central venous catheters (CVC) are generally considered an inevitable evil [1]. Their use is ever growing (see for instance DOPPS data from Germany: an increase from 5.3% in 2002 to 19.4% in 2010 despite all recommendations to limit it [2]). Many studies have demonstrated higher morbidity and mortality associated with CVC compared to permanent subcutaneous access types [3] and the effort to limit their use is thus fully understandable. On the other hand, CVC does not affect patient hemodynamics and bears no risk of hyperkinetic circulation.

Catheter Placement

In principle, there are two distinct CVC types: the temporary nontunneled CVC (ntCVC) and tunneled CVC (tCVC).

The ntCVC are quite short (10–20 cm) and are made of more rigid material (polyurethane, polyethylene, polyvinylchloride). It makes their insertion more straightforward, directly through the puncture site without a tunnel. The tip should not reach into the right atrium, and its position should always be verified. The ntCVC are intended for a short-term use only.

The tCVC are double-lumen lines for long-term use inserted via a subcutaneous tunnel and equipped with a polyester cuff, which allows a growth-through of the surrounding tissue effectively tamping the tunnel and preventing infections. Blood flow obtainable from the tCVC is higher due to a larger inner lumen. The tCVC materials are softer (silicone and other soft flexible polymers such as thin polyurethane/polycarbonate) reducing the risk of kinking, and more biocompatible (less thrombogenous, less prone to microbial colonization). The available tCVC differ in configuration of the inflow and outflow paths and design of the tip. Some tCVC are antibiotic bonded or heparin coated. All those

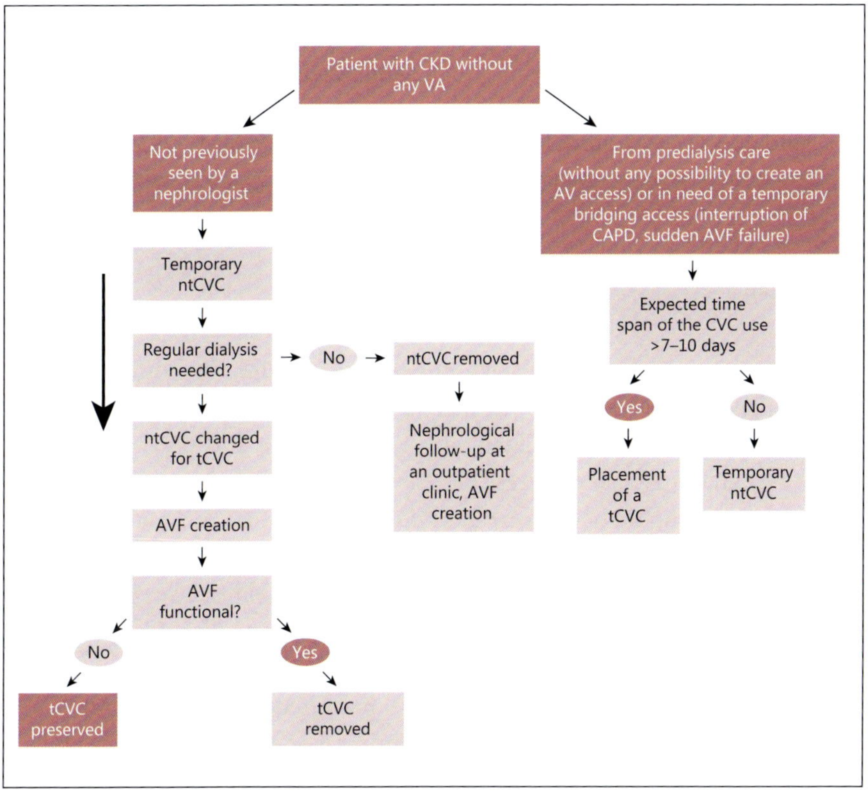

Fig. 1. Flowchart of the CVC type-selecting algorithm in patients with CKD.

variations have common goals – to enable high blood flows with virtually no recirculation, to prevent the tCVC tip obstruction and to reduce incidence of CVC-related infections. However, long-term trials are still needed to assess true benefits of those specific tCVC features.

The choice of the CVC type depends primarily on patient condition (fig. 1). An ntCVC is usually used to start dialysis in patients with acute renal failure, or in chronic kidney disease (CKD patients not previously seen by a nephrologist). It should be changed for a tCVC as soon as possible, see the K/DOQI [4] and EBPG [5]. Occasionally, an ntCVC can be changed once or twice along the guide wire as a slightly prolonged bridging solution [maturing arteriovenous fistula (AVF), infectious patient]. The tCVC is the access of choice for a long-term use or in specific cases of shorter expected period of use, e.g. as the only compromise achievable in a given moment (sudden loss of a subcutaneous access, interruption of CAPD, e.g. for a hernia operation or for severe peritonitis with a temporary transfer to hemodialysis, HD). It may also be the last rescue access when a vascular access (VA) fails, and there are no surgical possibilities to create a new one. Another reason to use a tCVC is a pre-existing severe congestive heart failure when creation of a VA would further worsen patient circulatory condition, or generally in patients with unfavorable life expectancy. Rather rare reasons for a tCVC use are 'needle phobia' [6] or patient refusal of AVF or arteriovenous graft (AVG).

Vein Choice

Theoretically, a CVC can be placed into any larger vein. Most often, the right internal jugular vein followed by the left jugular vein is used. The latter approach is, however, more often associated with complications and CVC dysfunction due to two anatomical curvatures (fig. 2), which makes the insertion more difficult. An X-ray should be done to check for guide wire or CVC malposition i.e. catheter tip in the brachiocephalic vein. Use of femoral vein is justified only in case of brachiocephalic vein or vena cava superior obliteration. The femoral CVC must be long enough to reach into vena cava inferior. The subclavian vein, often used in the past, is an acceptable site today only if neither jugular nor femoral access is possible. Its use is associated more frequently with stenoses and thromboses [7], which makes creation of an AVF or AVG on that side impossible.

A CVC used just to bridge the time for creation and/or maturation of a subcutaneous VA should be placed on the contralateral side. Safe CVC insertion by translumbal access into inferior vena cava with long-term patency in patients with no other options has also been described [8]. In patients with a cardiac pacemaker or implantable cardioverter-defibrillator placed under their clavicle, the contralateral approach should be preferred to avoid damage to the implanted device. Presence of such a device also hampers creation of a good subcutaneous tunnel.

Preinsertion Examinations

Before CVC placement, patient's detailed history should be taken. Information on previous CVC or interventions in the neck and thorax area (or inguinal one in case a femoral CVC) is of special importance. Adhesions and scars after previous operations (thyroidectomy, operations on carotid artery etc.) may have caused undesirable anatomical changes which would make CVC insertion difficult. Proper examination, X-ray and ECG record should also reveal rare anomalies, such as dextrocardia.

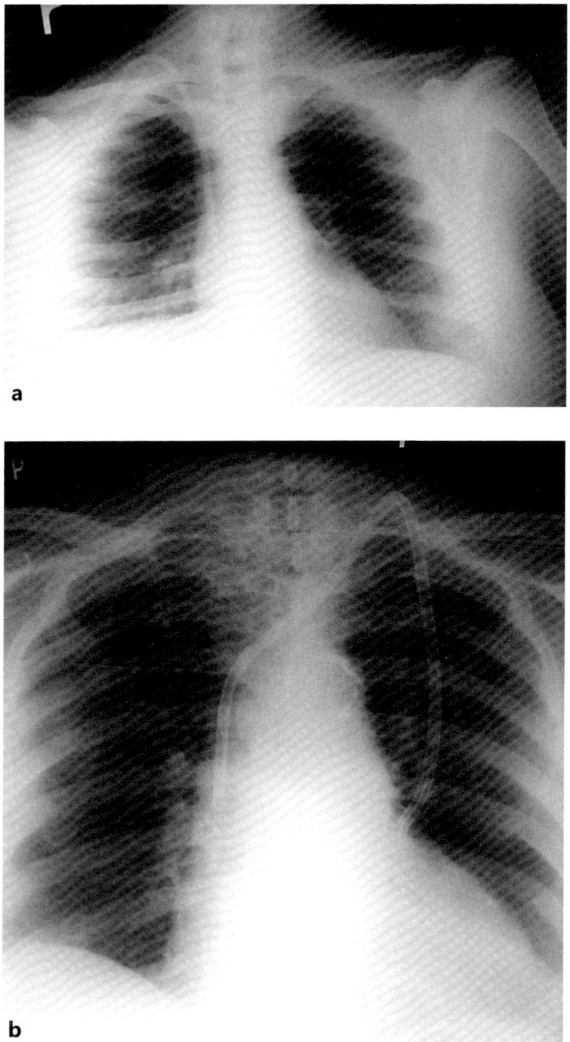

Fig. 2. Postinsertion X-ray check of the CVC showing a direct insertion path when using the right jugular vein (**a**) and an insertion path with two curvatures on the left jugular vein (**b**). X-ray images: Dialysis Department, Prague-Strahov.

It is important to check the whole planned tunnel area. Visible collateral circulation suggests vascular disorder which increases the risk of local bleeding. Immediate preoperative ultrasound examination of veins enables objective decision on the side and vein for the CVC placement.

Complete biochemical and hematological laboratory tests, including coagulation check-up, are mandatory. Prior to insertion, any anticoagulant medication should be stopped.

Skin lesions and infection should be looked for, as they could cause or contribute to infectious complications.

Informed Consent and Forensic Aspects

Catheter placement is an invasive procedure with unavoidable safety hazards. Life-threatening adverse events such as pneumothorax or cardiac tamponade are rare but not always avoidable. Each doctor should be well aware of such complications and know the clinical signs. Responsibility for the insertion and immediate postinsertion care stays with the inserting physician and comes over to the patient's attending or referring physician after patient discharge only. The patient should be informed about the indication, the steps of the procedure and their risks and a signed informed consent must be obtained from him. This helps the doctors to avoid later forensic problems [9]. A proper documentation of all subsequent steps with their date and time is an integral part of risk reduction strategy and also a decision-supporting tool.

Insertion

Both ntCVC and tCVC insertion is performed generally under local anesthesia by modified Seldinger's technique, adhering strictly to aseptic rules. Vein puncture should always be done under ultrasonic control [10, 11]. Using a micropuncture set may also help to avoid problems in case of an incidental puncture of the carotid artery. Guide wire location in the right atrium (or deep in vena cava inferior with a femoral CVC) should be checked by fluoroscopy immediately after insertion, before the CVC insertion itself (fig. 3). In tCVC, gentle creation of a tunnel minimizes bleeding risk with subsequent formation of hematoma prone to infection. Use of valved peal-away sheath or working without a sheath significantly decreases blood loss and also reduces risk of air embolism [12]. Trendelenburg position of the patients is an additional step to avoid air embolism. Insertion of the CVC through the tunnel can be either retrograde or antegrade. With the former approach, optimal placement of the CVC tip is easier to reach as it is done as the first step in the CVC placement (the outgoing part of the CVC is then shortened as needed). The latter one requires careful estimation of the necessary CVC length according to the expected tunnel path. Optimal CVC tip location can be assumed in the bottom half of the sternum. A CVC of corresponding length is then chosen, which enables to keep the CVC intact. The entire functional length of the CVC should be in the right atrium. Too deep insertion should, how-

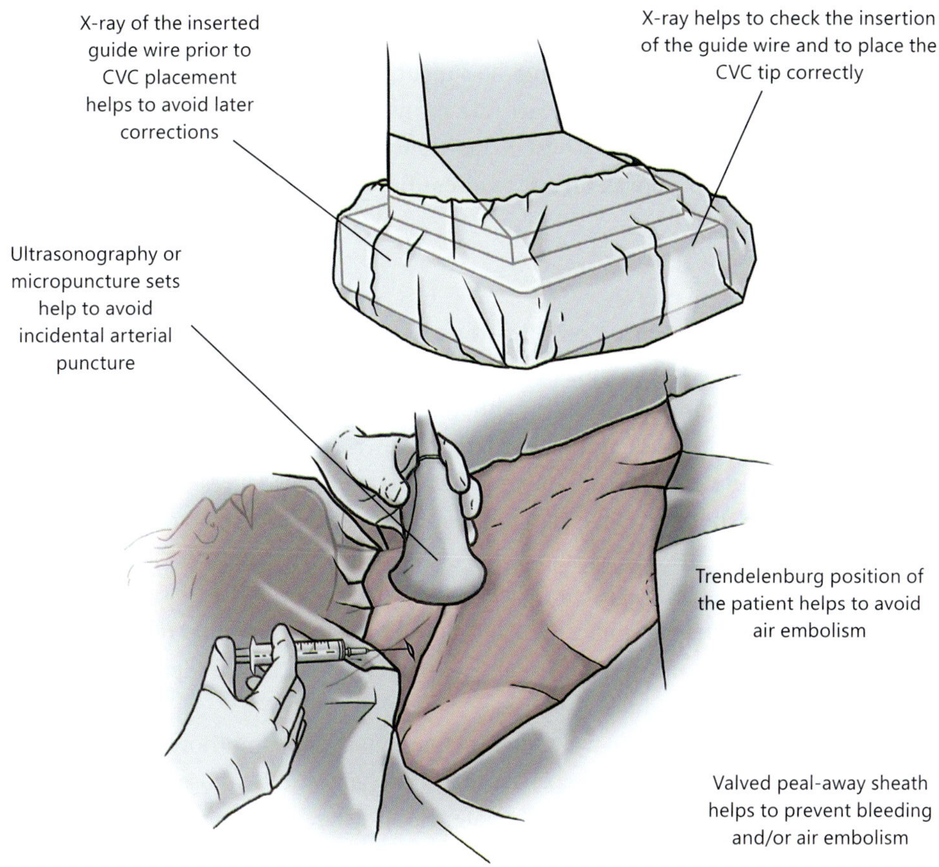

Fig. 3. Tools to avoid complications during a CVC placement.

ever, be avoided considering impact of postural changes upon the tip migration. After checking the correct catheter position by X-ray and filling and emptying a syringe several times quickly for each branch to check for undisturbed flow, the catheter should be blocked using a lock solution either with heparin or citrate.

Immediate Postinsertion Care

When HD is not required immediately after insertion (desirable to avoid bleeding risk associated with heparin administration), the patient should remain in supine or semi-supine position with a compression over the site of the CVC entry into the vein and along the subcutaneous tunnel. Careful supervision with blood pressure and heart rate monitoring is mandatory for timely detection of complications. Chest X-ray done after insertion excludes pneumothorax and hemothorax and should confirm the CVC tip position in the right atrium.

Troubleshooting in Acute Complications

Acute complications typically occur either during the insertion or within the following 24–48 h and are directly related to the experience of the physician inserting the CVC. Our rough estimate is not less than 20 procedures are needed to establish sufficient experience and another 20 per each following year to maintain it. Generally, the best is to place CVC in specialized centers with experienced staff and necessary instrumentation.

The most frequent complication is bleeding caused by puncture of an artery. An about 10-min compression usually helps. CVC insertion under ultrasonic control significantly reduces this risk.

Some complications are truly life threatening, e.g. pneumothorax (reported in up to 1% of cases), hemothorax (less than 1%), hemomediastinum, hemopericardium [13]. Onset of dyspnea, hypotension, tachycardia, etc. is typical for these complications, and immediate fluoroscopy or chest X-ray confirms the diagnosis.

If a CVC is erroneously inserted into carotid or femoral artery, it should be left in situ and further approach consulted with a vascular surgeon. The puncture hole caused by CVC is large; there is thus a risk of massive bleeding into the surrounding area after CVC removal.

Arrhythmias caused by the guide wires happen quite often (42% reported in Fiaccadori et al.) [14]. Usually, they are merely marked by benign extrasystoles. Occasionally, also serious ventricular tachycardia followed by asystolia can be evoked necessitating immediate guide wire removal.

A rare but serious iatrogenic complication is creation of an AV fistula [15]. It should be surgically closed.

Another serious complication is air embolism during CVC insertion into jugular or subclavian vein. As a prevention, mild Trendelenburg position and/or Valsalva maneuver is recommended.

Damage to ductus thoracicus with subsequent chylothorax or injury to neural branches is a rather rare early complication characterized by pain and/or neurological symptoms, mostly seen with CVC insertion into the subclavian vein.

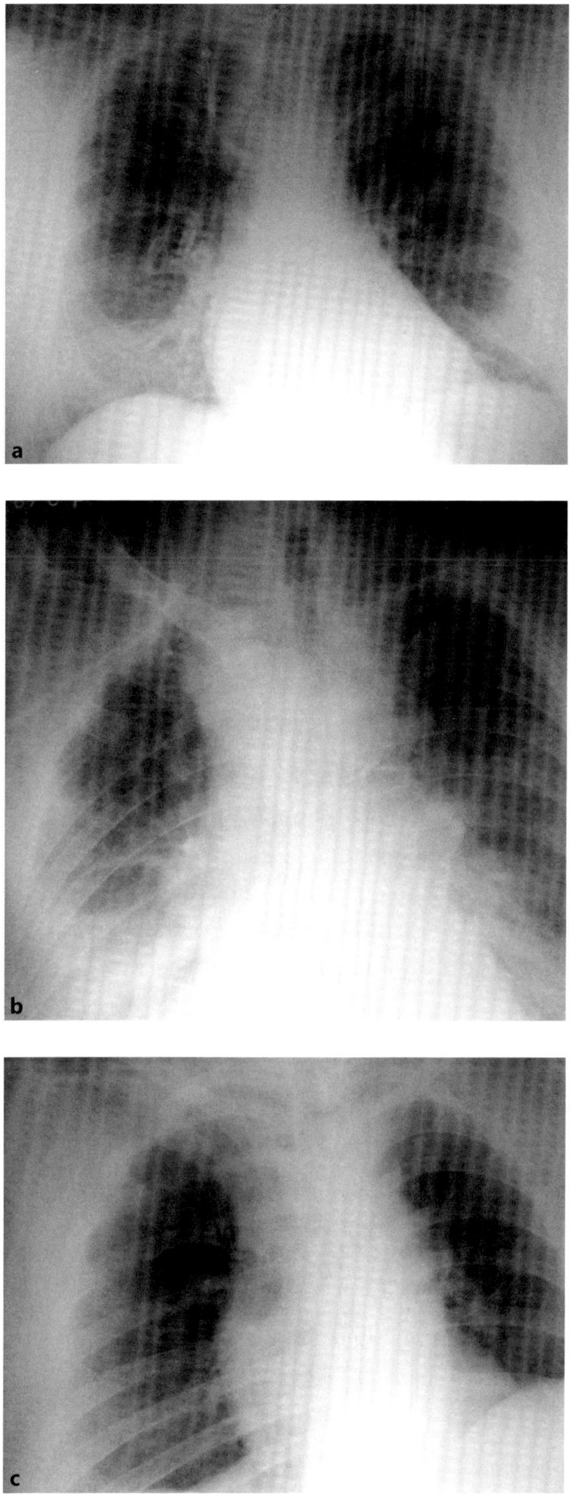

Fig. 4. Examples of CVC malposition. **a** The tip of the CVC introduced from the right jugular vein to the left-side vein. **b** The CVC introduced from the right jugular vein via the subclavian vein to the axillar vein. **c** Bended tip of the CVC. X-ray images: Dialysis Department, Prague-Strahov.

CVC malposition (CVC insertion into a wrong vein or penetration of the CVC tip outside the venous lumen) should be detected by fluoroscopy or immediate postinsertion X-ray (see examples in fig. 4). Malposition of CVC still inside the lumen can be solved by a fluoroscopy-controlled exchange. Insertion outside the venous lumen associated with vein perforation is a more serious complication, and vascular or cardiac surgeon cooperation is needed to solve this problem.

Safe and Effective Long-Term Catheter Use

Subsequent CVC Handling and Use

Follow-up care of the CVC after its insertion is equally if not more important for its long-term patency as the insertion itself. Use of the aseptic technique is a must [4, 5].

Disinfection and Disinfectants

Not all CVC types are made of the same material. During CVC care, the material comes in with applied disinfectant. CVC damage caused by nonadherence to the manufacturer's instructions on suitable disinfectant agents constitutes a typical preventable mistake. Table 1 gives principal information on the safety of use of the most often used disinfectant agents on the CVC material. Mixing of different disinfectant brands should generally never be attempted.

Regarding handling of the tCVC ports and exit site during personal hygiene (bath, shower), the CVC exit site should be always covered by a water-proof patch to avoid the CVC dressing material getting soaked. It is best to do it shortly before dialysis when the CVC dressing is changed.

Table 1. Applicability of the main disinfectant agents in the CVC materials

	Alcohol	Povidone-iodine
Polyurethane	no	yes
Silicon	yes	no
Polyurethane/polycarbonate copolymer	yes	yes

Risk of Blood Line Disconnection from the CVC Ports

The alarm system of current dialysis machines cannot reliably detect leaking connection(s) of the blood lines and the CVC ports or even their disconnection. This high safety thread can be significantly reduced by keeping the connectors visible during HD.

A detailed written history of each CVC must be maintained, starting with its insertion, immediate postinsertion care, changes of exit site dressing, description of all complications and provided treatment and interventions. Appointing a CVC coordinator simplifies all this. Each center should also have an internal written policy and procedure document on CVC insertion and subsequent care. It should provide detailed description of standard actions in CVC handling and care (exit site care, composition of the anticoagulation lock and its administration, etc.) as well as all interventions used in the particular center.

Anticoagulation Lock

An anticoagulation lock applied first immediately after insertion and then after each CVC use is necessary to prevent thrombosis. This area of CVC care is especially prone to errors classified as slip and lapses or commission errors in the introductory chapter. Currently, several solutions are used as anticoagulation lock differing both in the agent used and its concentration – heparin, trisodium citrate, taurolidine, antibiotics, etc. [16]. After proper flush-through with saline, the lock should be administered slowly to avoid partial entry into systemic circulation [17]. With heparin (concentrations in the lock 1,000–10,000 IU/l), it would lead to undesirable post-HD systemic anticoagulation. This lock is also suspected of contributing to biofilm formation. The 4% trisodium citrate provides comparable protection against intraluminal clotting, and inhibits biofilm formation (in vitro). Also decreased infection rate has been found with it [18]. High citrate concentration lock (30–46%) should be avoided because of a number of adverse events reported – from embolic complications [19, 20], catheter malfunctions up to fatal heart rhythm disruption caused by a change in blood calcium level when injected rapidly [21]. Contact of trisodium citrate with iodinated contrast media may also lead to precipitation reaction if the contrast media are not thoroughly flushed away before citrate injection [22]. Several alternative locks are now available, including combination of antiseptic solution or antibiotics with an anticoagulant [16] or recombinant tissue plasminogen activator (conventionally used as a thrombolytic agent). Novel CVC designs offer different coatings with antithrombotic and/or antiseptic effect (heparin, silver, bismuth), but their true benefits are still to be verified.

Special antimicrobial dressing materials are available, but studies with them have not shown any dramatic decrease in bloodstream infections [23, 24].

The recently introduced 'closed Luer-Lok access devices', sometimes called needle-free connectors may significantly reduce CVC bloodstream infections due to less manipulation with the ports. When there are no extracorporeal bloodlines connected to the CVC, the silicone seal automatically closes entry into it. With connection of the lines, a straight internal fluid path is created. Those devices make use of anticoagulant lock unnecessary and can thus be used in patients with heparin-induced thrombocytopenia. However, pressure drop over some types may decrease the blood flow obtainable from the CVC [25].

Monitoring Catheter Status and Function

K/DOQI guidelines on VA [5] say that 'dysfunctional catheter is usually easier to salvage than a nonfunctional one'. To detect a tCVC malfunction at its starting phase may be accomplished by regular monitoring. It can also serve as a supporting tool for decision on an intervention. For reliable detection of trends, monitoring should be done in a standardized way. The pressure/flow characteristics appear most suitable for this as both pre-pump pressure (PA) and pressure in the venous drip chamber (PV) and blood flow (Qb) are displayed on each dialysis machines.

The Hagen-Poiseuille's law postulates that the pressure drop along a tube is proportional to the flow through the tube and indirectly proportional to the fourth power of its inner diameter. In reality, the relation between Qb and PA or PV is slightly exponential [26] and relation of PA versus Qb is slightly steeper than that of PV versus Qb because of more turbulent flow in the 'arterial' CVC path. However, with intraluminal fibrin sheath formation (reduction in lumen), pressure drop increases indeed very steeply (with 4th power of decreasing CVC inner diameter). The sheath formation can thus be easily detected. In principle, the monitoring can use four different approaches looking at [27]:

- the Qb obtained at a predefined PA value
- the PA value reached at a predefined Qb value
- the Qb/PA ratio
- a complete graph of PA and PV versus Qb (PA and PV measured at several Qb values)

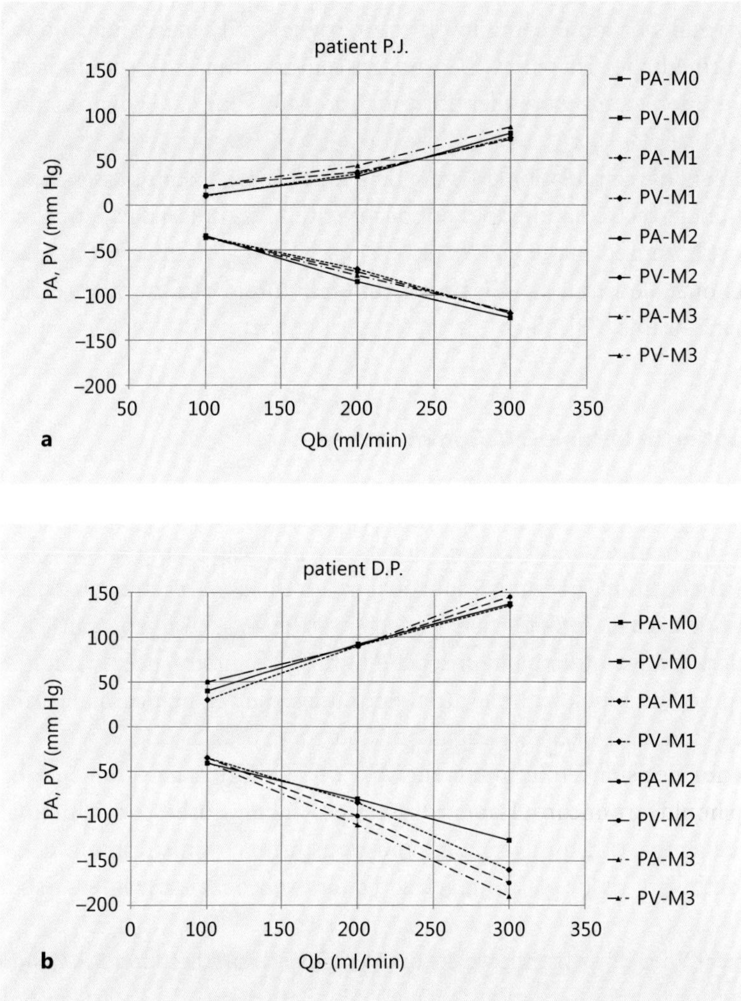

Fig. 5. The 'outward expanding' plot of in vivo measurements of PA, PV vs. Qb in several one-month intervals (M0, M1, M2, M3). **a** Well-functioning tCVC. **b** tCVC with gradually deteriorating arterial path. In vivo data from the Dialysis Department, Prague-Strahov.

The first three possibilities assess only the 'arterial' CVC path and provide basically the same information, although option 2 is the most practical of the three. Option 4 enables to assess status of both arterial and venous CVC path separately. Due to taking pressure values at several Qb, also the risk of incomparable slope evaluation inherent in option 3 is avoided.

Figure 5 shows an example of a well-functioning CV and a deteriorating CVC assessed in this way in several one-month intervals. In a small-scale analysis of preliminary results of monitoring in our unit, higher body mass index, lower blood flow through the vein with CVC, and low central venous pressure indicating poor hydration status were identified as risk factors for CVC malfunction development.

Measurement of recirculation does not help much in CVC status assessment. Cardiopulmonary recirculation does not occur with CVC unless the patient already has a still unused maturing AV access. Only CVC line reversal induces recirculation over 10%, and dialysis prolongation by 20–30 min may be needed to compensate for this [28].

Troubleshooting in Chronic CVC Complications

Causes of CVC malfunction (obtainable Qb <300 ml/min with PA = –250 mm Hg [29]) may be of mechanical nature, such as sharp CVC bending (kinking) or wrong CVC tip position (not in the right atrium). With CVC reaching just deep into superior vena cava, catheter may lean against the vessel wall and cause excessive suction. On the other hand, insertion of the CVC tip too deeply into the atrium bringing it in touch with the atrial floor may result in myocardial perforation.

CVC thrombosis may entirely disable CVC use. Unfortunately, none of the current approaches (anticoagulation locks, rapid saline flushes, intraluminal brushing, preventive oral anticoagulant and/or aspirin administration, weekly applied recombinant tissue plasminogen activator procedure) guarantees a success.

Fibrin sheath develops within weeks or even days (!) on the outer CVC surface and may act as a one-way valve when exceeding the CVC tip. Interventions include infusion of thrombolytics, endovascular fibrin sheath stripping using a snare catheter, disruption of the sheath by balloon angioplasty before the CVC exchange. In the case of CVC exchange, the catheter should be exposed near the neck, clamped and cut. In one lumen, a guide wire is inserted. After removing both parts of the old catheter, a new one is placed using a new subcutaneous tunnel to avoid infection.

Central vein stenosis is a frequent delayed complication (reported in 20–50% patients with CVC) eventually leading to thrombosis, especially in the subclavian vein. Sometimes, it is first diagnosed after the AVF creation, when the blood flow increases rapidly. A percutaneous balloon dilatation, other radiological interventions, stenting, or even surgery is needed.

In case of damaged parts of a catheter, catheter repair kits can be used so that catheter exchange is not necessary.

Conclusions

CVCs are special dialysis access type, very different from permanent AV accesses. On one side, patients with CVC exhibit higher morbidity and mortality, while on the other side CVC do not disrupt patient hemodynamics at all or to just a minor extent. Also risks and safety hazards associated with CVC use are different, often more serious than in AV accesses. CVC use and namely their insertion may thus have strong forensic implications. CVC status and patency monitoring is not yet properly developed and standardized. The ultimate solution may bring further development in CVC design [30] and use of less thrombogenic materials and coatings.

Acknowledgement

This work has been partly supported by the research project P25/LF1/2 of the Charles University Prague.

Disclosure Statement

The authors have no conflicts of interest to declare.

References

1 Schwab SJ, Beathard G: The hemodialysis catheter conundrum: hate living with them, but can't live without them. Kidney Int 1999; 56:1–17.

2 Rayner HC, Pisoni RL: The increasing use of hemodialysis catheters: evidence from the DOPPS on its significance and ways to reverse it. Semin Dial 2010;23:6–10.

3 Ocak G, Halbesma N, le Cessie S, et al: Haemodialysis catheters increase mortality as compared to arteriovenous accesses especially in elderly patients. Nephrol Dial Transplant 2011;26:2611–2617.

4 K/DOQI Clinical Practice Guidelines and Clinical Practice Recommendations 2006 Updates Vascular Access. Am J Kidney Dis 2006; 48(suppl 1):S176–S322.

5 Tordoir J, Canaud B, Haage P, Konner K, Basci A, Fouque D, Kooman J, Malo AM, Pedrini L, Pizzarelli F, Tattersall J, Vennegoor M, Wanner Ch, ter Wee P, Vanholder R: EBPG on Vascular Access. Nephrol Dial Transplant 2007;22(suppl 2):ii88–ii117.

6 McLaughlin K, Manns B, Mortis G et al: Why patients with ESRD do not select self-care dialysis as a treatment option. Am J Kidney Dis 2003;41:380–385.

7 Schillinger F, Schillinger D, Montagnac R, et al: Post catheterization vein stenosis in hemodialysis – comparative angiographic study of 50 subclavian and 50 internal jugular accesses. Nephrol Dial Transplant 1991;6:722–724.

8 Power A, Singh S, Ashby D, et al: Translumbar central venous catheters for long-term haemodialysis. Nephrol Dial Transpl 2010; 25:1588–1595.

9 Gallieni M: Central venous catheters: legal issues. J Vasc Access 2011;12:273–279.
10 Geddes CC, Walbaum D, Fox JG, Mactier RA: Insertion of internal jugular temporary hemodialysis cannulae by direct ultrasound guidance – a prospective comparison of experienced and inexperienced operators. Clin Nephrol 1998;50:320–325.
11 Keenan SP: Use of ultrasound to place central lines. J Crit Care 2002;17:126–137.
12 Polakovič V, Švára F, Dvořáková M: Dialysis catheter insertion with and without peel-away sheaths. Nephrol Dial Transplant 2007; 22:2359.
13 Vats HS: Complications of catheters: tunneled and nontunneled. Adv Chronic Kidney Dis 2012;19:188–194.
14 Fiaccadori E, Gonzi G, Zambrelli P, Tortorella G: Cardiac arrhythmias during central venous catheter procedures in acute renal failure: a prospective study. J Am Soc Nephrol 1996;7:1079–1084.
15 Gong Y, Xu HX, Lin M, Gu Y: An iatrogenic complication of internal jugular vein catheterization for hemodialysis. Ir J Med Sci 2012;181:135–137.
16 Niyyar VD: Catheter dysfunction: the role of lock solutions. Sem Dial 2012;25:693–699.
17 Polaschegg HD: A novel method for measuring catheter lock spillage: an in vitro study. Artif Organs 2012;36:824–829.
18 Zhao Y, Li Z, Zhang L, Yang J, Yang Y, Tang Y, Fu P: Citrate versus heparin lock for hemodialysis catheters: a systematic review and metaanalysis of randomized controlled trials. Am J Kidney Dis 2014;63:479–490.
19 Willicombe MK, Vernon K, Davenport A: Embolic complications from central venous hemodialysis catheters used with hypertonic citrate locking solution. Am J Kidney Dis 2010;55:348–351.
20 Schilcher G, Scharnagl H, Horina JH, et al: Trisodium citrate induced protein precipitation in haemodialysis catheters might cause pulmonary embolism. Nephrol Dial Transplant 2012;27:2953–2957.
21 FDA warning on Tricitrasol. http://www.hdcn.com/00/004fdci.htm.
22 Delcour C, Bruninx G: Incompatibility of contrast medium and trisodium citrate. Cardiovasc Intervent Radiol 2013;36:237–238.
23 Camins BC, Richmond AM, Dyer KL, et al: Crossover intervention trial evaluating the efficacy of a chlorhexidine-impregnated sponge in reducing catheter-related bloodstream infections among patients undergoing hemodialysis. Infect Control Hosp Epidemiol 2010;31:1118–1123.
24 Banton J: Techniques to prevent central venous catheter infections: products, research, and recommendations. Nutr Clin Pract 2006; 21:56–61.
25 Eloot S, De Vos JY, Hombrouckx R, Verdonck P: How much is catheter flow influenced by the use of closed luer lock access devices? Nephrol Dial Transplant 2007;22:3061–3064
26 Twardowski ZJ, Haynie JD: Measurements of hemodialysis catheter blood flow in vivo. Int J Artif Organs 2002;25:276–280.
27 Besarab A, Pandey R: Catheter management in hemodialysis patients: delivering adequate flow. Clin J Am Soc Nephrol 2011;6:227–234.
28 Twardowski ZJ, Van Stone JC, Jones ME, et al: Blood recirculation in intravenous catheters for hemodialysis. J Am Soc Nephrol 1993;3:1978–1981.
29 Niyyar VD, Chan MR: Interventional nephrology: catheter dysfunction – prevention and troubleshooting. Clin J Am Soc Nephrol 2013;8:1234–1243.
30 Ash SR: Advances in tunneled central venous catheters for dialysis: design and performance. Semin Dial 2008;21:504–515.

Vladimír Polakovič, MD, MBA
Department of Internal Medicine
General University Hospital
Šermířská 5, CZ–16900 Prague 6 – Strahov (Czech Republic)
E-Mail vladimir.polakovic@vfn.cz

Widmer MK, Malik J (eds): Patient Safety in Dialysis Access.
Contrib Nephrol. Basel, Karger, 2015, vol 184, pp 205–221
DOI: 10.1159/000366120

Nosocomial Infections in Dialysis Access

Alexander Schweiger[a] • Sergio Trevino[b] • Jonas Marschall[a, b]

[a]Department of Infectious Diseases, Bern University Hospital, Bern, Switzerland; [b]Division of Infectious Diseases, Washington University School of Medicine, St. Louis, Mo., USA

Abstract

Nosocomial infections in patients requiring renal replacement therapy have a high impact on morbidity and mortality. The most dangerous complication is bloodstream infection (BSI) associated with the vascular access, with a low BSI risk in arteriovenous fistulas or grafts and a comparatively high risk in central venous catheters. The single most important measure for preventing BSI is therefore the reduction of catheter use by means of early fistula formation. As this is not always feasible, prevention should focus on educational efforts, hand hygiene, surveillance of dialysis-associated events, and specific measures at and after the insertion of catheters. Core measures at the time of insertion include choosing the optimal site of insertion, the use of maximum sterile barrier precautions, adequate skin antisepsis, and the choice of catheter type; after insertion, access care needs to ensure hub disinfection and regular dressing changes. The application of antimicrobial locks is reserved for special situations. Evidence suggests that bundling a selection of the aforementioned measures can significantly reduce infection rates. The diagnosis of central line-associated BSI (CLABSI) is based on clinical signs and microbiological findings in blood cultures ideally drawn both peripherally and from the catheter. The prompt installation of empiric antibiotic treatment covering the most commonly encountered organisms is key regarding CLABSI treatment. Catheter removal is recommended in complicated cases or if cultures yield *Staphylococcus aureus*, enterococci, *Pseudomonas* or fungi. In other cases, guide wire exchange or catheter salvage strategies with antibiotic lock solutions may be acceptable alternatives.

Recommendations to Improve Patient Safety

- The implementation of a multidisciplinary team and so-called prevention bundles can decrease infections and improve safety in dialysis patients.
- The most effective preventive measure for vascular access infections is using a fistula instead of a catheter.
- Surveillance of dialysis-associated events is necessary to develop and measure the effectiveness of preventive measures.
- Infectious Diseases Society of America and European Renal Best Practice have developed guidelines for the management of hemodialysis catheter-associated infections.

Introduction

Health care-associated infections (HAIs) are one of the major threats to patient safety, yet they have not been widely perceived as such before the advent of the patient safety movement. Between one and two third of HAIs are thought to be preventable [1], which would translate into ten thousands of saved lives and billions of dollars in expenses avoided in US hospitals alone each year. A number of entities such as the Centers for Disease Control and Prevention (CDC), the Society for Healthcare Epidemiology of America (SHEA), the European Renal Association (ERA), and also the patient safety-oriented Institute for Healthcare Improvement (www.ihi.org) therefore publish HAI prevention guidelines to advance implementation of best practices [2, 3]. The incidence of central line-associated bloodstream infections (CLABSIs), which exhibit higher mortality than most other HAIs, may drop to rates as low as zero with a robust infection prevention program [4].

Hemodialysis (HD) catheter-associated bloodstream infections (BSIs) are a type of CLABSI due to a central venous catheter (CVC) specifically designed for HD. In 2002, it was estimated that 50,000 CLABSIs occur in dialysis patients in the US annually. A more recent surveillance study found the rate of access-related BSIs to be 0.73 events per 100 patient-months [5]. Aside from catheters, patients in need of renal replacement therapy should eventually use arteriovenous fistula (AVF) or arteriovenous grafts (AVG) for HD, or alternatively, may receive peritoneal dialysis. All renal replacement therapies are associated with a risk of infection; however, this risk varies with the method selected. Data from a CDC surveillance program display nicely how the type of access influences the BSI rate per 100 patient-months: 0.5 (for AVFs), 0.9 (AVG), 4.2 (permanent CVCs), and an impressive 27.1 for temporary CVCs [6]. Another, more practical effect of an infection is that the vascular access is (at least temporarily) lost, thereby complicating care further. Therefore, the single most important preventive measure for CLABSI is using a fistula instead of a catheter. However, an AVF requires maturation before it can be accessed the first time. Temporary catheterization for HD may be necessary in cases where renal function deteriorates quickly and the fistula is not functional yet. An emphasis for early planning of vascular surgery has been made by the Centers for Medicare and Medicaid Services' Fistula First initiative. The goal of having a ready-to-use fistula in 66% of patients meeting dialysis criteria for the first time, however, has not yet been reached.

In the following text, we will discuss the current management and prevention strategies for HD catheter-associated BSIs. Because the population of patients requiring renal replacement therapy in the US is expected to grow from approximately 600,000 today to 750,000 in the year 2020 [7], implementing evidence-based infection prevention strategies now will spare our patients much suffering in the future.

Prevention

There is relatively little research on CLABSI in dialysis patients; nevertheless, several authorities have issued guidelines concerning the prevention of (dialysis-associated) CLABSI, including the CDC, SHEA and the ERA [2, 3, 8]. Major recommendations are summarized in table 1. In addition, a bundled approach for prevention of BSI in dialysis facilities was proposed by the CDC [9]; key interventions are listed in table 2.

Before Insertion

Staff Education and Competency

All staff need to receive education upon entry into the facility, which has to be repeated in regular intervals (at least annually), and should be accompanied by regular audits to ensure sustained compliance. Education should focus on knowledge about nosocomial infections at dialysis centers, infection control best practices, including access care and aseptic technique, and how to educate patients and other caregivers [9].

Table 1. Overview of specific recommendations for the prevention of CLABSIs as applicable to HD patients

Intervention	CDC [3]	SHEA [4]	ERA [5]
Before insertion			
Staff education and periodic assessment	Yes	Yes	Establishment of standard protocols in each center
Patient education	No recommendation	No recommendation	Yes
Reduction of catheter use	Yes Remove nonessential catheters	Remove nonessential catheters	Yes
At insertion			
Tunneled catheters	No recommendation	No recommendation	Preferred except in acute kidney injury
Hand hygiene	Yes	Yes	Yes
Coated catheters	CHSS or minocycline/rifampin for dwelling times >5 days if lack of control despite basic practices	Lack of control despite basic practices	No recommendation
Insertion site	Avoid femoral site in adults Avoid subclavian site in dialysis patients Tunneled CVC: no recommendation	Avoid femoral site in adults	Jugular vein preferred (right > left) Femoral and subclavian discouraged
Skin antisepsis	Alcoholic CHG >0.5%, alternatives if contraindicated: iodophore, tincture of iodine, or 70% alcohol CHG age <2 months: unresolved issue Alcoholic CHG vs. alcoholic PVI: unresolved issue	CHG based (age <2 months)	No specific recommendation
Maximum sterile barrier precautions	Yes	Yes	Yes
Checklist/CVC-cart	No recommendation	Yes/yes	No recommendation

Table 1 (continued)

Intervention	CDC [3]	SHEA [4]	ERA [5]
After insertion Dressing changes			
– Interval	Short-term CVCs: – Gauze: 2 days – Transparent ≤7 days Tunneled or implanted: – Transparent ≥7 days until site healed – No recommendation if exit site healed Replace if loose, soiled or damp	Nontunneled: – Transparent: 5–7 days – Site care with CHG-based solution (adults and adolescents) – Gauze: 2 days Replace if loose, soiled or damp	Replace on a routine base if not clean or intact
– Type of dressing	Gauze or transparent-semipermeable Gauze if patient diaphoretic or site is oozing/bleeding	No recommendation	Gauze preferred
Antimicrobial ointments/ impregnated dressings	PVI or polysporin ointment in HD patients CHG sponge for short-term catheters if lack of control despite basic practices	Antimicrobial ointments CHG sponges (>2 months) if lack of control despite basic practices	To consider until insertion site has healed
Antimicrobial locks	Patients with long-term catheters and multiple CLABSI despite aseptic technique	Consider if CLABSI rates are high despite basic practices	Use advocated, citrate 4% preferred
Needleless connectors	Split septum preferred over some mechanical valves	No routine use of mechanical valves and only after risk-analysis and education on proper use	No recommendations
Hub disinfection	Yes	Yes	No specific recommendation
Scheduled catheter changes	Not recommended	Not recommended	No recommendation
Guide wire exchange	Nontunneled: not in case of suspected infection	No recommendation	In infected catheters if successful antibiotic treatment for 3 days
Surveillance	Yes	Yes	No recommendation

CHG = Chlorhexidine gluconate; CHSS = chlorhexidine-silver sulfadiazine; PVI = povidone iodine.

Table 2. Core interventions for dialysis BSI prevention [16]

Key intervention	Contents
Surveillance and feedback	– Conduct monthly surveillance for BSIs and other dialysis events using CDCs National Healthcare Safety Network (NHSN) – Calculate facility rates and compare to rates in other NHSN facilities – Actively share results with front-line clinical staff
Hand hygiene observations	– Perform observations of hand hygiene opportunities monthly and share results with clinical staff
Catheter/vascular access care observations	– Perform observations of vascular access care and catheter accessing quarterly – Assess staff adherence to aseptic technique when connecting and disconnecting catheters and during dressing changes – Share results with clinical staff
Staff education and competency	– Train staff on infection control topics, including access care and aseptic technique – Perform competency evaluation for skills such as catheter care and accessing every 6–12 months and upon hire
Patient education/ engagement	– Provide standardized education to all patients on infection prevention topics including vascular access care, hand hygiene, risks related to catheter use, recognizing signs of infection, and instructions for access management when away from the dialysis unit
Reduction of catheter use	– Incorporate efforts (e.g., through patient education, vascular access coordinator) to reduce catheters by identifying and addressing barriers to permanent vascular access placement and catheter removal
Chlorhexidine for skin antisepsis	– Use an alcohol-based chlorhexidine (>0.5%) solution as the first-line skin antiseptic agent for central line insertion and during dressing changes – Povidone-iodine (preferably with alcohol) or 70% alcohol alternatives for patients with chlorhexidine intolerance
Catheter hub disinfection	– Scrub catheter hubs with an appropriate antiseptic after cap is removed and before accessing – Perform every time catheter is accessed or disconnected – If closed needleless connector device is used, disinfect connector device per manufacturer's instructions
Antimicrobial ointment	– Apply antibiotic ointment or povidone-iodine ointment to catheter exit sites during dressing change – Use of chlorhexidine-impregnated sponge dressing might be an alternative

Patient Education

In its core interventions for BSI reduction, the CDC advocates patient education. Main components are (1) hand hygiene and basic infection control practices during catheter accessing process (e.g., aseptic technique, masks, hub disinfection), (2) access care at home, (3) role of and risks associated with catheters, and (4) knowing signs and symptoms of infection and when to notify the physician. Despite mixed results in other studies, Cheng et al. [10] described a 40% lower risk of hospitalization due to infection and a 51% mortality reduction in patients with chronic kidney disease who received a multidisciplinary education prior to dialysis onset. We conclude that patient education is a valuable tool in the prevention of CLABSIs.

Hand Hygiene of Staff

Hand washing, or preferably hand disinfection reduces HAIs in different settings, and is one of the key measures for preventing CLABSI. Regular audits on compliance with hand hygiene should be performed. Alcohol-based waterless products or the combination of antiseptic soap and water are preferred. The use of gloves does not obviate hand hygiene [11].

At Insertion

Insertion Site

HD catheters are inserted in the internal jugular vein (IJV) or femoral vein (FV). The subclavian site should be avoided due to the risk of stenosis formation, which may only manifest after AVF creation [3]. No significant differences in CLABSI rates were found between IJV and FV with short-term dialysis (median 5 days). But with longer dwelling time, the FV site carries a 5 times higher risk for bacteremia in dialysis patients than the IJV [12]. The likelihood of bacteremia for the FV site increases by catheterization weeks 1–2, whereas for the IJV the risk increase comes at a later time, around weeks 3–4. Both CDC and ERA recommend using the IJV first for HD.

In addition, maximum sterile barrier precautions for catheter insertion should be meticulously applied as they reduce the incidence of CLABSIs [4].

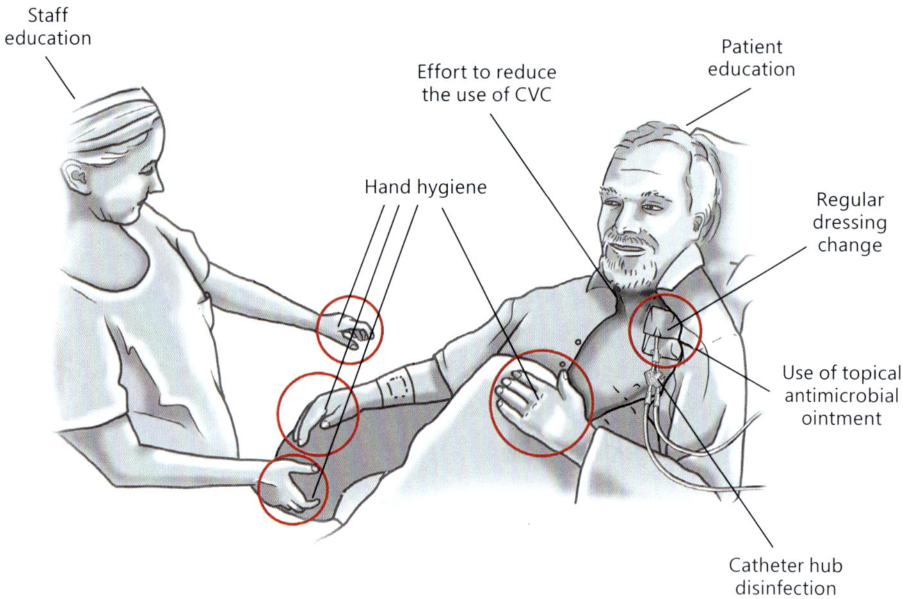

Fig. 1. Strategies to prevent CLABSIs.

Coated Catheters

The efficacy of antimicrobial coating of CVCs in the acute setting has been thoroughly evaluated. Coatings with chlorhexidine-silver sulfadiazine and minocycline/rifampin have been proven to significantly reduce the risk of CLABSI. In situations of high CLABSI rates and short-term dwelling times, these catheters can be cost-efficient. In HD patients, high-level evidence for significant reduction of the infection risk only exists for catheters coated with minocycline/rifampin [13]. Catheters solely coated with silver were not superior to untreated catheters in dialysis patients. Although some coated catheters will influence the CLABSI risk in dialysis patients, the additional cost has to be factored in.

Skin Antisepsis

Chlorhexidine gluconate (CHG) for skin antisepsis is superior to aqueous povidone iodine (PVI) for prevention of CLABSI [14]. In comparison to *alcoholic* PVI, no clear evidence exists as to the superiority or inferiority of CHG solutions. The optimal concentration of CHG remains unclear. The CDC advocate the use of alcoholic CHG >0.5%, although this recommendation is mainly based on the fast bactericidal activity, longer-lasting antimicrobial effect, and the low rate of CHG inactivation by protein-rich materials (e.g., blood) [2]. Octenidine 0.1% in propranolol, which is not FDA approved, showed mixed results when compared with ethanol/propranolol or CHG. Further trials are needed to clarify its efficacy.

Whereas no reactions of polyurethane catheters to either of the aforementioned disinfectants are reported in the literature, PVI may adversely affect silicone tubing. Therefore, its compatibility with silicone catheters should be verified according to the manufacturer's recommendations prior to use.

After Insertion

As the risk of CLABSI increases in function of dwelling time [12, 15], catheter care after insertion is of paramount importance (fig. 1).

Dressing Changes

Dressing changes should be performed at regular intervals of up to 7 days for transparent dressings, which is not inferior to changes every 3 days [16]. Gauze dressings should be changed every other day, but with tunneled catheters the interval can be as long as 7 days [2]. Dressings should be changed earlier when loose, damp or soiled [2, 8]. CHG-impregnated dressings or sponges significantly reduced the rate of CLABSIs when compared with standard dressings in nondialysis studies [16].

Camins et al. [17] evaluated the efficacy of CHG sponges (Biopatch®) compared to standard of care (sodium-hypochlorite solution 0.114%) in dialysis patients. No significant differences in terms of CLABSI rates were found. The authors suspected that the infection risk in their patient collective was more likely to have originated from the hub than from the insertion site.

The main adverse event of CHG is contact dermatitis (~5% rate), although 96% of these events occurred in neonates. Reduced susceptibility to CHG has been documented, but its clinical impact is unclear. In summary, the use of CHG-impregnated dressings reduced the CLABSI risk in short-term nontunneled CVCs, but as of yet no sound evidence supports its application in dialysis patients.

Topical Compounds (for CLABSI Prevention)

Topical antimicrobial ointments (mupirocin, polysporin, PVI) can reduce CLABSI rates in HD patients. Specifically, mupirocin ointment significantly reduced CLABSIs (OR: 0.17, 95% CI 0.07–0.43). No serious adverse events were reported in all studies included in this meta-analysis [18], nor are there reports of mupirocin resistance in studies involving dialysis patients. Polysporin antibiotic ointment (bacitracin/gramicidin/polymyxin B) was evaluated in a double-blind, placebo-controlled, randomized trial including 162 dialysis patients, yielding a significantly lower rate of bacteremia [0.63 catheter-days (treatment group) vs. 2.48/1,000 (placebo group); $p = 0.0004$]. The time to first bacteremia, infection-related morbidity, and mortality rates also scored favorably in the treatment group [19]. Topical PVI significantly reduced CLABSI incidence as compared to sterile gauze alone (2 vs. 17%, $p < 0.01$), and this risk reduction was most evident in nasal *Staphylococcus aureus* carriers [20]. Topical Medhoney (a medicinal honey formulation) did not reduce the risk of infectious complications [18].

In conclusion, evidence exists for the topical use of mupirocin, polysporin B, and to a lesser degree PVI for CLABSI prevention. The potential for mupirocin resistance development has to be considered. Currently, while gramicidin is not available in the US, a similar preparation in the form of bacitracin/neomycin/polymyxin B is commonly used.

Hub Disinfection

All hubs should be disinfected prior to and after accessing. The efficacy of different disinfection times (3, 10, 15 s) with 70% ethanol on deliberately *S. aureus*-contaminated hubs was evaluated. Although no significant difference in reduction of contamination was found, the number of colony-forming units was markedly lower after 15 s. The authors posited a protecting role of longer disinfection [21]. No data exist for HD catheters.

More data are needed regarding the role of needleless connectors in the prevention of CLABSI. The safety of mechanical valve systems has been questioned in several studies on CLABSIs [22, 23]. If needleless connectors are used, split-septum devices are preferred to devices with mechanical valves. Currently, there is no sound evidence supporting or opposing the use of closed luer access devices to prevent CLABSI.

Antimicrobial Lock Solutions

Antimicrobial lock solutions (ALS) containing antibiotics (vancomycin, minocycline, gentamicin, cefazolin, and cefotaxim alone or in combination with gentamicin) decrease CLABSI rates in HD patients. Studies have shown that ALS containing gentamicin were more efficient than those without, but there is concern for publication bias. Other lock solutions with antimicrobial properties, such as citrate- and taurolidine-containing locks have showed mixed results regarding the impact on CLABSI incidence in dialysis patients. A novel catheter lock solution containing 7.0% sodium citrate, 0.15% methylene blue, 0.15% methylparaben, and 0.015% propylparaben (C-MB-P) was superior to standard heparin lock in a randomized controlled trial of 407 HD patients [24]. Thrombolytic locking solution has also shown promise in reducing bacteremias. The use of recombinant tissue plasminogen activator (rt-PA) substituting heparin at the midweek dialysis session significantly reduced the incidence of catheter malfunction and bacteremia [25]. When used for prevention, ALS significantly lowers CLABSI risk. In our opinion, antibiotics used in the treatment of systemic infections should not be routinely used for prevention purposes in form of ALS due to the risk of antimicrobial resistance development. In contrast, citrate, C-MB-P and rt-PA are not used for infection therapy and are therefore valuable alternatives. Nevertheless, the safety, applicability and cost of the latter two strategies still require further studies.

Bundles

The implementation of bundles containing various key interventions for infection prevention as discussed earlier has been advocated by the CDC initiative for reducing CLABSI in HD patients (table 2). The implementation of these key interventions or select elements thereof in a bundled approach has been shown to reduce CLABSI rates by 21–100% [5, 26, 27].

Prevention and Surveillance at a Facility Level

As mentioned above, prevention and management of CLABSIs in dialysis patients requires a multidisciplinary effort as suggested by the CDC core interventions. The most effective intervention for reducing CLABSIs is avoiding the placement of a CVC. The implementation of a multidisciplinary CVC team or designating a vascular access nurse in conjunction with evidence-based guidelines has multiple benefits; but when it pertains to prevention, it has been shown to achieve the following goals [28, 29]:

- Increase the use of AVF as the first vascular access
- Reduce the total number of CVC days
- Reduce the rate of CVC loss due to infection
- Decrease the rate of treatment failure in CLABSI
- Lower the rate of death due to sepsis.

In order to track catheter infections over time and correlate them with preventive measures, the facility must perform CLABSI surveillance. Currently, all outpatient HD facilities in the US are required to conduct monthly surveillance using the NHSN Dialysis Event Manual (available at: http://www.cdc.gov/nhsn/dialysis/dialysis-event.html). The facility has 60 days to submit the surveillance report with data about the three types of dialysis events: (1) intravenous antimicrobial starts – all intravenous antibiotics and antifungals; (2) positive blood culture, categorized by source as vascular access, other source or contaminant; (3) pus, redness, or increased swelling at the vascular access site.

Surveillance and prevention of drug-resistant organisms (DRO) such as MRSA and vancomycin-resistant *Enterococcus* (VRE) are still an unresolved issue without specific recommendations from the Infectious Diseases Society of America (IDSA) or European Renal Best Practice (ERBP). MRSA colonization in a high-prevalence country was found to be 2–4% in HD patients and 4–6% in dialysis unit personnel. Patients that require HD and are MRSA carriers have a 2.5-fold increase in all-cause mortality [30]. Decolonization techniques including nasal mupirocin and whole body chlorhexidine wash may achieve elimination of *Staphylococcus* and a risk reduction for major infections in the short term, but development of resistance has been documented. VRE colonization prevalence in HD patients can be up to 3–9%, depending on geographical region. Of note, there is a significant potential for MRSA and VRE transmissions between HD patients in the dialysis setting [31]. The unique situation of dialysis patients (relative immunosuppression, frequent exposure to antibiotics, and repeated exposure to health care settings) exposes them to multiple opportunities to acquire DROs outside the dialysis setting and introduce it to the unit. The transmission dynamics of a dialysis unit are complex and involve large open rooms, shared treatment environment, and contact with multiple inanimate surfaces in common areas. Contact isolation of known DRO-colonized or -infected patients is difficult to achieve in outpatient HD centers, but effective when correctly implemented. Organizational strategies from other industries such as Toyota production systems (TPS) and positive deviance (PD) are being studied and have demonstrated a reduction of MRSA colonization, infection and BSI rates in a dialysis setting [32]. TPS involves the continuous identification of problem processes (e.g., inconveniently located alcohol dispensers for hand hygiene) and the standardization of solutions (e.g., placement of dispensers to optimize access). PD is a systems and behavior change strategy that recognizes exceptional progress or 'positive deviants' in a certain process (e.g., a specific nursing unit that achieved 100% hand hygiene rates) by studying their process and sharing it with the rest of the organization.

Management of BSIs

Recommendations for diagnosis and management of CLABSIs associated with HD catheters are based on IDSA [33] and ERBP [3] guidelines. Local signs may include erythema, warmth, swelling, tenderness, and purulent discharge, and may be found both in exit site infections and in BSIs, although the absence of local signs does not rule out bacteremia. The diagnosis of HD catheter-associated BSIs rests on blood culturing just like it does for CLABSIs outside the dialysis unit. If CLABSI is suspected (e.g., fever, sepsis, purulent discharge from the catheter exit site), at least two sets of blood cultures should be obtained, ideally pairing a catheter culture with another one drawn peripherally. If a fistula has yet to be created, peripheral cultures in that extremity may not be in order. It is recommended to apply a disinfectant to both catheter hub and skin before drawing these cultures. Also, intravenous antibiotics should be held until cultures have been taken. Common pathogens are *Staphylococcus aureus*, coagulase-negative staphylococci, and to a lesser degree, Gram-negative bacteria, enterococci and *Candida*. The formation of biofilm plays a major role in the pathophysiology and treatment of CLABSIs. In patients with bacteremia, the outer surface of the extravascular segment of the tunneled dialysis catheters has the thickest measured biofilm and is most likely to have an organism cultured [34]. The presence and location of the biofilm contributes to the need for catheter removal in certain infections. The management of CLABSIs is summarized in the flowchart (fig. 2). Infections are considered 'complicated' if any of the characteristics in table 3 is present.

Empiric therapy should be tailored to each institution's resistance profile, but usually will include vancomycin (or cefazolin if low prevalence of MRSA) plus another antibiotic with Gram-negative coverage (e.g., third-generation cephalosporin, carbapenem, or β-lactam/β-lactamase inhibitor). If methicillin-susceptible *S. aureus* is found as the causative pathogen, then cefazolin or flucloxacillin/oxacillin should be the treatment of choice. In general, we prefer antibiotics that need to be administered after dialysis only. The most commonly utilized postdialysis antibiotic regimens include vancomycin, teicoplanin, cefazolin,

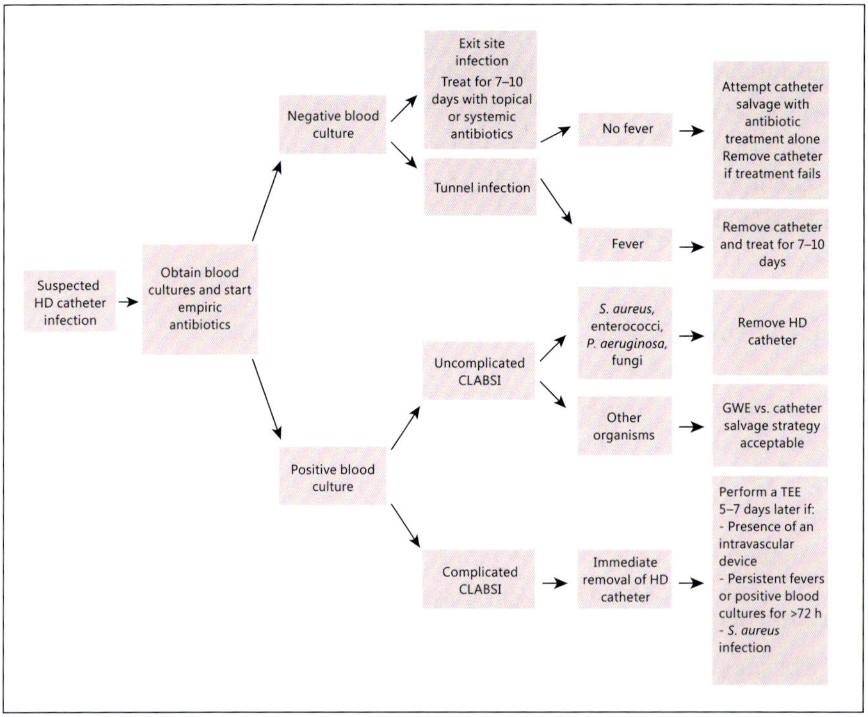

Fig. 2. Treatment algorithm for suspected HD catheter infection. TEE = Transesophageal echocardiography; GWE = guidewire exchange.

Table 3. The presence of any of these criteria should prompt the classification of a CLABSI as 'complicated CLABSI' and it should be managed accordingly

Criteria for complicated CLABSI
Severe sepsis
Thrombophlebitis
Metastatic infection
Tunnel infection with fever
Persistent signs and symptoms or positive blood culture after >48–72 h of appropriate antimicrobial therapy

ceftazidime and daptomycin. The duration of antibiotic therapy for HD catheter infections is summarized in table 4.

A frequently encountered clinical scenario in CLABSIs with HD catheters is the decision to perform a guide wire exchange (GWE) versus changing the access site. Immediate catheter removal is preferable in complicated infections.

Table 4. Duration of antibiotic treatment for CLABSI after blood cultures are negative

Tunnel infection and negative blood culture	7–10 days
Uncomplicated CLABSI	2–3 weeks
Uncomplicated CLABSI with *S. aureus*	4 weeks[a]
CLABSI with positive blood culture >48–72 h after catheter removal	6 weeks
CLABSI with metastatic infection	6 weeks
CLABSI and osteomyelitis	8 weeks

[a] 2–3 weeks should suffice if transesophageal echocardiogram fails to show vegetations.

Performing GWE is acceptable with uncomplicated CLABSIs or when other access sites are unavailable. If clinical symptoms resolve within 2–3 days and there is no evidence of metastatic infection, GWE is associated with comparable cure rates to those encountered after immediate removal and delayed placement of a new catheter. If catheter removal or GWE is deemed unnecessary, undesirable or impossible, catheter salvage with antibiotic lock solution along with systemic antibiotics can be considered. In our personal experience, only a small number of dialysis patients qualify for lock therapy. Also, the logistics of administering lock therapy have to be considered. Both GWE and catheter salvage strategies are associated with (unacceptably) high treatment failure rate when *S. aureus*, *Pseudomonas aeruginosa*, enterococci or fungi are involved. If a GWE or catheter salvage strategy is chosen but the patient has ongoing symptoms for >72 h or blood cultures are persistently positive, the catheter has to be removed. Surveillance blood cultures should be obtained one week after completion of antibiotic therapy in the setting of GWE or catheter salvage; if positive, catheter removal is indicated.

Infections of AVF are less frequent than CLABSI, and usually occur at the cannulation site. Vascular surgeons should evaluate the AVF to determine the need for surgical resection. Regardless, these infections should be treated for 6 weeks, in analogy to subacute bacterial endocarditis. Antibiotic therapy should be guided by culture results and resistance profiles. AVG infections usually require surgical revision with either partial, subtotal or total excision of the graft.

Disclosure Statement

A.S. and S.T. have no conflict of interest to report. Over the past 5 years, J.M. has been supported by the NIH CTSA (UL1RR024992) and is a recipient of a KL2 career development award (KL2RR024994). Via the NIH NCATS, he received support from the Building Interdisciplinary Research Careers in Women's Health program, a career development award (5K12HD001459-13). Currently, he is the section leader for a subproject of the CDC Prevention Epicenters Program grant (U54 CK000162; PI: Fraser). In addition, J.M. received funding from the Barnes-Jewish Hospital Patient Safety & Quality Fellowship Program and a research grant from the Barnes-Jewish Hospital Foundation & Washington University's Institute for Clinical and Translational Science. He has received funding for speaking at and attending an international conference from Gilead Sciences, Switzerland.

References

1 Umscheid CA, et al: Estimating the proportion of healthcare-associated infections that are reasonably preventable and the related mortality and costs. Infect Control Hosp Epidemiol 2011;32:101–114.
2 O'Grady NP, et al: Guidelines for the prevention of intravascular catheter-related infections. Clin Infect Dis 2011;52:e162–e193.
3 Vanholder R, et al: Diagnosis, prevention and treatment of haemodialysis catheter-related bloodstream infections (CRBSI): a position statement of European Renal Best Practice (ERBP). NDT Plus 2010;3:234–246.
4 Pronovost P, et al: An intervention to decrease catheter-related bloodstream infections in the ICU. N Engl J Med 2006;355: 2725–2732.
5 Patel PR, et al: Bloodstream infection rates in outpatient hemodialysis facilities participating in a collaborative prevention effort: a quality improvement report. Am J Kidney Dis 2013;62:322–330.
6 Klevens RM, et al: Dialysis Surveillance Report: National Healthcare Safety Network (NHSN)-data summary for 2006. Semin Dial 2008;21:24–28.
7 Camins BC: Prevention and treatment of hemodialysis-related bloodstream infections. Semin Dial 2013;26:476–481.
8 Yokoe DS, et al: A compendium of strategies to prevent healthcare-associated infections in acute care hospitals. Infect Control Hosp Epidemiol 2008;29(suppl 1):S12–S21.
9 Centers for Disease Control and Prevention: CDC Approach to BSI Prevention in Dialysis Facilities (i.e., the Core Interventions for Dialysis Bloodstream Infection (BSI) Prevention). 2013. http://www.cdc.gov/dialysis/prevention-tools/core-interventions.html.
10 Cheng SY, et al: Evaluation of inpatient multidisciplinary palliative care unit on terminally ill cancer patients from providers' perspectives: a propensity score analysis. Jpn J Clin Oncol 2013;43:161–169.
11 Boyce JM, Pittet D: Guideline for Hand Hygiene in Health-Care Settings: recommendations of the Healthcare Infection Control Practices Advisory Committee and the HICPAC/SHEA/APIC/IDSA Hand Hygiene Task Force. Infect Control Hosp Epidemiol 2002;23(12 suppl):S3–S40.
12 Lemaire X, et al: Analysis of risk factors for catheter-related bacteremia in 2000 permanent dual catheters for hemodialysis. Blood Purif 2009;28:21–28.
13 Chatzinikolaou I, et al: Antibiotic-coated hemodialysis catheters for the prevention of vascular catheter-related infections: a prospective, randomized study. Am J Med 2003; 115:352–357.
14 Maiwald M, Chan ES: The forgotten role of alcohol: a systematic review and meta-analysis of the clinical efficacy and perceived role of chlorhexidine in skin antisepsis. PLoS One 2012;7:e44277.
15 Oliver MJ, et al: Risk of bacteremia from temporary hemodialysis catheters by site of insertion and duration of use: a prospective study. Kidney Int 2000;58:2543–2545.
16 Timsit JF, et al: Chlorhexidine-impregnated sponges and less frequent dressing changes for prevention of catheter-related infections in critically ill adults: a randomized controlled trial. JAMA 2009;301:1231–1241.
17 Camins BC, et al: A crossover intervention trial evaluating the efficacy of a chlorhexidine-impregnated sponge in reducing catheter-related bloodstream infections among patients undergoing hemodialysis. Infect Control Hosp Epidemiol 2010;31:1118–1123.

18 McCann M, Moore ZE: Interventions for preventing infectious complications in haemodialysis patients with central venous catheters. Cochrane Database Syst Rev 2010; CD006894.
19 Lok CE, et al: Hemodialysis infection prevention with polysporin ointment. J Am Soc Nephrol 2003;14:169–179.
20 Levin A, et al: Prevention of hemodialysis subclavian vein catheter infections by topical povidone-iodine. Kidney Int 1991;40:934–938.
21 Simmons S, Bryson C, Porter S: 'Scrub the hub': cleaning duration and reduction in bacterial load on central venous catheters. Crit Care Nurs Q 2011;34:31–35.
22 Maragakis LL, et al: Increased catheter-related bloodstream infection rates after the introduction of a new mechanical valve intravenous access port. Infect Control Hosp Epidemiol 2006;27:67–70.
23 Jarvis WR, et al: Health care-associated bloodstream infections associated with negative- or positive-pressure or displacement mechanical valve needleless connectors. Clin Infect Dis 2009;49:1821–1827.
24 Maki DG, et al: A novel antimicrobial and antithrombotic lock solution for hemodialysis catheters: a multi-center, controlled, randomized trial. Crit Care Med 2011;39:613–620.
25 Hemmelgarn BR, et al: Prevention of dialysis catheter malfunction with recombinant tissue plasminogen activator. N Engl J Med 2011; 364:303–312.
26 Rosenblum A, et al: Hemodialysis catheter care strategies: a cluster-randomized quality improvement initiative. Am J Kidney Dis 2014;63:259–267.
27 Bren V, et al: Getting to zero: outpatient hemodialysis catheter-associated bloodstream infections; in Fifth Decennial International Conference on Healthcare-Associated Infections, Atlanta, March 2010.
28 Polkinghorne KR, Seneviratne M, Kerr PG: Effect of a vascular access nurse coordinator to reduce central venous catheter use in incident hemodialysis patients: a quality improvement report. Am J Kidney Dis 2009;53: 99–106.
29 Mokrzycki MH, et al: An interventional controlled trial comparing 2 management models for the treatment of tunneled cuffed catheter bacteremia: a collaborative team model versus usual physician-managed care. Am J Kidney Dis 2006;48:587–595.
30 Lai CF, et al: Nasal carriage of methicillin-resistant *Staphylococcus aureus* is associated with higher all-cause mortality in hemodialysis patients. Clin J Am Soc Nephrol 2011;6: 167–174.
31 Lee SC, et al: An outbreak of methicillin-resistant *Staphylococcus aureus* infections related to central venous catheters for hemodialysis. Infect Control Hosp Epidemiol 2004; 25:678–684.
32 Ellingson K, et al: Sustained reduction in the clinical incidence of methicillin-resistant *Staphylococcus aureus* colonization or infection associated with a multifaceted infection control intervention. Infect Control Hosp Epidemiol 2011;32:1–8.
33 Mermel LA, et al: Clinical practice guidelines for the diagnosis and management of intravascular catheter-related infection: 2009 Update by the Infectious Diseases Society of America. Clin Infect Dis 2009;49:1–45.
34 Ramanathan V, et al: Characteristics of biofilm on tunneled cuffed hemodialysis catheters in the presence and absence of clinical infection. Am J Kidney Dis 2012;60:976–982.

Jonas Marschall, MD
Department of Infectious Diseases
Bern University Hospital
Friedbühlstrasse 51, CH–3010 Bern (Switzerland)
E-Mail jonas.marschall@insel.ch

Widmer MK, Malik J (eds): Patient Safety in Dialysis Access.
Contrib Nephrol. Basel, Karger, 2015, vol 184, pp 222–233
DOI: 10.1159/000366121

How to Improve Vascular Access Care

Magda van Loon
University Medical Center, Maastricht, The Netherlands

Abstract
Preservation of a well-functioning vascular access (VA) is one of the most important and problematic areas in the care of dialysis patients. Providing high quality of care can reduce morbidity, improve quality of life and reduces costs. Given the increased complexity and the multidisciplinary character of VA care, it is a prerequisite to establish a dedicated multidisciplinary approach. An essential part of VA care is the management of the process before, during and after cannulation. A lack of knowledge and skills can have major implications for dialysis patients and may be related to VA outcome. Therefore, VA care requires continuous education of staff and patients, timely referral, adequate planning, and early identification or prevention of complications with elective treatment. Furthermore, access care data should be measured to continuously improve VA quality and measure the effects of the performance and effort.

Recommendations to Improve Patient Safety

- Education of patients and caregivers is an essential aspect for the successful creation and maintenance of a vascular access (VA).
- VA care requires an integrated, multidisciplinary approach including all parties involved in VA care, with close cooperation and clear, effective communication between team members to ensure patient safety and outcome.
- The VA coordinator works as part of the integrated, multidisciplinary team and plays a pivotal role in providing continuity and coordinated care.

- Cannulation of the VA requires a high level of awareness, specific knowledge and skills of the dialysis nurse.
- Each center should establish a computerized database for continuous data collection that is focused on indicators related to improve VA outcome.

Introduction

Vascular access (VA) care requires an integrated multidisciplinary approach including all parties involved in VA care, with close cooperation and clear, effective communication between team members to ensure patient safety and outcome.

Education of patients and caregivers is an essential aspect for successful creation and maintenance of the VA. Patient education programs on VA are associated with increased use of arteriovenous fistula (AVF) at dialysis initiation [1].

Due to the ongoing contact with patients, dialysis nurses play a pivotal role in the education of (pre-)dialysis patients and their family on all aspects of VA care such as VA types, vein protection for future fistula construction, the risk of adverse events with catheters, monitoring and surveillance, and complications. Patient education should be multidisciplinary and tailored to the needs of the patient with the aim of optimizing patient involvement in their own care. Because patients differ in their learning style, a variety of educations materials should be available, in combination with individual conversations, and access to expert patients.

High-quality VA care with creation of a safe care environment can only be achieved if all professionals involved are well educated on the VA standards, guidelines, policies, and procedures (fig. 1).

Education initiatives should include all multidisciplinary team members on VA (dialysis nurses/vascular access coordinator (VAC), nephrologists, surgeons, radiologists, and ultrasound technicians), emphasizing the importance of multidisciplinary care to achieve successful VA outcome. Education programs should be incorporated into the curriculum of the physicians and dialysis nurses. A structured curriculum should focus on core concepts such as (a) an understanding of the pros and cons of different VA types, (b) individualization of patient VA choice and peritoneal dialysis options, and (c) physical examination of a VA including a thorough understanding of the interpretation of the physical examination and subsequent actions required. These skills could be acquired through (a) a dedicated dialysis access lecture series, (b) a nephrologists and radiologist should observe endovascular procedures and learn the physical examination of the VA, (c) communication with a dedicated VA surgeon to understand the issues involved in access selection and placement, and

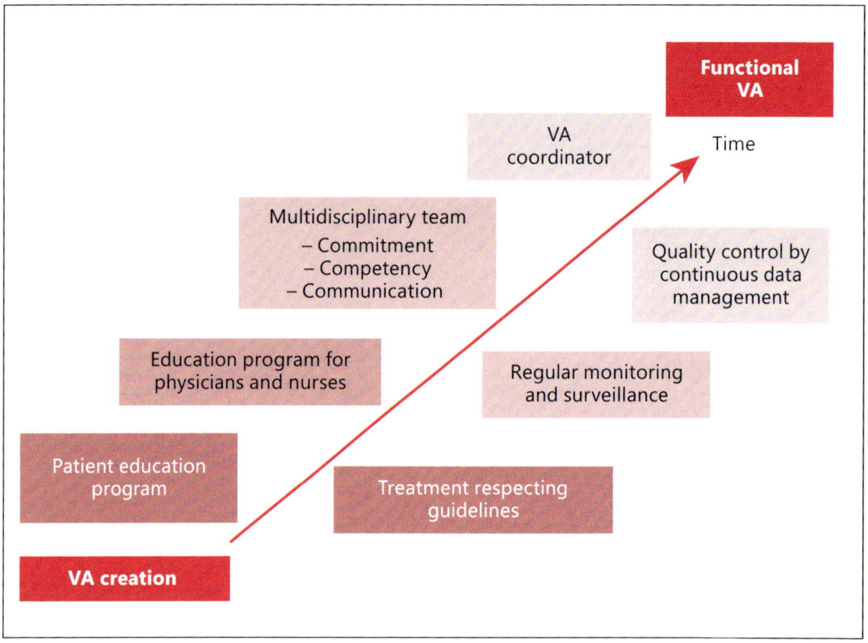

Fig. 1. Aspects that may help to create more functional VA.

(d) rotations at outpatient dialysis units with a skilled dialysis nurse to learn the challenges of cannulation of VA [2, 3]. Several ways of learning can contribute to improve VA outcomes such as didactic lectures, visual teaching (http://www.fistulafirst.org/HealthcareProfessionals/FFBIChangeConcepts/ChangeConcept8.aspx), e-learning (www.fistulafirst.org/Home/VascularAccessAtlas.aspx), simulation training, and use of cadavers and animal models. Surgical experience and skills are associated with failure or success of fistulas. Studies showed that the probability of primary failure is strongly related to the center of access creation, suggesting an important role for the vascular surgeon's skills and decisions [4].

Maturation

Assessment of the VA is the key to determine the usability for cannulation with a minimal risk for complications and the ability to deliver the prescribed blood flow during dialysis. After creation, the VA should be monitored on a regular basis for maturity by a thorough physical examination of the fistula according to a standardized protocol (table 1).

Table 1. Physical examination of new AVF

	Evaluation	Procedure	Normal	Abnormal
Inspection	Each treatment	Inspection of arm (hand and fingers), shoulder, breast, neck and face Always compare with contralateral arm	Normal healing of incision lines Patient has no complaints or symptoms related to AVF	Signs of infection/occlusion (phlebitis); redness, warmth, swelling, erythema, pain Edema of limb, chest, neck or face Hematoma Collateral veins of neck, upper arm or shoulder Accessory veins Signs of steal syndrome; pale, cyanotic, cold, decreased sensation, decreased function, absence of radial pulse Aneurysm
Palpation	Each treatment	Palpation of the thrill by placing fingers up the vein from the anastomosis along the drainage vein to the chest wall	A palpable continuous thrill felt through the entire vein, with higher intensity at the anastomosis The entire fistula is soft and easily compressible Presence of arterial pulse distal of the VA	Absence of thrill; occlusion of fistula Hyperpulsatile and firm/water – hammer; compressed or occluded Weak thrill; weak inflow Absence of radial pulse
	After 4–6 weeks	Caliber of the vessel	Vein depth <0.6 cm Vein diameter >0.6 cm Area of straight vein >10 mm	Small-caliber AVF Deep AVF >0.6 mm Limited straight portion for cannulation
Augmentation test	Each treatment	Complete occlusion of the inflow several cm beyond the arterial anastomosis to evaluate the inflow segment With side to side upper arm fistula; manually occlude one vein in order to detect presence of outflow stenosis	Major augmentation of pulse	Weak augmentation of pulse between anastomosis and compressed area; poor quality of inflow Thrill does not disappear; collaterals or side branches accessory veins
Capillary refill	Each treatment	Blanching the nail bed, and measure time interval until normal coloration	Capillary refill of the nail bed is <3 s	Signs of cyanosis of the finger tips and delayed refill of the nail beds of >3 s
Elevation test	Each treatment	Elevation of the extremity for examination of the normal collapse	Flattening and collapse of the entire fistula	Partial vein collapse; fistula distal to the point of stenosis remains distended No collapse of the venous segment upon arm elevation; outflow stenosis
Auscultation	Each treatment	Listen with stethoscope from the anastomosis moving upwards the drainage vein, paying attention to changes and the quality of the bruit (frequency and duration)	A low pitch, continuous bruit and audible on diastole and systole, with higher intensity near the anastomosis	High-pitched and only systolic component (discontinuous, systolic thrill); outflow stenosis Weak systolic thrill; inflow stenosis Intense and continuous bruit along the vessel until a root of the arm and in the precordial region; high flow

Physical examination of the VA is essential to identify complications or dysfunction during the maturation process or during HD. Assessment of an AVF is more difficult than assessment of an arteriovenous graft (AVG).

Physical examination includes inspection (arm, shoulder, breast, neck, and face), palpation (from artery graft anastomosis to chest wall), and auscultation. Pulse augmentation and arm elevation tests, to evaluate the inflow and outflow tract, is also recommended [5]. Physical examination requires training, but is easily performed and has a high level of accuracy [5]. Robbin et al. [6] showed that an experienced hemodialysis nurse is able to predict the likelihood of AVF maturity with 80% accuracy with physical examination.

No consensus has been reached concerning the timing of first cannulation of the VA. The K/DOQI practice guidelines state that a good functioning access has a flow of approximately 600 ml/min, is less than 6 mm below the surface of the skin, and has a minimum diameter of 6 mm [7]. However, the changing demographics of the ESRD population, makes it difficult to create and maintain a well-functioning fistula that can meet these criteria. In clinical practice, the definition of maturation varies by local practice, and VA cannulation is based on the experience and skills of dialysis staff. In addition to physical examination, these parameters should be measured by Doppler ultrasound and finger pressure measurement at 6–8 weeks postoperatively to evaluate the blood flow and vessel diameter in the maturing AVF and prosthetic VA, and to identify complications such as hand ischemia, accessory veins, stenosis, high-output cardiac failure, aneurysms or venous hypertension. It also enables to determine the best cannulation sites. Depending on the fistula configuration, a mature forearm AVF will have a blood flow between 600 and 1,200 ml/min, while an upper arm AVF will have a flow of 600–2,000 ml/min.

Which Needles Do Best?

Hemodialysis adequacy depends – among other factors – on the effective blood flow through the dialyzer. The blood is pumped to and from the VA through dialysis needles; smaller needles have a larger flow resistance that decrease delivered Qb (table 2).

Therefore, it is critical to adjust the appropriate needle according to the desired blood pump speed and the available access flow rate in the VA in order to achieve dialysis efficiency (Kt/V). It is important to match needle gauge with blood flow rate (table 2). If the negative arterial pressure falls below –200 to –250 mm Hg, and the venous outflow pressure above +250 mm Hg, the needle size should be increased (i.e. smaller gauge number should be used). For can-

Table 2. Recommended needle size for the state blood flow rate settings

Blood flow rate	Needle gauge	Inner diameter, mm
200 ml/min	18	0.838
<300 ml/min	17	1.067
300–350 ml/min	16	1.194
350–450 ml/min	15	1.372
>450 ml/min	14	1.600

nulation of AVG, the smallest gauge needle can be used that will achieve the desired blood flow. Needles are available from 14 to 18 gauge. Progression of needle size should be based on the assessment of adequate vessel size and intra-access flow (Q) [7].

One method used to select the appropriate needle size is a visual and tactile examination, which depends on the experience. This examination allows the cannulator to determine which needle gauge would be most appropriate, based on the size of the vessels in the fistula. Alternately, place 17- and 16-gauge needles with the protective cap in place (prevents a needle stick) over the cannulation site. Use the needle size that is equal to or smaller than the vein (without the tourniquet) for the cannulation [7].

To reduce needle penetration of the back wall of the vessel, the shortest needle length should be chosen (20–32 mm). The dialysis staff may alter needle lengths in order to reach deep accesses. The arterial needle should always have a back eye to ensure that the optimal flow is achieved; this prevents suction of the needle to the inner vessel wall and therefore reduces the rate for rotation of the needle.

Needles are available as sharp or blunt ones. Sharp needles have a cutting edge and a silicone coating for optimum insertion, and low flow resistance. Blunt needles are designed/developed for the buttonhole cannulation technique; they are rounded on the top and do not have a sharp, cutting edge like traditional needles. Two specific embodiments are described: an all stainless-steel version and a plastic version with a sharp or a blunt mandrin, which is removed after cannulation.

The venous needle must always point toward the venous return (antegrade) to encourage better venous return. Arterial needle placement can be antegrade (in the direction of the blood flow) or retrograde (against the direction of the blood flow). The antegrade puncture of the arterial needle would not increase the risk of recirculation if the access blood flow is significantly greater than the blood pump flow [7, 8]. There is no evidence that retrograde cannulation in grafts leads to 'flap' creation that may be kept open with the blood flow after needle removal, and delay hemostasis or contribute to insertion-related complications.

Once the needle is cannulated, it is crucial to tape and monitor dialysis needles and blood lines securely to prevent complication such as infiltration and completely or partially needle dislodgement. Needle dislodgement is a serious potential complication of hemodialysis therapy. Especially, venous needle dislodgement can give injury or can be fatal. Therefore, every dialysis unit should develop clear guidelines for securing the needles and blood lines to reduce the risk. VA and needle sites should be visible at all times during hemodialysis. Staff and patients should be aware of the risk and consequences for needle dislodgement. Additional protection can be provided by devices intended to detect blood loss to the environment [9].

The technique of needle removal is as important as cannulation to protect the VA from damage and to facilitate proper hemostasis. Needles should be removed at the same angle as they were inserted. When the needles are removed, hemostasis should be obtained by applying mild, digital direct pressure over the needle sites, using two-digit technique, one finger at the skin (external), and one finger at the blood vessel wall (internal), for at least 10 min. In general, prosthetic grafts require a longer time to achieve hemostasis. Prolongation of the compression time is suspect from a proximal stenosis.

Cannulation Technique

Cannulation of the VA is a basic but essential part of the dialysis treatment, and remains stressful to patients and medical staff. With today's population, cannulation of the VA requires a high level of awareness, specific knowledge and skills of the dialysis nurse. A deficit in cannulation skills can have negative consequences for patients' VA. Studies showed that a great percentage of patients encounter cannulation-related problems such as infiltrations, hematoma formation, infections and aneurysms resulting in catheter use and single-needle dialysis. Needle infiltration due to a fragile vessel wall, is a relatively frequent complication in newly mature fistulas, which occurs most commonly in older patients [10, 11]. Single-needle dialysis may be a valuable option for patients with an immature fistula or cannulation-related complications, although the single needle technique requires careful monitoring of the dialysis dose.

Many of the cannulation-related problems can be prevented with proper cannulation techniques. Therefore, it is important that only an experienced dialysis nurse with excellent cannulation skills cannulates newly matured fistulas. Every

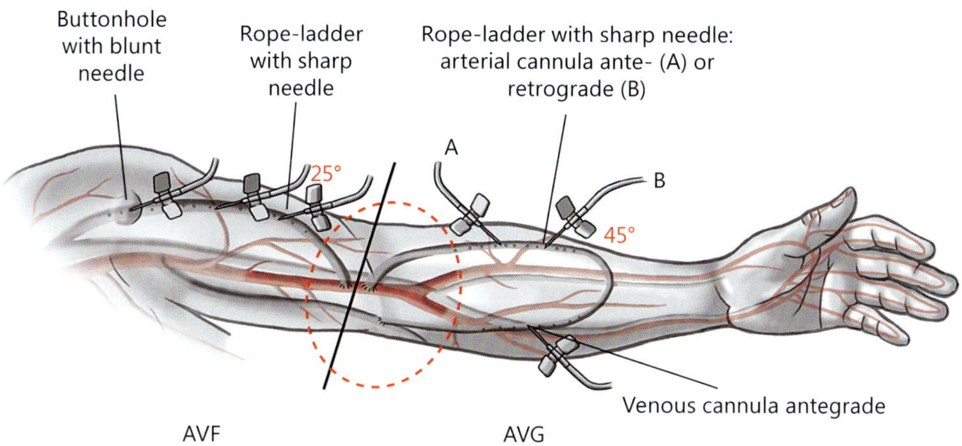

Fig. 2. Ideal cannulation technique for AVFs and AVGs.

dialysis department should develop and implement a standardized protocol for cannulation of the VA, in particular 'new fistulas'. The evidence-based practice protocols should be with clear and detailed instructions about the cannulation procedure and interventions for complications. Ultrasound-guided cannulation may facilitate successful cannulation of difficult accesses.

There are two methods for cannulation of the VA (fig. 2).

The conventional cannulation method is the rope-ladder technique (RL). For every dialysis, two new sites are chosen for needle placement and the whole access length is used for cannulation, with a minimum of 2–3 cm between the tips of the arterial and venous needles, at least 3 cm from the anastomosis, and avoiding the previous sites. Based on the assessment of the VA, the unique angle of insertion is chosen, which is generally 25° for the AVF and 45° for the AVG [7]. To allow rotation of the needle sites, a cannulation segment of 10 cm is required [10]. The RL is advised for the cannulation of AVG, to avoid graft disintegration. In daily practice, often the same area of the VA is cannulated (so called area technique), for reasons of comfort and ease, a complicated cannulation route, or a short length of vein segment, which weakens the fistula wall and leads to formation of pseudoaneurysms and stenosis [12]. Although it is not preferable, the area technique is very often used.

Another cannulation method, the buttonhole technique (BH), was first used with patients who had limited AVF cannulation sites [13]. It requires repeated cannulation with sharp needles at exactly the same spot, using the same angle and same depth of penetration to create a tunnel track, preferably performed by a single cannulator to prevent the risk of multitrack formation. Because creation of the BH track can be difficult, especially in units with multiple cannulators, various devices can be used to assist BH track creation, such as the polycarbonate peg (BH Stick®, Nipro Corporation, Osaka, Japan) [12] and the recently developed surgical implanted vascular needle guide VWING [14]. With the use of the polycarbonate peg, a sterile 5-mm-long thumbtack-shaped polycarbonate peg is inserted toward the tunnel created by the removed dialysis needle once hemostasis has been achieved. For a period of 2 weeks, the peg is left in place between dialysis treatments and is removed before the next cannulation [15]. The VWING is a subcutaneous titanium needle guide sutured directly on the top of the AVF to guide the needle [14]. These approaches might be effective in the creation of tunnel tracks for buttonhole cannulation.

Once the track is formed (8–12 times), subsequent cannulators should use blunt needles, and must follow exactly the direction and angle of the developed track to minimize vessel trauma, which may extend VA lifespan [16–18]. A recent article reported that the concept of the BH is to create a 'vasculocutaneous fistula' of a very narrow diameter. Obliquity and length, between 5 and 10 mm, are two key components that help hemostasis and function [19].

The BH is not just a variation on the RL, but is an entirely different way of performing cannulation and requires different attitudes and skills of the dialysis nurse. Several studies have compared the cannulation of the BH versus the RL technique and showed potential benefits of the BH with reduced risk of access-related complications such as needle infiltration and subsequent hematoma formation, aneurysm formation, and cosmetic appearance, cannulation ease and less pain.

However, recent randomized studies found that the BH is associated with an increased risk of infectious complications [20–23]. Infection induced by the BH should not be underestimated, and requires an aseptic and correct technique of the procedure with careful attention to scab removal to reduce the infection risk. Although in the last years much has been published about the BH versus RL, best practices have not been determined. Further research is required to provide information regarding the long-term outcome of the BH compared to the RL technique. The BH may have advantage for patients with a short or complicated cannulation segment or for self-cannulation. Continuous training, education and evaluation of the VA technique to prevent or minimize complications are mandatory.

When choosing the most appropriate cannulation technique, it is important that the specific AVF, patient characteristics, patient preference and nursing experience are taken into account.

Multidisciplinary Approach

VA care requires continuous education of staff and patients, timely referral, adequate planning, early identification or prevention of complications with elective treatment. Given the increased complexity and the multidisciplinary character of VA care, it is a prerequisite to establish a dedicated multidisciplinary approach involving the patient, dialysis nurses/VAC, nephrologists, surgeons, radiologists, and ultrasound technicians. The fact that different professionals are involved may lead to fragmentation of management and care, with a lack of overview and insufficient knowledge about VA standards or responsibility of the different professionals. To prevent this, it is a prerequisite to establish a dedicated approach by implementing structured multidisciplinary quality improvement program based on international guidelines, in every dialysis facility. Close collaboration, commitment, competency and communication between the team members, are mandatory to deliver the highest quality of care and improved VA outcomes. A regular multidisciplinary access meeting to discuss relevant issues, find solutions and evaluate outcome data is essential. Studies demonstrated that the implementation of a VA care pathway to streamline the processes increased patient satisfaction and reduced hospital days and costs while achieving acceptable outcomes for access surgery [24].

Vascular Access Coordinator

The VAC works as part of the integrated, multidisciplinary team and plays a pivotal role to provide continuity and coordinated care by being an advocate and liaison between all the involved parties.

The responsibilities of the VAC are:

- maintain collaborative relationships and streamline communication between the multidisciplinary team;
- support staff to ensure ongoing monitoring and surveillance of the VA, and coordinate intervention if necessary;
- troubleshooting for all VA-related problems;
- ensure the practice is evidence based and identifies quality improvement;
- ensure quality education and competency of staff/patients;
- oversee data collection and management.

To achieve this goal, it is important that the VAC is a dedicated person who has the ability to be flexible, to organize, and effectively communicate and collaborate with all members of the VA team. A coordinated multidisciplinary approach proved to be effective with improvement of patient outcomes in VA care such as greater patient satisfaction, reduced number of hospitalizations and reduction of the average waiting time for treatment [25, 26]. Overall, this strategy enables the delivery of an individualized plan of VA care, with emphasis on patient safety and outcome.

Data Collection and Management

Access care data are measured to continuously improve VA quality process and measure the effects of the performance and effort. Each center should establish a computerized database for continuous collection that is focused on indicators related to improvement of VA outcome including the number and types of VA placement, hospital admissions (and days), waiting time for VA construction, catheter use, results of surgical/ radiological procedures and complication rates. Data should be reviewed weekly/monthly at multidisciplinary meetings.

These data allow multidisciplinary evaluation and review of outcomes and if necessary to make adjustments to the VA process. Clinical outcomes enable to improve decision making and benchmarking to the national and international standards. Furthermore, it is valuable for research to discover relevant knowledge and improve VA care.

Disclosure Statement

The author has no conflict of interest to declare.

References

1 Lacson E, Wang W, DeVries C, et al: Effects of a nationwide predialysis educational program on modality choice, vascular access, and patient outcomes. Am J Kidney Dis 2011;58:235–242.
2 Roy-Chaudhury P, Yevzlin A, Bonventre JV, et al: Academic interventional nephrology: a model for training, research, and patient care. Clin J Am Soc Nephrol 2012;7:521–524.
3 Moist LM, Lee TC, Lok CE, et al: Education in vascular access. Semin Dial 2013;26:148–153.
4 Huijbregts HJTAM, Bots ML, Moll FL, Blankestijn PJ: Hospital specific aspects predominantly determine primary failure of hemodialysis arteriovenous fistulas. J Vasc Surg 2007;45:962–967.
5 Asif A, Leon C, Orozco-Vargas LC, et al: Accuracy of physical examination in the detection of arteriovenous fistula stenosis. Clin J Am Soc Nephrol 2007;2:1191–1194.
6 Robbin ML, Chamberlain NE, Lockhart ME, et al: Hemodialysis arteriovenous fistula maturity: US evaluation. Radiology 2002;225:59–64.

7 Clinical practice guidelines for vascular access. Am J Kidney Dis 2006;48(suppl 1): S176–S247.
8 Ozmen S, Kadiroglu K, Ozmen C, et al: Does the direction of arterial needle in AV fistula cannulation affect dialysis adequacy? Clin Nephrol 2008;70:229–232.
9 Van Waeleghem J-P, Chamney M, Lindley EJ, Pancírová J: Venous needle dislodgement: how to minimise the risks. J Ren Care 2008; 34:163–168.
10 Van Loon MM, Kessels AGH, Van der Sande FM, Tordoir JHM: Cannulation and vascular access-related complications in hemodialysis: factors determining successful cannulation. Hemodial Int 2009;13:498–504.
11 Lee T, Barker J, Allon M: Needle infiltration of arteriovenous fistulae in hemodialysis: risk factors and consequences. Am J Kidney Dis 2006;47:1020–1026.
12 Kronüng G: Plastic deformation of Cimino fistula by repeated puncture. Dial Transplant 1984;13:635–638.
13 Twardowski Z: Different sites versus constant sites of needle insertion into arteriovenous fistulas for treatment by repeated dialysis. Dial Transplant 1979;8:978–980.
14 Hill A, Vasudevan T, Young NP, et al: Use of an implantable needle guide to access difficult or impossible to cannulate arteriovenous fistulae using the buttonhole technique. J Vasc Access 2013;14:164–169.
15 Toma S, Shinzato T, Fukui H, et al: A timesaving method to create a fixed puncture route for the buttonhole technique. Nephrol Dial Transplant 2003;18:2118–2121.
16 Ball LK, Treat L, Riffle V, Scherting D, Swift L: A multi-center perspective of the buttonhole technique in the Pacific Northwest. Nephrol Nurs J 2007;34:234–241.
17 Verhallen AM, Kooistra MP, van Jaarsveld BC: Cannulating in haemodialysis: rope-ladder or buttonhole technique? Nephrol Dial Transplant 2007;22:2601–2604.
18 Van Loon MM, Goovaerts T, Kessels AGH, van der Sande FM, Tordoir JHM: Buttonhole needling of haemodialysis arteriovenous fistulae results in less complications and interventions compared to the rope-ladder technique. Nephrol Dial Transplant 2010;25: 225–230.
19 Wilson NA, Shenoy S: Managing 'buttonhole' complications. J Vasc Access 2014;15(suppl 7):91–95.
20 Chow J, Rayment G, San Miguel S, Gilbert M: A randomised controlled trial of buttonhole cannulation for the prevention of fistula access complications. J Ren Care 2011;37:85–93.
21 Macrae JM, Ahmed SB, Atkar R, Hemmelgarn BR: A randomized trial comparing buttonhole with rope ladder needling in conventional hemodialysis patients. Clin J Am Soc Nephrol 2012;7:1632–1638.
22 Vaux E, King J, Lloyd S, et al: Effect of buttonhole cannulation with a polycarbonate PEG on in-center hemodialysis fistula outcomes: a randomized controlled trial. Am J Kidney Dis 2013;62:81–88.
23 Struthers J, Allan A, Peel RK, Lambie SH: Buttonhole needling of ateriovenous fistulae: a randomized controlled trial. ASAIO J 2010; 56:319–322.
24 Becker BN, Breiterman-White R, Nylander W, et al: Care pathway reduces hospitalizations and cost for hemodialysis vascular access surgery. Am J Kidney Dis 1997;30:525–531.
25 Dwyer A, Shelton P, Brier M, Aronoff G: A vascular access coordinator improves the prevalent fistula rate. Semin Dial 2012;25: 239–243.
26 Polkinghorne KR, Seneviratne M, Kerr PG: Effect of a vascular access nurse coordinator to reduce central venous catheter use in incident hemodialysis patients: a quality improvement report. Am J Kidney Dis 2009;53: 99–106.

Magda van Loon, NP, PhD
University Medical Center
P. Debeyelaan 25, Postbus 5800
NL–6202 AZ Maastricht (The Netherlands)
E-Mail magda.van.loon@mumc.nl

Widmer MK, Malik J (eds): Patient Safety in Dialysis Access.
Contrib Nephrol. Basel, Karger, 2015, vol 184, pp 234–250
DOI: 10.1159/000366107

The Patient's Role in Patient Safety and the Importance of a Dedicated Vascular Access Team

David Shemesh[a] · Oded Olsha[a] · Ilya Goldin[a] · Sigalit Danin[b]

[a]Department of Surgery and Hemodialysis Access Center and [b]Hemodialysis Unit, Shaare Zedek Medical Center, Jerusalem, Israel

Abstract

The role of dialysis patients in ensuring their own safety throughout the process of vascular access construction should be far from negligible. Patients can make important contributions to their safety starting in the predialysis stage, via vascular access construction and through the experience of chronic hemodialysis. Currently, patients assume a passive role and their empowerment requires both patients and caregivers to overcome many personal and cultural barriers, thus encouraging safety-related behavior. There are many opportunities for end-stage renal failure patients to be involved in every stage of their disease. In this chapter, we discuss how hemodialysis patients can participate in patient safety, including some of the main opportunities for involvement along the care pathway from the point at which the decision is made that the patient requires vascular access surgery.

Recommendations to Improve Patient Safety

- Patients can make important contributions to their own health care safety.
- In order to enable patients to contribute to increasing their safety, they should not be sidelined into a passive role.
- Hemodialysis patients can and should participate in patient safety, and there are many opportunities for them to be involved in every stage of their disease.

- Empowerment should be a fundamental feature of any intervention aimed at increasing the patient's level of confidence in performing safety-related behaviors.
- Caregivers should set aside traditional patronizing roles in order to bridge personal and cultural barriers enabling themselves and their patients to assume their individual roles in safety-related relationships.

Introduction

In medical care in general, patients can make important contributions to their own health care safety [1–4], reducing their susceptibility to medical errors by practicing safety-related behaviors to reduce the risk of or even prevent medical errors. In addition to any information about their medical history, they or their accompanying caregivers or relatives can (and should be encouraged to) discuss their concerns about the care they receive, oversee care processes, and report on complications [1]. This type of patient-based behavior has the potential to prevent errors in medical management. Types of behavior that have the potential to prevent errors should be collaborative between patients and the dialysis team, encouraging patients to ask questions about their condition, its treatment, complications, expected outcomes and prognosis. The knowledge gained by patients in this type of interaction can enable awareness of untoward and unexpected events in order to alert the staff, or in the early stages of an adverse process or complication. In surgical patients, up to half of all adverse events may be associated with surgical procedures, and 30–50% of major complications occurring in patients undergoing general surgical procedures are thought to be preventable [5, 6]. Some types of safety-related behaviors will necessarily be specific to surgical procedures.

The type of involvement by the patient, for example asking questions, and the relative importance for such involvement in reducing patients' susceptibility to medical errors or facilitating optimal surgical health outcomes, is discussed. Some examples include asking health care staff if they have washed their hands before treatment to reduce susceptibility to infection, checking medication to prevent drug prescribing or administration errors, and checking medical notes to identify errors or omissions in the records such as incorrect medication (fig. 1).

The dialysis access center is a multidisciplinary facility that includes a dedicated vascular access team for the creation and maintenance of AV access according to the 'one stop shop' model. Planning, constructing and maintaining the access with continuous surveillance is carried out by the same surgeon who

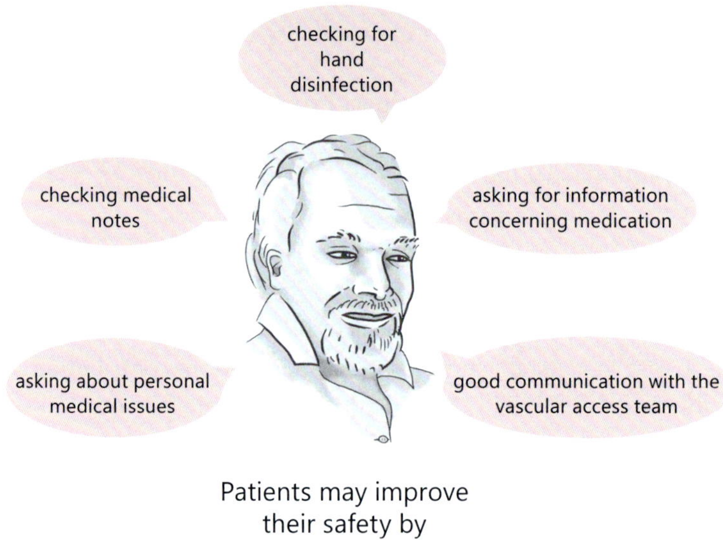

Fig. 1. Empowerment of hemodialysis patients can improve the safety process. Communication between the health care team and the patient is key to overcome intrapersonal, interpersonal and cultural barriers.

performs the preoperative mapping and planning using physical examination, Doppler ultrasound scan and venography when needed. The vascular access team is made up of dedicated vascular surgeons, radiologists, nephrologists and a nurse coordinator. This dedicated team can give vascular access services to one or more dialysis units in close cooperation with the responsible nephrologists of every referring unit. An ideal access center team should involve all the professionals' activities centering on the patient himself, enfolding and accompanying the patient through the 'via dolorosa' of stepping into hemodialysis.

The types of opportunity for patient participation, both to prevent medical errors and to optimize health outcome, will vary along the care pathway. However, for any patient to participate in any behavior at any stage of his care, 3 things will consistently be required: knowledge on how to participate; ability to participate – derived, in part, from the patient's knowledge but also largely dependent on the patient's physical and cognitive capacity; and his/her willingness to participate. Unfortunately, many dialysis patients are not able to participate, but a family member may represent the patient or take his place, thus preserving patient participation in patient safety management.

Safety-Related Behaviors, Barriers to Patient Involvement and Clinical Implications

Five types of safety-related behaviors have been defined by Davis et al. [7]: continuous versus on-off; proactive versus reactive; interactive versus noninteractive; confrontational versus nonconfrontational; and behaviors to prevent errors of omission versus errors of commission. For example, a patient asking a health care professional to check that they have received the correct medication involves the patient asking a question to prevent a medication error. The action comprises the following characteristics: continuous, proactive, interactive, confrontational, and preventing a potential error of commission. In this example, patient participation could be facilitated by encouragement to challenge the clinician's competence, and there is evidence in the context of medication safety and infection control that provides some support for this view [8].

Patient involvement in safety depends on their interactions with health care professionals. Barriers affecting patient involvement need to be overcome in order to encourage patient involvement [9, 10]. These consist of: intrapersonal factors (such as the patient's degree of comfort in questioning staff about treatment); interpersonal factors impacting on how the two sides interact (such as the surgeon encouraging the patient to challenge medical decisions); and cultural factors (for example, whether staff are willing to have their judgment questioned in the first place) [9–13]. Communication between health care professionals is the key to overcoming these intrapersonal, interpersonal, and cultural barriers that impede participation and may vary from behavior to behavior and from patient to patient.

Empowerment should be a fundamental feature of any intervention aimed at increasing the patient's level of confidence in performing safety-related behaviors. A major cultural barrier to patient empowerment and, in turn, patient involvement is professional defensiveness and resistance to the move away from the paternalistic viewpoint that the 'physician knows best' [12, 13]. For example, physicians may be antagonistic to increasing patient involvement because of a cultural outlook that discussion of risk may have a negative psychological impact. Cultural interventions aimed at health workers within the organization are imperative to make patient involvement in safety realistic. This includes educational approaches aimed at changing stereotypical assumptions and to increase staff compliance to being openly questioned and challenged by patients. Patients should be given the means to increase their knowledge of the illness, the points at which they can participate in the delivery of their health care and to express their views without concern, without increasing their anxiety at a time when they may already feel vulnerable. Steps should be taken by the caregiver to bridge

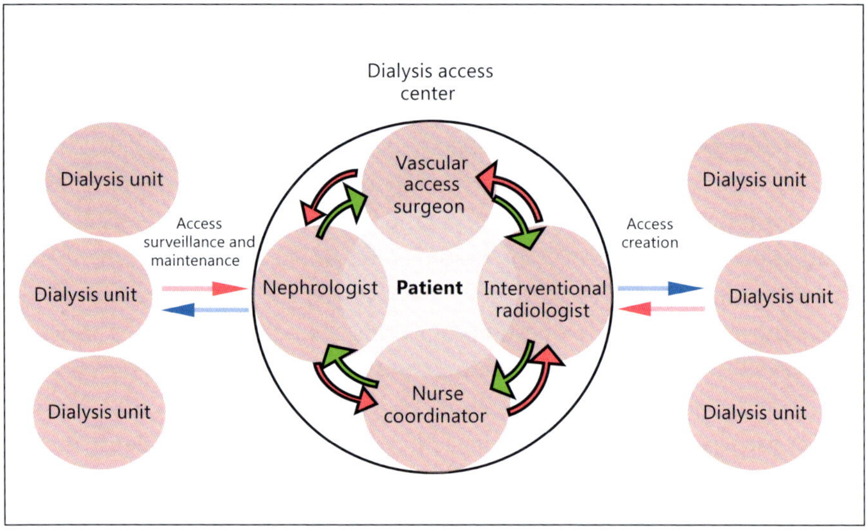

Fig. 2. Patient-centered approach with close collaboration between members of the access center team.

the intrapersonal, interpersonal and cultural barriers, while setting aside traditional patronizing roles, to the benefit of both the caregiver and the patient.

Patients have much to contribute to increase their safety and they should not be sidelined into a passive role.

The Role of the Access Center and Stages in Hemodialysis Access Management

The center effect has been discussed in conferences, but there has been no clinical trial that has reported on the advantages of the vascular access center. Although highly recommended by many leading surgeons, there are no quantitative data demonstrating its success or justifying its existence.

Patient referral by the nephrologist to the access surgeon or center should be done at an early stage of the disease (stage 2–3) [14]. Clear transfer of information between all the members of the team is mandatory (fig. 2). For example, on referral for vascular access construction, the nephrologist should inform the surgeon of the patient's anticipated date for starting on hemodialysis (even though that date may change) so that the surgeon can plan the surgery accordingly. The referral letter should also include a comprehensive report of the diagnosis, risk factors, list of medications (specifically anticoagulant medication) and allergies. Included in the report should be recent blood tests such as blood count, electrolytes and coagulation profile. If a hypercoagulability state exists, this should be noted, so the surgeon can avoid using grafts in such patients.

The conceptual structure of an ideal, patient-centered access center is one where all the professionals act proactively and cooperatively. Patients are referred by many dialysis units and the best possible access is created in each individual patient by the team. Surveillance and maintenance are similarly carried out with patients referred between the various professionals immediately on encountering problems.

Patients should have preoperative evaluation using Doppler ultrasound-enhanced physical examination for vascular access planning, preferably in the nondominant arm. The mapping should be performed by the surgeon who will do the actual surgery, taking into account patient age, medical conditions and other risk factors mentioned in the nephrologist's report. When the same person plans and carries out the surgery, the plan is tailored for the patient's benefit according to the surgeon's capabilities. For example, a surgeon who is not experienced in femoral vein transposition may choose to do a graft instead for the benefit of both patient and surgeon [14]. The surgeon who does the planning informs the nephrologist of his recommendation for a specific patient using a drawing of the hand vasculature and the planned access surgery. Similarly, the surgeon should inform the nephrologist and the patient of his recommendation and of the optimal timing for construction of the access.

The access is preferably performed by a dedicated vascular access surgeon, who is a member of the team, in a center equipped with a dedicated operating room with a dedicated angiography suite. After the surgery, the access team is responsible for fistula maturation using exercise with rubber ball and venous tourniquet starting 5 days postoperatively. Suture removal is done by the team as a first surveillance station in the postoperative access follow-up process.

A Doppler ultrasound-enhanced physical examination is performed for fistulas 4–6 weeks postoperatively to assess maturation [14]. In case of nonmaturation, the cause of nonmaturation should be identified and treated by the surgeon or the interventional radiologist, who are both part of the access team.

When the fistula is established as mature, the patient is referred back to the nephrologist and dialysis staff equipped with a clear letter and a drawing of the access, including accurate data such as flow, vein diameter and vein depth. The best location for the puncture sites should be clearly marked on the skin over the access.

Decisions regarding fistula adequacy and removal of a central vein catheter are made by the access team to ensure access patency by minimizing the risk of central vein complications, mainly infection or occlusion.

Access surveillance and maintenance are carried out according to the principles of the dedicated access team, preferably in an access center setting. Patients with symptomatic stenosis should be referred for treatment armed with a clear drawing of the access to enable tailoring of the procedure to the specific problem. All team members surrounding the patient share the goal of keeping the access patent for the entire period of the patient's life from diagnosis of renal failure until death.

There are many opportunities along this path for the patient to be engaged in safety behaviors and for the access team to ensure such behaviors.

The Patient's Role in Patient Safety in the Process of Access Construction

The stages of the care pathway in end-stage kidney disease are defined as follows (table 1).

Predialysis Period

The predialysis period is the time between the diagnosis of renal failure to the time of dialysis initiation. During this period, the patient is referred to a surgeon to construct vascular access in preparation for hemodialysis.

Patient education should be started in the predialysis period if possible to increase the rates of early access placement [15]. During the predialysis period, the patient should be aware of vein preservation, avoiding puncturing of veins in the nondominant arm for any reason including blood sampling, intravenous lines and administration of medication.

According to the results of the preoperative evaluation, the surgeon should educate the patient to preserve the veins of the arm selected for surgery with the best access possible for the patient. Sometimes, the best arm is the dominant arm, and blindly preserving the veins of the nondominant arm is useless. During this encounter, there is a role for both the patient and the surgeon in overcoming the inhibitions between the caregiver and the patient, thus creating the first step towards a healthy interactive relationship between them.

Preoperative Planning

All patients should undergo Doppler ultrasound vascular examination, and planning of the best possible access prior to construction of a fistula [14].

Table 1. Surgical care algorithm and key opportunities for patient involvement along the pathway

Stage of the care pathway	Key opportunities for patient involvement
Predialysis period	Asking questions about vein preservation: the patient should be aware of venous preservation avoiding puncturing the vein in the nondominant arm for any reason including blood sampling, intravenous lines and administration of medications.
	Asking questions about preemptive access planning: during preoperative evaluation with Doppler ultrasound for access planning, the need to preserve the veins of the arm with the best potential for access construction should be discussed. Sometimes, the best arm is not the nondominant arm and preserving the veins of that arm is useless.
Preoperative planning	Selecting the nondominant hand: the patient should inform the surgeon about the side of the dominant arm and ask to do the access in the nondominant arm if possible [14].
	Selecting the type and location of access: patients should be involved in the decision about the type of access and ask the surgeon about the consequences for each access. For example, patients should enquire why native fistula construction is not possible if this is better than graft, or why an upper arm access is to be created when starting in the forearm is more likely to preserve the vasculature [14].
Decision to operate (initial consultation with the access surgeon)	Consenting to the procedure: knowledge of risks and benefits of as well as alternatives to the medical intervention enables fully informed consent to be given and reduces the possibility of an inappropriate decision being made. This knowledge can also influence compliance to recommendations resulting in better health outcomes [1, 12, 13].
	Choosing an access surgeon: patients should choose (when possible) a high-volume surgeon to reduce the risk of primary fistula failure, which may be 34% lower when placed by a surgeon who created 25 or more fistulas during training [17].
	Asking questions about surgery: patients should be fully informed about their surgery and what to expect from the subsequent recovery process to make them more likely to understand how to adhere to their treatment regime. This heightened understanding can increase compliance to improve outcomes and facilitate the recovery process.
Preoperative assessment clinic	Discussion of preexisting conditions: nearly all patients have a preexisting condition such as diabetes, hypertension, or cardiac disease; they should discuss the effects of the new access on their current illness with their surgeon, such as the effect of access surgery on cardiac function in patients with congestive heart failure.
	Discussion of current medication regimen: patients should make staff aware of their medication regimen. For example, patients on anticoagulant therapy should discuss when to stop the treatment if at all, possible replacement therapy and the consequences of stopping the medication.
Time between preoperative assessment clinic and hospitalization	Fasting before surgery: the patient should understand the importance of fasting for 6 h prior to the operation to reduce the risk of perioperative vomiting with its potentially serious consequences.

Table 1 (continued)

Stage of the care pathway	Key opportunities for patient involvement
During hospitalization: at admission	Medications: health care staff should be informed of drug allergies and bad reactions to anesthesia.
	Patient identification wristbands: patients should notify staff at any stage of hospitalization if the information on their wristband is incorrect or if they have no wristband to prevent errors related to patient misidentification.
During hospitalization: preoperative stage	Site identification: patients should ensure the surgeon clearly marks the extremity that is to be operated on and verify that this is the correct surgical site to prevent wrong site surgery (wrong person, wrong organ or limb, or wrong procedure).
	Telling the anesthetist about medications: information about current medication, drug allergies, and any bad reactions to anesthesia reduces the likelihood of a medication error including undesirable drug interactions.
	Asking questions about recovery: if patients ask questions and know what to expect in their recovery, they can alert a member of staff if they think there is a problem.
During hospitalization: postoperative stage	Problems with the surgical dressing: notifying staff could help to reduce the likelihood of infection or other wound complications.
	Deterioration in condition: chest pain or difficulty breathing, suggesting deterioration in the renal function and threatening of dialysis initiation, should be reported.
During hospitalization: discharge stage	Postdischarge treatment plan: patients who know what to expect from their treatment plan are more likely to adhere to the plan; this can help increase compliance, which positively affects the recovery process and can reduce the likelihood of a readmission due to postoperative treatment complications.
Posthospital discharge stage	Wound infection: patients should notify a member of the outreach health care team. This can help to prevent the spread of infection and can speed up the recovery process.
	Verification of access function: patients should know how to check for thrill and who should be called in case the thrill is not palpated.
	Patient should be aware of late complications: patients should know whether to expect edema of the arm or at the wounds. In the case of AV graft, edema may be a normal outcome of weeping from the graft.
Fistula maturation	Asking questions about the condition of the access: patients should understand the concept of fistula maturation, including flow and diameter, and ask when the fistula will be ready for cannulation. For AV graft, there needs to be an understanding of early cannulation of regular grafts. Patients should ask what to expect at the initiation of cannulation and when any central venous catheter should be removed.
Fistula adequacy	Asking questions about the condition of the access: during dialysis patients should ask about the adequacy of dialysis and the need for assessment by Duplex ultrasound, or intervention.

Before surgery, the patient should be prepared for the surgical process including the type of anesthesia for the surgery and should be informed of the risks of the surgery and how to minimize them. Patients should be encouraged to ask others on dialysis about the surgery and their experience of it. They should be supported and counselled in obtaining information from the Internet.

Decision to Operate

The timing and type of vascular access should be undertaken by the nephrologist in coordination with the vascular access surgeon.

Assessment Clinic

The patient should be examined before surgery to assess the patient risk for surgery. Ideally, this should be done together with the access planning. In the time between the assessment clinic and hospitalization, the patient should be prepared for surgery by performing blood tests, electrocardiogram and other tests as indicated.

Hospitalization Period

This is the period from patient admission through the preoperative stage continuing in the postoperative stage and concluding in the discharge stage. Patients should receive specific instructions regarding wound care, exercising the hand to encourage maturation of fistulas, and an appointment for follow-up examination. It is critical that the staff ensure that the patient and his/her representative comprehend these instructions before discharge.

Postoperative Period

The postoperative period is one of the most precarious periods influencing the success of surgery and patient safety. Patients should be instructed about all the common complications including pain, bleeding, hematoma and false aneurysm.

The patient should be informed about what to do about each complication, and the surgeon should provide a phone number where the patient will be able to report when necessary.

Clear reporting to the nephrologist about the operation is essential.

Posthospital Discharge Stage

This is the time after the patient is discharged. Exercises with a rubber ball are started after suture removal (preferably by the vascular access surgeon who operated on the patient), which is the first surveillance point, and additional exercises with a venous tourniquet are prescribed.

Fistula Maturation

This is the process by which a fistula becomes suitable for cannulation. The rule of sixes states that a mature fistula must be a minimum of 6 mm in diameter with discernable margins when a tourniquet is in place, less than 6 mm deep, have a blood flow greater than 600 ml/min, and the fistula should be evaluated for non-maturation if, after 6 weeks from surgical creation, it does not meet these criteria [14].

Fistula Adequacy

A fistula is considered adequate if it supports a blood flow of ≥350 ml/min in at least 6 dialysis sessions in one month [16].

Maintaining Access Function

Problems in access function should be detected by clinical surveillance and promptly referred for further evaluation and treatment.

Post-Kidney Transplantation Period

Hemodialysis is no longer necessary but plasmapheresis may be required for high antibody levels, and rejection may lead to hemodialysis in the future. Patients should be instructed to care for the fistula in the same fashion as during the dialysis phase, and blood sampling should be from native fistulas, if present, to preserve the contralateral arm for future access surgery.

Table 2. Hemodialysis care and key opportunities for patient involvement along the pathway

Stage of the care pathway	Key opportunities for patient involvement
Preparation for hemodialysis	Discussion of current medication regimen and medical update: patients should update the staff on every change in their medical condition, new medication prescribed to them and ask questions about the influence of these changes on hemodialysis. This should be an interactive and proactive discussion if feasible.
	Discussion of fluid balance: the patients' role is the most important factor in the prevention of this problem. Strict fluid intake limitation mitigates the risk of pulmonary edema between dialysis sessions.
	Discussion of hypertension: it is the patients' responsibility to monitor their blood pressure and to take their medication regularly.
Cannulation	Ensure dialysis staff performs a precannulation access physical examination: patients should be involved in avoiding cannulation of occluded accesses or complicated aneurysms.
	Alert dialysis staff if the distance between cannulation sites is too close: it should be 6 cm according to guidelines.
	Discussion of the cannulation technique: the area technique versus buttonhole technique for fistulas, and in grafts the rope ladder technique, should be used to prevent accelerated destruction of the graft.
During dialysis	Ensure dialysis staff pay attention to alarms on the dialysis machine: this could be a sign of a problem in the access or clotting of the coil.
	Discussion of the progress of dialysis: patients should discuss with the dialysis staff the significance of every alarm during the hemodialysis session and understand the significance of each alarm. Patients should participate in ensuring proper treatment if there is a persistent alarm.
Termination of dialysis session	Notify staff if there is prolonged bleeding from puncture sites or bleeding at home: this is highly suspicious for draining vein stenosis, and patients should be referred to a vascular access surgeon.
Patient discharge	Notify staff if there is weakness or dizziness: these could be symptoms of hypotension and can be alleviated by rest and drinking coffee.
	Discussion of the weight after dialysis: patients should discuss whether the target weight has been achieved and what their ideal dry weight is. Patients should inform staff how they feel with this weight and if they are too dry.

The Patient's Role in Patient Safety in the Hemodialysis Unit

Table 2 details some of the key opportunities for patient involvement along the hemodialysis care pathway from the point at which the decision to start hemodialysis is made. The nature of the activity required (such as asking questions) and the importance for such involvement in reducing patients' susceptibility to medical errors or facilitating optimal surgical health outcomes is discussed.

Choosing a Dialysis Unit

Patients can choose a dialysis unit according considerations such as proximity to home and being familiar with and trusting the nephrologists and their staff.

Patient Safety in the Dialysis Unit

The patient should be encouraged to be engaged in every step of his treatment during dialysis. Vascular access for hemodialysis is the renal failure patient's life line. Inadequate dialysis [low Kt/V (<0.8)] significantly correlates with increased mortality rate [18]. Protection and supervision of the vascular access is a multidisciplinary task, where the patient has a major role together with the dialysis nurse, nephrologist and vascular access surgeon.

Education is extremely important for dialysis patients (or their carers for patients who are not competent). Patient education has been shown to prevent complications such as infection and may improve access survival [19]. The patient should keep the vascular access area clean and wash it daily, avoid shaving near the puncture sites and avoid tattoos. In addition to personal hygiene, all patients should be taught self-examination, including where and how to feel for a thrill, how to recognize infection, and to notify a member of the dialysis staff in case of abnormal or suspicious findings.

Patients should have a supervisory role in ensuring that the staff use proper aseptic techniques whenever the access is palpated, inspected, or cannulated. Patients should be taught about puncturing techniques to avoid 'one-site-itis' using the rotation technique or the buttonhole method in native fistula, or by using the rope ladder cannulation technique in grafts [14].

For patients with central vein catheters, they should be educated in keeping the dressing sealed, clean and dry, especially when taking a shower. In case of bleeding or catheter withdrawal, the patient should press on the exit site and be admitted to the emergency room. In case of fever, pain or swelling, patients should immediately notify a member of the outreach health care team.

The stages of the care pathway in the dialysis unit are defined as follows.

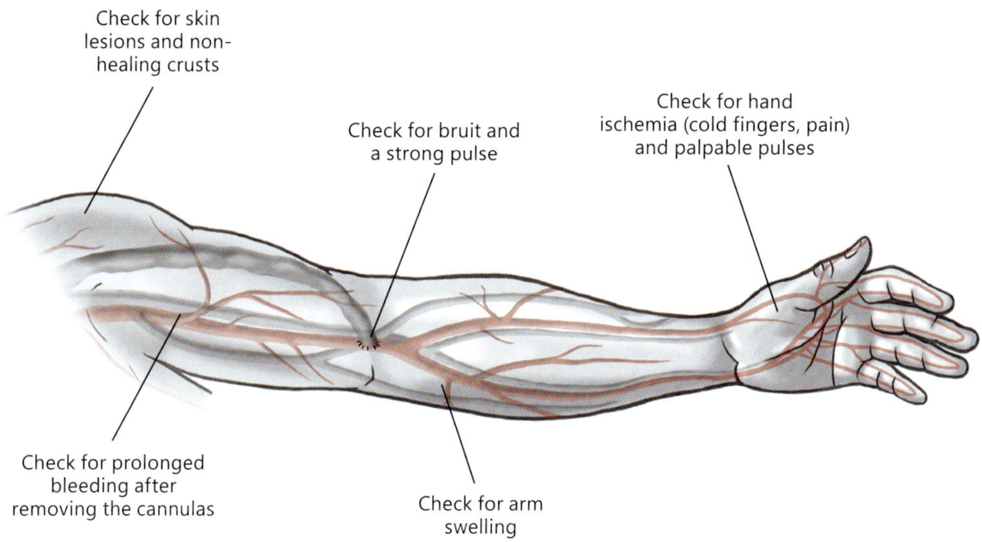

Fig. 3. Each vascular access should be checked before every hemodialysis session.

Preparation for Hemodialysis

(1) Receiving updated medical information about the patient's condition or new medicines. Symptom assessment such as cramps, prolonged bleeding from puncture sites, or fluid loss due to diarrhea. If the patient complains of cold fingers on the side of the access, a glove should be used during the winter.
(2) Evaluation for fluid overload. The patient is weighed in the dialysis unit. The patient should be responsible for fluid balance, avoiding excessive fluid and salt intake.
(3) Hemodynamic assessment including blood pressure and pulse rate.

Cannulation

(1) The limb with the access is gently scrubbed with antiseptic soap.
(2) Access physical examination (fig. 3) is carried out for infection and function, presence of thrill and absence of strong pulse over the puncture sites. Avoid cannulation of aneurysm when possible and change the puncture site. Inspect for local skin ischemia and the presence of nonhealing crust. Swelling

of the arm indicates draining vein stenosis and should be explored. When signs of hand ischemia and nonhealing finger ulcer and necrosis are present, the patient should be referred urgently to a vascular surgeon.
(3) For all vascular accesses, aseptic technique with sterile gloves and face masks for the patient and the nurse should be used for all cannulation procedures. The dialysis nurses cleanse the skin by facility-approved antimicrobial preparation [14].
(4) There must be a sufficient distance between the puncture sites to prevent recirculation.
(5) Fixation of the needles is essential.
(6) Cannulation techniques are important: area versus buttonhole in fistulas, and using the rope ladder technique in grafts [20, 21].

During Hemodialysis

The patient should be involved in the dialysis process and not allow alarms to be ignored. High venous pressure may indicate clotting of the coil leading to blood loss. Persisting high venous pressure is suspicious for the presence of outflow vein stenosis. Blood pressure should be kept stable during dialysis.

At the End of Dialysis Session

With guidance from the dialysis nurse, the needles are withdrawn first from the venous and then the arterial puncture sites. Prolonged bleeding from puncture sites is highly suspicious for draining vein stenosis, and the patient should be referred to vascular access surgeon.

Patient Discharge

The patient is weighed to assess if the target weight was achieved.

Conclusions

The access center concept is to follow the patient from access planning and creation to maturation and maintenance of the access until the patient dies. Full cooperation and teamwork are essential for success. Protocols to ensure patient safety are well established; however, the professionals making up the access team are in a unique position to influence patients to take responsibility for their own safety as part of access center policy.

Disclosure Statement

The authors have no conflicts of interest to declare.

References

1 Coulter A, Ellins J: Patient-Focused Interventions: A Review of the Evidence. London, Picker Institute Europe/Health Foundation, 2006.
2 Darzi A: High Quality Care for All: NHS Next Stage Review Final Report. London, Department of Health, 2008.
3 Vincent C, Coulter A: Patient safety: what about the patient? Qual Saf Health Care 2002; 11:76–80.
4 Davis RE, Jacklin R, Sevdalis N, Vincent CA: Patient involvement in safety: what factors influence patient participation and engagement? Health Expect 2007;10:259–267.
5 Weingart SN, Wilson R, Gibberd RW, et al: Epidemiology of medical errors. BMJ 2000; 320:774–777.
6 Vincent C, Moorthy K, Sarker SK, et al: Systems approaches to surgical quality and safety; from concept to measurement. Ann Surg 2004;239:475–482.
7 Davis RE, Sevdalis N, Jacklin R, Vincent CA: An examination of opportunities for the active patient in improving patient safety. J Patient Saf 2012;8:36–43.
8 Davis R, Koutantji M, Vincent C: How willing are patients to question healthcare staff on issues related to the quality and safety of their healthcare? An exploratory study. Qual Saf Health Care 2008;17:90–96.
9 Howe A: Can the patient be on our team? An operational approach to patient involvement in interprofessional approaches to safe care. J Interprof Care 2006;20:527–534.
10 Mishler EG: The Discourse of Medicine, Dialectics of Medical Interviews. Norwood, Ablex, 1984.
11 Barry C, Bradley C, Britten N, et al: Patients' unvoiced agendas in general practice consultations: qualitative study. BMJ 2000;320: 1246–1250.
12 Arnstein SR: A ladder of participation. J Am Inst Planners 1969;35:218–224.
13 O'Keefe D, Hogg C: Public participation and marginalised groups: the community development model. Health Expect 1999;2:245–254.
14 NKF: KDOQI Clinical Practice Guidelines and Clinical Practice Recommendations for 2006 Updates: Hemodialysis Adequacy, Peritoneal Dialysis Adequacy and Vascular Access. Am J Kidney Dis 2006;48:S1–S322.
15 Lindberg JS, Husserl FE, Ross JL, Jackson D, Scarlata D, Nussbaum J, Cohen A, Elzein H: Impact of multidisciplinary, early renal education on vascular access placement. Nephrol News Issues 2005;19:35–36, 41–43.
16 Miller PE, Tolwani A, Luscy CP, Deierhoi MH, Bailey R, Redden DT, Allon M: Predictors of adequacy of arteriovenous fistulas in hemodialysis patients. Kidney Int 1999;56: 275–280.
17 Saran R, Elder SJ, Goodkin DA, Akiba T, Ethier J, Rayner HC, Saito A, Young EW, Gillespie BW, Merion RM, Pisoni RL: Enhanced training in vascular access creation predicts arteriovenous fistula placement and patency in hemodialysis patients: results from the Dialysis Outcomes and Practice Patterns Study. Ann Surg 2008;247:885–891.

18 Parker TF 3rd, Husni L, Huang W, Lew N, Lowrie EG: Survival of hemodialysis patients in the United States is improved with a greater quantity of dialysis. Am J Kidney Dis 1994; 23:670–680.
19 Deaver K: Preventing infections in hemodialysis fistula and graft vascular accesses. Nephrol Nurs J 2010;37:503–505.
20 Dinwiddie LC: Vascular access for hemodialysis; in Counts CS (ed): Core Curriculum for Nephrology Nursing, ed 5. Pitman, American Nephrology Nurses' Association, 2008, pp 735–752.
21 White JJ, Olvier MJ, Schwab SJ: Temporary vascular access for hemodialysis; in Nissenson AR, Fine RN (eds): Handbook of Dialysis Therapy, ed 4. Philadelphia, Saunders Elsevier, 2008, pp 23–35.

David Shemesh, MD, RVT
Department of Surgery and Hemodialysis Access Center
Shaare Zedek Medical Center
12 Bayt Street, PO Box 3235
Jerusalem 91031 (Israel)
E-Mail shemeshd@szmc.org.il

Widmer MK, Malik J (eds): Patient Safety in Dialysis Access.
Contrib Nephrol. Basel, Karger, 2015, vol 184, pp 251–263
DOI: 10.1159/000366465

Patient Safety in Dialysis Access: Education and Research

Jan H.M. Tordoir[a] · Matthias K. Widmer[b]

[a]Department of Surgery, MUMC, Maastricht, The Netherlands; [b]Department of Cardiovascular Surgery, Bern University Hospital, Bern, Switzerland

Abstract

Today, a growing activity to improve patient safety in all domains of medicine is reality. This chapter deals with patient safety research in general, but is also about strategies to implement this evidence in the daily clinical work treating patients on dialysis. Good clinical research practice has been well established for some years. In the domain of dialysis access, further basic, clinical, epidemiological and health service research will be important to further improve patient safety as a whole.

Recommendations to Improve Patient Safety

- The specialization today and fragmentation of our work time have to be counterbalanced by better lifelong learning and continuous communication.
- Dialysis access patient-centered organization is a key issue, and daily effort in education to sensitize staff and patients to change their behavior is important.
- A teaching culture including knowledge transfer, simulation and team training allows a feedback culture using workplace assessment and is the fundament to establish a safety culture where critical incidence reporting systems and morbidity and mortality conferences are instruments to improve organizational learning in the health care system.

- Research about issues of patient safety (health service research) with a focus on dialysis access needs further investigation.
- Basic and clinical research in relation to dialysis access needs more well-designed multicenter randomized controlled trials with enough power and international collaboration.

Introduction

The patient safety aspect in the daily business of health care professionals is interconnected with the health care system, educational behaviors of staff and patients and finally efforts in research. The latter is on one hand extremely important to show the evidence of a treatment strategy or to evaluate the efficacy of new devices. On the other hand research is by itself a very sensitive domain in which unexpected adverse events can become a major issue for patients with end-stage renal disease (ESRD) under investigation.

In this chapter, we will focus on steps in research concerning patient safety and what kind of educational efforts are necessary to implement patient safety strategies especially in the population of patients on dialysis. We will also reflect and give some input concerning research aspects in the field of dialysis access.

Research Topics in Patient Safety

In 2011, Shekelle et al. [1] stated in their paper about advancing the science of patient safety that the theory behind should be more enlightened and that the patient safety practice should be assessed more in respect of outcomes and possible unexpected effects. Topics that should be addressed in future research are external factors (i.e. regulatory requirements, public reporting, pay-for-performance), organization structural characteristics (i.e. size, complexity, financial status or strength), teamwork, leadership and patient safety culture and finally management tools (training resources, internal organization incentives, audit and feedback). In conclusion, the authors claim for more measurement and reporting in order to show that the benefits of a safety intervention in medicine compensate for the costs.

Today, more than 10 patient safety strategies are strongly recommended that should be implemented and others are potentially valuable. Table 1 summarizes some of those topics which are especially relevant in patients with ESRD [2].

Table 1. Patient safety strategies with focus on ESRD patients with dialysis access [2]

Patient safety strategies worthwhile to be implemented
Preoperative and intraoperative checklists (WHO)
Bundles that include checklists to prevent central line-associated infections
Hand hygiene
Barrier precautions to prevent health care-associated infections
Use of real-time ultrasonography for central line placement
Patient safety strategies with a potential benefit
Multicomponent interventions to reduce falls
Use of clinical pharmacists to reduce adverse drug events
Documentation of patient preferences for life-sustaining treatment
Obtaining informed consent to improve patients' understanding of the potential risks of procedures
Team training
Practice to reduce radiation exposure from fluoroscopy and CT
Use of simulation exercises in patient safety efforts

As clinicians involved in the education process, during the last years we have been facing working hour restrictions, a trend for a new work life balance, the specialization of health care professionals and a progression in the complexity of patient care. These realities are responsible for more interfaces between health care professionals. We therefore need a systematic hand-over system in order to facilitate a continuous and lasting communication. As for other specialties documented, we have to assume that the quality of outcome in vascular access creation is directly correlated with the case load of the surgeons [3].

Patient Safety and Organization

Changes in the organization towards a patient-centered process in dialysis access centers with well-defined treatment algorithm helps, thanks to standardized procedures, to avoid mistakes especially those by omission. Another important fact is to recruit for these dialysis access team persons with specific competences who have an interest to improve the care of patients with ESRD. Last but not least, a big issue to optimize patient safety is engaging the patient to be more responsible for themselves. The patient has to get involved in the treatment process and has to ask critical and therefore important questions. Only a few centers have experiences with vascular access coordinators, but it seems that this model is effective and successful [4].

Patient Safety and Education Efforts

Patient safety is a big deal in concerns of staff education. We need nurses and doctors capable of anticipating problems and willing to change their behavior if the evidence shows that a patient safety strategy is beneficial. Leadership by a crew of an institution but also an established teaching culture is key to develop a feedback culture. This culture allows a no-blame atmosphere to create a safety culture in which everybody is interested to improve the system by reporting critical events. Simulation and team training should become more and more popular supported in practice by workplace assessment to check for standard procedures but also to improve the performance of each health care professional. Morbidity and mortality conferences but also critical reporting systems are instruments to push the safety culture. It is without doubt that change management is extremely important to introduce patient safety strategies.

Patient Safety and Clinical Research

Good Clinical Practice

Clinical patient-related research is necessary to establish the safety and effectiveness of specific health and medical products in hemodialysis vascular access practices. Adherence to the principles of good clinical practice, including adequate human subject protection is universally recognized as a critical requirement to the conduct of research involving human subjects (World Medical Association Declaration of Helsinki) [5]. Much of what is known today about the safety and efficacy of specific treatments has come from randomized controlled clinical trials (RCTs) that are designed to answer important scientific health care questions. RCTs form the foundation for 'evidence-based medicine', but such research can be relied upon only if it is conducted according to principles and standards collectively referred to as 'good clinical practice'. This contains a good and understandable research question with one primary end point and one or two well-defined secondary end points. Each study needs a clear study design with a correct power calculation, an ethical approval and a study registration number so that also studies with a negative outcome will be published. RCTs are the fundament for further meta-analysis using tools like PRISMA and STROBE [6, 7]. In order to propagate among health care professionals the evidence for a treatment concept, societies and organizations invest time and money to write guidelines screening the literature for specific, up to now nonanswered research questions [8, 9].

How to Build and Organize a Research Unit

Basic and clinical studies are the fundamentals of good dialysis access research. Access to the animal lab and the possibility to include large patient populations are essential prerequisites to design studies according to good clinical research guidelines. Therefore, most of fundamental and clinical research studies are performed in university medical centers. For large clinical patient-related studies, cooperation between university centers and multiple dialysis facilities is mandatory.

These studies require the participation of trained clinical research personnel with the ability to accurately collect data (maintenance of databases) under the supervision of an investigator experienced in clinical research methodologies. Basic and clinical research in hemodialysis vascular access benefits from a multidisciplinary approach, particularly in the context of collaborations with basic sciences such as vascular biology, physiology, biomedical technology, and clinical specialties like nephrology, surgery, radiology and pathology. In addition, an important interaction at the clinical and basic science levels would be the relationship between large dialysis facilities and the university medical center.

Fundamentals of Vascular Access Research

Basic Research

Basic medical research includes animal experiments, cell studies, biochemical, genetic and physiological investigations, and studies on the properties of drugs and materials. In almost all experiments, at least one independent variable is varied and the effects on the dependent variable are investigated. The procedure and the experimental design can be precisely specified and implemented. For example, the population, number of groups, case numbers, treatments and dosages can be exactly specified. It is also important that confounding factors should be specifically controlled or reduced. In experiments, specific hypotheses are investigated and causal statements are made.

Clinical Studies

Clinical studies include both interventional studies and noninterventional (or observational) studies. The aim of an interventional clinical study is to compare treatment procedures within a dialysis patient population, which should exhibit as few as possible internal differences, apart from the treatment. This is to be achieved by appropriate measures, particularly by random allocation of the dialysis patients to the groups, thus avoiding bias in the result. Possible therapies include treatment with drugs, for instance anticoagulants or cell cycle blockers, the performance of a novel operative technique or the use of new prosthetic grafts or stents. Most studies require a favorable evaluation from the responsible medical ethics committee. For clinical studies, it is absolutely essential that the patient signs an informed consent form. A control group is included in most clinical studies. This group receives another treatment regimen and/or placebo – a therapy without substantial efficacy. The selection of the control group must not only be ethically defensible, but also be suitable for answering the most important questions in the study. Clinical studies should ideally include randomization, in which the patients are allocated by chance to the therapy arms. This procedure is performed with random numbers or computer algorithms. Randomization ensures that the patients will be allocated to the different groups in a balanced manner and that possible confounding factors – such as risk factors, comorbidities and genetic variability – will be distributed by chance between the groups. Randomization is intended to maximize homogeneity between the groups and prevent, for example, a specific therapy being reserved for patients with a particularly favorable prognosis. A well-designed clinical study must include case number planning. This ensures that the assumed therapeutic effect can be recognized as such, with a previously specified statistical probability (statistical power). If patient populations are exposed to drugs (i.e. anticoagulants, cell cycle inhibitors) or implantation of novel devices (stent, vascular graft), adverse effects should be registered and published. The RCT with case number planning is accepted as the gold standard for testing the efficacy and safety of therapies or drugs and together with meta-analyses regarded as level A evidence. Level B evidence concerns data from a single randomized clinical trial or large nonrandomized studies. Level C is consensus of opinion of experts and/or small studies, retrospective studies and registries.

The assessment of patency of an implanted vascular graft or operation technique is a special modality of a clinical study. Valid comparisons on vascular access patency rates can be made only if patency is defined in a way that can be universally used by all specialties in a consistent manner [10]. Kaplan-Meier analysis is the most commonly used life table method in medical practice. It adequately copes with the issues such as patients for whom the event has not yet occurred and for those lost to follow-up. The data required by the method include the time of commencement of the treatment and the time the measured event occurred (e.g. thrombosis, infection). Patients who dropped out of treatment and those who are still alive at the end of the study period are 'censored', but the contribution that they have made to the event probability is fully accounted for. The method records the time since initiation of treatment at which an event occurs and counts the number of patients at risk of the event at that time. The rate of the event at that time is then one divided by the number at risk. This is repeated for each event at each time. By multiplying the rate at each time by that for the time of the previous event, a cumulative rate and probability can be calculated. Patients who do not experience the event contribute to the number at risk but not to the event rate for as long as they remain on treatment. The time intervals with number of patients at risk and standard errors are indispensable to the life tables.

Epidemiological Studies

The main point of interest in epidemiological studies is to investigate the distribution and historical changes in the frequency of diseases and the causes for these. Observational studies can be subdivided into cohort studies (follow-up studies), case-control studies and cross-sectional studies (prevalence studies). In the simplest case, cohort studies involve the observation of two groups of HD patients over time. It is recorded prospectively (into the future) how often a specific complication and/or event occurs in the two groups. The incidence for the occurrence of the event can be determined for both groups. Moreover, the relative risk (quotient of the incidence rates) is a very important statistical parameter which can be calculated in cohort studies. Patient population studies from large databases are very popular, and recently the relative risk of death in patients with central vein catheters versus arteriovenous fistulas (AVFs) and arteriovenous grafts (AVGs) or the risk of death in hemodialysis versus peritoneal dialysis patients, has been investigated in several studies [11–13].

Health Services Research

Health services research (HSR) is concerned with how health care is provided and covers research into the organization of health care provision and patient safety.

HSR is a relatively new multidisciplinary scientific field with a focus on the social science perspectives investigating how to organize, manage, finance and deliver high-quality care. HSR is particularly important to ensure that advances in clinical care reach patients in reality. Research in this area can give an answer which safety strategies are successful in preventing adverse events and errors. In the field of dialysis access, HSR has to be pushed further. The International Association of Risk Management in Medicine (www.iarmm.org) is an organization that makes an effort to discuss the results of HSR during their annual meetings.

Pooling of Studies

Following a systematic review, data from individual studies may be pooled quantitatively and reanalyzed using established statistical methods. This technique is called meta-analysis. The rationale for a meta-analysis is that, by combining the samples of the individual studies, the overall sample size is increased, thereby improving the statistical power of the analysis as well as the precision of the estimates of treatment effects.

Meta-analysis is a two-stage process. The first stage involves the calculation of a measure of treatment effect with its 95% confidence intervals (CI) for each individual study. The summary statistics that are usually used to measure treatment effect include odds ratios (OR), relative risks, and risk differences. In the second stage of meta-analysis, an overall treatment effect is calculated as a weighted average of the individual summary statistics. Greater weights are given to the results from studies that provide more information, because they are likely to be closer to the 'true effect' we are trying to estimate. The odds for a group are defined as the number of patients in the group who achieve the stated end point divided by the number of patients who do not. An OR or relative risk greater than 1 indicates increased likelihood of the stated outcome being achieved in the treatment group. If the OR or relative risk is less than 1, there is a decreased likelihood in the treatment group. A ratio of 1 indicates no difference – that is, the outcome is just as likely to occur in the treatment group as it is in the control group. As in all estimates of treatment effect, ORs or relative risks reported in meta-analysis should be accompanied by CIs. Risk, as opposed to odds, is calculated as the number of patients in the group who achieve the stated end point divided by the total number of patients in the group. Recently, a systematic search of the literature was used to identify RCTs evaluating the effect of antiplatelet agents in AVG and AVF [14]. Ten trials were included in the analysis, 9 of which reported outcomes on AVG and AVF thrombosis. Antiplatelet agents reduced the rate of AVF thrombosis (OR 0.54, 95% CI 0.31–0.94; fig. 1) but not grafts (OR 0.50, 95% CI 0.16–1.53). Both analyses had a moderate degree of statistical heterogeneity, likely because of differences in study design, antiplatelet agent and dose, as well as other possible factors.

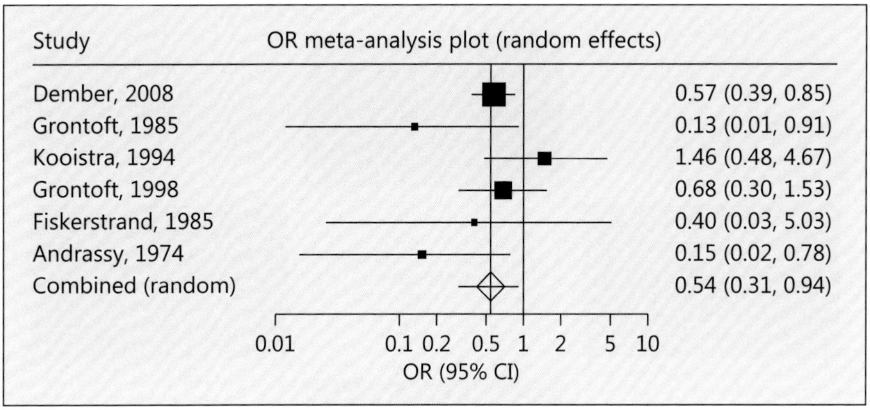

Fig. 1. Meta-analysis of RCTs on the effect of anticoagulants on the thrombosis rate of AVFs. The pooled OR is <1, meaning a favorable effect of the drug on AVF thrombosis [6].

Publications

After submission of a paper, the editors of a journal will start the review process in order to critically investigate the paper and to improve its quality. For publication about hemodialysis vascular access, one can publish in different papers depending on the research question of the paper and the methodological quality. Table 2 summarizes the impact factor of journals in which peer-reviewed papers can be found dealing with dialysis accesses [15]. The table further shows clearly a lack in RCTs in the domain of vascular access and that more well-designed studies are mandatory to improve patient safety in regard of treatment strategies.

Research Domains in Dialysis Access

Patient safety depends directly on research. As described above, different methods are known in the field of dialysis access. Figure 2 gives an overview of research activities in basics, clinics epidemiology and health services.

In basic research today, the evaluation to find local agents (drugs, genes, cells, chemicals and devices) to inhibit myointimal hyperplasia in the process of vessel remodeling after vascular access surgery is still under investigation. A direct connection of artery and vein without a capillary bed, results in instantaneous large hemodynamic changes in terms of high blood flows and shear stress on the vessel wall with usually accelerated development of myointimal proliferation. Therefore, research of computational fluid dynamics to study and understand

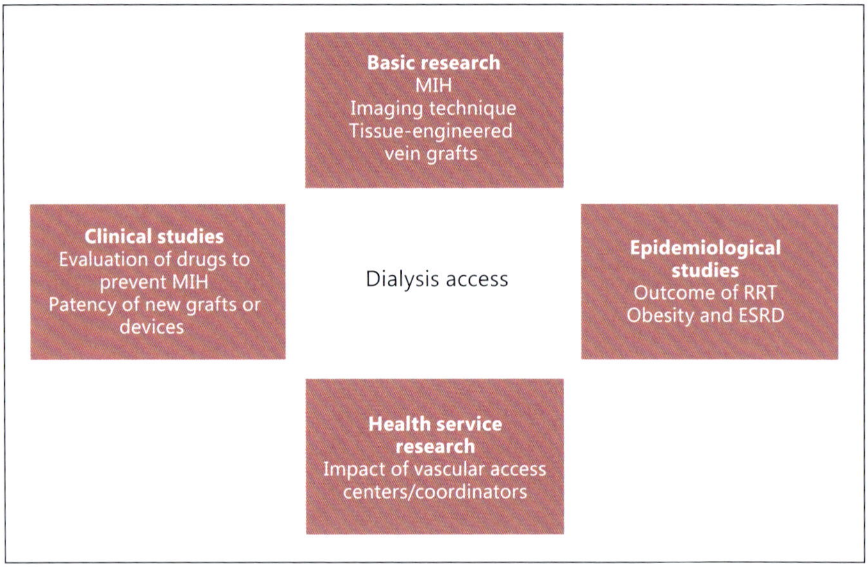

Fig. 2. Research domains in dialysis access with some examples of topics. MIH = Myointimal hyperplasia; RRT = renal replacement therapy.

Table 2. Journals publishing regularly about vascular access with an update of the impact factor for 2012 [15]

Abbreviated journal title	Specialty	Number of articles (in 2010)	Number of RCTs (in 2010)	Journal's impact factor (in 2012)
J Am Soc Nephrol	nephrology	69	9	8.98
Kidney Int	nephrology	123	11	7.916
Am J Kidney Dis	nephrology	161	5	5.294
Clin J Am Soc Nephrol	nephrology	23	1	5.068
Nephrol Dial Transplant	nephrology	260	3	3.371
Semin Dial	nephrology	172	0	2.247
ASAIO	nephrology	55	1	1.491
Radiology	radiology	52	4	6.339
J Vasc Interv Radiol	radiology	206	9	2.002
Cardiovasc Intervent Radiol	radiology	61	2	2.138
AJR	radiology	40	0	2.90
J Vasc Surg	surgery	145	9	2.879
Eur J Vasc Endovasc Surg	surgery	54	1	2.820
Ann Vasc Surg	surgery	69	1	0.985
J Vasc Access	surgery	218	2	0.97
Vasc Endovasc Surg	surgery	39	0	0.880
Total		1,747	57	

this problem is important [16]. The development of a tissue-engineered vein conduit is another hot topic of research [17].

In clinical studies, a lot of underpowered and often not randomized trials were published to show the benefit of a new device/product. Vessel modeling by means of computational simulation may have the potential to improve outcome of AVF creation and to determine strategies for intervention in complicated access, and larger patient studies are underway [16]. Phase 1 studies on the effect and dose of drug administration (in particular sirolimus or paclitaxel and drug-eluting stents) in animals showed favorable results in terms of lower incidence of myointimal proliferation coupled to less vessel wall thickening and intimal/media area. Although in most animal studies, favorable effects of systemic drug administration or local drug-eluting balloons, AVGs, stents (usually coated by sirolimus or paclitaxel) in vascular access constructions were seen, in humans most of these positive outcomes could not been mimicked [18, 19]. The American Dialysis Access Consortium has recently performed a number of studies on the effect of drug administration in HD patients. Some of these studies showed favorable effects on vascular access outcome and patient health in terms of less cardiovascular events [20, 21].

In epidemiology, it will be very important in the future to have an overview how the still growing diabetic population and the avalanche of patients with obesity will influence the practice in renal replacement therapy and the outcome of dialysis access procedures. Another hot and permanent topic is the use of central venous lines and the monitoring and control of infections in patients with ESRD [13]. The last topic is also addressed in the field of health service research in addition to the discussion about the implementation of vascular access centers and/or a vascular access coordinator.

Conclusions

Patient safety research needs further progress especially related to dialysis access patients. In the implementation of the results, staff and patient education is key. With regard to clinical research questions, more RCTs are mandatory, and therefore multicenter studies are important, and international collaboration like the Kidney Health Initiative (www.asn-online.org/khi) should be established [22].

Acknowledgement

We thank David Schwappach, Swiss Patient Safety Foundation, for his critical review of the manuscript.

Disclosure Statement

The authors have no conflicts of interest to declare.

References

1 Shekelle PG, Pronovost PJ, Wachter RM, Taylor SL, Dy SM, Foy R, et al: Advancing the science of patient safety. Ann Intern Med 2011;154:693–696.

2 Shekelle PG, Pronovost PJ, Wachter RM, McDonald KM, Schoelles K, Dy SM, et al: The top patient safety strategies that can be encouraged for adoption now. Ann Intern Med 2013;158:365–368.

3 Konner K, Hulbert-Shearon TE, Roys EC, Port FK: Tailoring the initial vascular access for dialysis patients. Kidney Int 2002;62:329–338.

4 van Loon M, van der Mark W, Beukers N, de Bruin C, Blankestijn PJ, Huisman RM, et al: Implementation of a vascular access quality programme improves vascular access care. Nephrol Dial Transplant 2007;22:1628–1632.

5 World Medical Association Declaration of Helsinki. www.wma.net/en/30publications/10policies/b3/ (accessed July 12, 2014).

6 Moher D, Altman DG, Liberati A, Tetzlaff J: PRISMA statement. Epidemiology 2011;22:128; author reply.

7 Ebrahim S, Clarke M: STROBE: new standards for reporting observational epidemiology, a chance to improve. Int J Epidemiol 2007;36:946–948.

8 Development and validation of an international appraisal instrument for assessing the quality of clinical practice guidelines: the AGREE project. Qual Saf Health Care 2003;12:18–23.

9 Lameire N, Van Biesen W: Clinical practice guidelines: an important tool in improving dialysis quality; in Ronco C, Rosner MH, Crepaldi C (eds): Peritoneal Dialysis – State-of-the-Art 2012. Contrib Nephrol. Basel, Karger, 2012, vol 178, pp 58–67.

10 Sidawy AN, Gray R, Besarab A, Henry M, Ascher E, Silva M Jr, et al: Recommended standards for reports dealing with arteriovenous hemodialysis accesses. J Vasc Surg 2002;35:603–610.

11 Perl J, Wald R, McFarlane P, Bargman JM, Vonesh E, Na Y, et al: Hemodialysis vascular access modifies the association between dialysis modality and survival. J Am Soc Nephrol 2011;22:1113–1121.

12 Ocak G, Halbesma N, le Cessie S, Hoogeveen EK, van Dijk S, Kooman J, et al: Haemodialysis catheters increase mortality as compared to arteriovenous accesses especially in elderly patients. Nephrol Dial Transplant 2011;26:2611–2617.

13 Ravani P, Palmer SC, Oliver MJ, Quinn RR, MacRae JM, Tai DJ, et al: Associations between hemodialysis access type and clinical outcomes: a systematic review. J Am Soc Nephrol 2013;24:465–473.

14 Coleman CI, Tuttle LA, Teevan C, Baker WL, White CM, Reinhart KM: Antiplatelet agents for the prevention of arteriovenous fistula and graft thrombosis: a meta analysis. Int J Clin Pract 2010;64:1239–1244.

15 Kian K, Asif A: Status of research in vascular access for dialysis. Nephrol Dial Transplant 2010;25:3682–3686.

16 Caroli A, Manini S, Antiga L, Passera K, Ene-Iordache B, Rota S, et al: Validation of a patient-specific hemodynamic computational model for surgical planning of vascular access in hemodialysis patients. Kidney Int 2013;84:1237–1245.

17 McAllister TN, Maruszewski M, Garrido SA, Wystrychowski W, Dusserre N, Marini A, et al: Effectiveness of haemodialysis access with an autologous tissue-engineered vascular graft: a multicentre cohort study. Lancet 2009;373:1440–1446.

18 Baek I, Bai CZ, Hwang J, Park J, Park JS, Kim DJ: Suppression of neointimal hyperplasia by sirolimus-eluting expanded polytetrafluoroethylene (ePTFE) haemodialysis grafts in comparison with paclitaxel-coated grafts. Nephrol Dial Transplant 2012;27:1997–2004.

19 Paulson WD, Kipshidze N, Kipiani K, Beridze N, DeVita MV, Shenoy S, et al: Safety and efficacy of local periadventitial delivery of sirolimus for improving hemodialysis graft patency: first human experience with a sirolimus-eluting collagen membrane (Coll-R). Nephrol Dial Transplant 2012;27:1219–1224.
20 Dixon BS, Beck GJ, Vazquez MA, Greenberg A, Delmez JA, Allon M, et al: Effect of dipyridamole plus aspirin on hemodialysis graft patency. N Engl J Med 2009;360:2191–2201.
21 Lok CE, Moist L, Hemmelgarn BR, Tonelli M, Vazquez MA, Dorval M, et al: Effect of fish oil supplementation on graft patency and cardiovascular events among patients with new synthetic arteriovenous hemodialysis grafts: a randomized controlled trial. JAMA 2012;307:1809–1816.
22 Archdeacon P, Shaffer RN, Winkelmayer WC, Falk RJ, Roy-Chaudhury P: Fostering innovation, advancing patient safety: the kidney health initiative. Clin J Am Soc Nephrol 2013;8:1609–1617.

Jan H.M. Tordoir, MD
Department of Surgery, Maastricht University Medical Center
P. Debijelaan 2
NL–6202 AZ Maastricht (The Netherlands)
E-Mail j.tordoir@mumc.nl

Author Index

Subject Index